DATE DUE

			PRINTED IN U.S.A.

Pain

SOURCEBOOK

Fifth Edition

Health Reference Series

Fifth Edition

Pain
SOURCEBOOK

Basic Consumer Health Information about Causes and Types of Acute and Chronic Pain and Disorders and Injuries Characterized by Pain, Including Arthritis, Back Pain, Burns, Carpal Tunnel Syndrome, Headaches, Fibromyalgia, Neuropathy, Neuralgia, Sciatica, Shingles, and More

Along with Facts about Over-the-Counter and Prescription Analgesics, Physical Therapy, and Complementary and Alternative Medicine Therapies, Tips for Managing Pain, a Glossary of Related Terms, and a Directory of Additional Resources

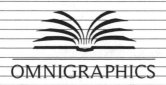

OMNIGRAPHICS

615 Griswold, Ste. 901, Detroit, MI 48226

Bibliographic Note

Because this page cannot legibly accommodate all the copyright notices, the Bibliographic Note portion of the Preface constitutes an extension of the copyright notice.

* * *

Health Reference Series
Siva Ganesh Maharaja, *Managing Editor*
***

OMNIGRAPHICS
A PART OF RELEVANT INFORMATION
***

Copyright © 2017 Omnigraphics
ISBN 978-0-7808-1571-1
E-ISBN 978-0-7808-1572-8

Library of Congress Cataloging-in-Publication Data

Title: Pain sourcebook: basic consumer health information about causes and types of acute and chronic pain and disorders and injuries characterized by pain, including arthritis, back pain, burns, carpal tunnel syndrome, headaches, fibromyalgia, neuropathy, neuralgia, sciatica, shingles, and more; along with facts about over-the-counter and prescription analgesics, physical therapy, and complementary and alternative medicine therapies, tips for managing pain, a glossary of related terms, and a directory of additional resources.

Description: Fifth edition. | Detroit, MI: Omnigraphics, [2017] | Series: Health reference series | Includes bibliographical references and index.

Identifiers: LCCN 2017029185 (print) | LCCN 2017029343 (ebook) | ISBN 9780780815728 (eBook) | ISBN 9780780815711 (hardcover: alk. paper)

Subjects: LCSH: Pain--Popular works.

Classification: LCC RB127 (ebook) | LCC RB127.P332123 2017 (print) | DDC 616/.0472--dc23

LC record available at https://lccn.loc.gov/2017029185

Table of Contents

Part II: Musculoskeletal Pain

Part III: Other Pain-Related Injuries and Disorders

Part IV: Medical Management of Pain

Part V: Additional Help and Information

Preface

About This Book

According to the National Institutes of Health (NIH), pain affects more Americans than diabetes, heart disease, and cancer combined, and chronic pain is the most common cause of long-term disability in the United States. During the past few decades, medical researchers have learned a great deal about how pain is induced and experienced, but a cure remains elusive. Pain-relieving medications are often insufficient, and many carry the risk of serious side effects, including addiction and death. Other conventional, surgical, and complementary and alternative medicine (CAM) approaches to pain management offer varying degrees of relief, but so far nothing has been discovered that fully addresses the diverse needs of people experiencing pain. Nevertheless, millions of people are able to lessen their suffering and enjoy a better quality of life by taking advantage of medications, therapies, and techniques that can provide some relief.

Pain Sourcebook, Fifth Edition provides updated information about the many ways people encounter pain and the steps they can take to avoid it. It explains the different ways people experience pain and how pain affects mental health, sleep patterns, and everyday tasks. Details about the causes and treatments of the most common types of musculoskeletal pain—including arthritis and back pain—and many other pain-related injuries and disorders, such as burns, headaches, neuropathy, and postoperative pain, are included. A section on pain management offers tips for working with a healthcare provider or pain management team, facts about diagnostic procedures, and information about the most commonly used conventional and CAM therapies for pain relief. The book concludes with a glossary and a directory of resources for additional help and information.

How to Use This Book

This book is divided into parts and chapters. Parts focus on broad areas of interest. Chapters are devoted to single topics within a part.

Part I: Encountering and Avoiding Pain examines the phenomenon of pain, the various ways people experience it, and the differences in pain perception among specific subpopulations. It offers strategies for coping with chronic pain and provides tips for avoiding pain.

Part II: Musculoskeletal Pain describes what is known about disorders and injuries that can cause pain in the joints, tendons, ligaments, bones, and muscles. Individual chapters examine the most common acute and chronic conditions associated with musculoskeletal pain, including arthritis and other rheumatic disorders, back and neck pain, foot pain, and sports injuries.

Part III: Other Pain-Related Injuries and Disorders provides information about conditions of the body's organs, systems, and tissues where pain is the primary symptom or a common complication. These include complaints defined by pain—such as headaches and somatoform pain disorder—and a wide variety of diseases associated with pain, such as cancer, heart disease, appendicitis, sickle cell anemia, sinusitis, and kidney stones. Painful injuries and wounds to the body, such as burns, amputations, and surgical incisions, are also discussed.

Part IV: Medical Management of Pain offers tips about effectively communicating pain-related symptoms to a healthcare provider, and it describes the tools that are used to diagnose the sources of acute and chronic pain. It recounts various approaches to pain management and discusses the benefits and risks associated with some of the most commonly used pain relievers. Invasive, implanted, and surgical interventions are also addressed, and the part concludes with information about palliative care.

Part V: Additional Help and Information includes a glossary of terms related to pain and pain management and a directory of resources for readers seeking more details or assistance.

Bibliographic Note

This volume contains documents and excerpts from publications issued by the following U.S. government agencies: Agency for Healthcare Research and Quality (AHRQ); Centers for Disease Control and Prevention (CDC); Centers for Medicare and Medicaid Services (CMS); Chemical Hazards Emergency Medical Management (CHEMM); ClinicalTrials.gov; Division of Occupational Health and Safety (DOHS); *Eunice Kennedy Shriver* National Institute of Child Health and Human Development (NICHD); Genetic and Rare Diseases Information Center (GARD); Genetics Home Reference (GHR); National Center for Complementary and Integrative Health (NCCIH); National Heart Lung and Blood Institute (NHLBI); National Institute of Arthritis and Musculoskeletal and Skin Diseases (NIAMS); National Institute of Dental and Craniofacial Research (NIDCR); National Institute of Diabetes and Digestive and Kidney Diseases (NIDDK); National Institute of General Medical Sciences (NIGMS); National Institute of Neurological Disorders and Stroke (NINDS); National Institute of Nursing Research (NINR); National Institute on Aging (NIA); National Institute on Alcohol Abuse and Alcoholism (NIAAA); National Institute on Drug Abuse (NIDA); National Institutes of Health (NIH); National Wildfire Coordinating Group (NWCG); *NIH News in Health*; NIHSeniorHealth; Office on Women's Health (OWH); Rhode Island Judiciary; Substance Abuse and Mental Health Services Administration (SAMHSA); U.S. Department of Health and Human Services (HHS); U.S. Department Of Transportation (DOT); U.S. Department of Veterans Affairs (VA); U.S. National Library of Medicine (NLM); and the U.S. Food and Drug Administration (FDA).

It may also contain original material produced by Omnigraphics and reviewed by medical consultants.

About the Health Reference Series

The *Health Reference Series* is designed to provide basic medical information for patients, families, caregivers, and the general public. Each volume takes a particular topic and provides comprehensive coverage. This is especially important for people who may be dealing with a newly diagnosed disease or a chronic disorder in themselves or in a family member. People looking for preventive guidance, information about disease warning signs, medical statistics, and risk factors for health problems will also find answers to their questions in the *Health*

Reference Series. The *Series*, however, is not intended to serve as a tool for diagnosing illness, in prescribing treatments, or as a substitute for the physician/patient relationship. All people concerned about medical symptoms or the possibility of disease are encouraged to seek professional care from an appropriate healthcare provider.

A Note about Spelling and Style

Health Reference Series editors use *Stedman's Medical Dictionary* as an authority for questions related to the spelling of medical terms and the *Chicago Manual of Style* for questions related to grammatical structures, punctuation, and other editorial concerns. Consistent adherence is not always possible, however, because the individual volumes within the *Series* include many documents from a wide variety of different producers, and the editor's primary goal is to present material from each source as accurately as is possible. This sometimes means that information in different chapters or sections may follow other guidelines and alternate spelling authorities.

Medical Review

Omnigraphics contracts with a team of qualified, senior medical professionals who serve as medical consultants for the *Health Reference Series*. As necessary, medical consultants review reprinted and originally written material for currency and accuracy. Citations including the phrase, "Reviewed (month, year)" indicate material reviewed by this team. Medical consultation services are provided to the *Health Reference Series* editors by:

Dr. Vijayalakshmi, MBBS, DGO, MD
Dr. Senthil Selvan, MBBS, DCH, MD
Dr. K. Sivanandham, MBBS, DCH, MS (Research), PhD

Our Advisory Board

We would like to thank the following board members for providing initial guidance on the development of this series:

- Dr. Lynda Baker, Associate Professor of Library and Information Science, Wayne State University, Detroit, MI

- Nancy Bulgarelli, William Beaumont Hospital Library, Royal Oak, MI

- Karen Imarisio, Bloomfield Township Public Library, Bloomfield Township, MI

- Karen Morgan, Mardigian Library, University of Michigan-Dearborn, Dearborn, MI

- Rosemary Orlando, St. Clair Shores Public Library, St. Clair Shores, MI

Health Reference Series *Update Policy*

The inaugural book in the *Health Reference Series* was the first edition of *Cancer Sourcebook* published in 1989. Since then, the *Series* has been enthusiastically received by librarians and in the medical community. In order to maintain the standard of providing high-quality health information for the layperson the editorial staff at Omnigraphics felt it was necessary to implement a policy of updating volumes when warranted.

Medical researchers have been making tremendous strides, and it is the purpose of the *Health Reference Series* to stay current with the most recent advances. Each decision to update a volume is made on an individual basis. Some of the considerations include how much new information is available and the feedback we receive from people who use the books. If there is a topic you would like to see added to the update list, or an area of medical concern you feel has not been adequately addressed, please write to:

Managing Editor
Health Reference Series
Omnigraphics
615 Griswold, Ste. 901
Detroit, MI 48226

Part One

Encountering and Avoiding Pain

Chapter 1

Pain: The Universal Disorder

Pain in its most benign form warns us that something isn't quite right, that we should take medicine or see a doctor. At its worst, however, pain robs us of our productivity, our well-being, and, for many of us suffering from extended illness, our very lives. Pain is a complex perception that differs enormously among individual patients, even those who appear to have identical injuries or illnesses.

The burden of pain in the United States is astounding. More than 100 million Americans have pain that persists for weeks to years. The financial toll of this epidemic cost $560 billion to $635 billion per year according to *Relieving Pain in America: A Blueprint for Transforming Prevention, Care, Education, and Research*, a report from an Institute of Medicine (IOM). Pain is ultimately a challenge for family, friends, and healthcare providers who must give support to the individual suffering from the physical as well as the emotional consequences of pain.

A Pain Primer: What Do We Know about Pain?

What is pain? The International Association for the Study of Pain (IASP) defines it as: An unpleasant sensory and emotional experience associated with actual or potential tissue damage or described in terms of such damage. The IASP definition means that pain is a subjective experience; one that cannot be objectively measured and depends on

---

This chapter includes text excerpted from "Pain: Hope through Research," National Institute of Neurological Disorders and Stroke (NINDS), January 2014.

the person's self-report. As will be discussed later, there can be a wide variability in how a person experiences pain to a given stimulus or injury.

Pain can be classified as acute or chronic, and the two kinds differ greatly.

- **Acute pain**, for the most part, results from disease, inflammation, or injury to tissues. This type of pain generally comes on suddenly, for example, after trauma or surgery, and may be accompanied by anxiety or emotional distress. The cause of acute pain can usually be diagnosed and treated. The pain is self-limiting, which means it is confined to a given period of time and severity. It can become chronic.

- **Chronic pain** is now believed to be a chronic disease condition in the same manner as diabetes and asthma. Chronic pain can be made worse by environmental and psychological factors. By its nature, chronic pain persists over a long period of time and is resistant to many medical treatments. It can—and often does—cause severe problems. People with chronic pain often suffer from more than one painful condition. It is thought that there are common mechanisms that put some people at higher risk to develop multiple pain disorders. It is not known whether these disorders share a common cause.

We may experience pain as a prick, tingle, sting, burn, or ache. Normally, acute pain is a protective response to tissue damage resulting from injury, disease, overuse, or environmental stressors. To sense pain, specialized receptors (called nociceptors) which are found throughout the body, trigger a series of events in response to a noxious (painful) stimulus. The events begin with conversion of the stimulus to an electrical impulse that travels through nerves from the site of injury or disease process to the spinal cord. These signals are transmitted to a specialized part of the spinal cord called the dorsal horn.

Anatomy of Pain

Pain signals from the head and face directly enter the brainstem where they join the pain pathways that travel from the spinal cord to the brain. One central place these signals travel to is the thalamus. The thalamus is a relay station that distributes sensory signals to many other brain regions—including the anterior cingulate cortex, somatosensory cortex, insular cortex, and prefrontal cortex. These cortical brain regions process the nociceptive (pain causing or reacting to pain) information from the body and generate the complex experience of pain. This pain experience has multiple components that include the:

- sensory-discriminative aspect which helps us localize where on our body the injury occurs,

- affective-motivational aspect which conveys just how unpleasant the experience is,

- cognitive-evaluative which involves thoughtful planning on what to do to get away from the pain.

Many of these characteristics of pain have been associated with specific brain systems, although much remains to be learned. Additionally, researchers have found that many of the brain systems involved with the experience of pain overlap with the experience of basic emotions. Consequently, when people experience negative emotions (e.g., fear, anxiety, anger), the same brain systems responsible for these emotions also amplify the experience of pain.

Fortunately, there are systems in the brain that help to dampen or decrease pain. Descending signals from the brain are sent back to the spinal cord and can inhibit the intensity of incoming nociceptive signals, thereby reducing the pain experience.

Neurochemistry of Pain

This complicated process by which we perceive pain involves intricate connections among multifaceted brain regions. The nervous system uses a set of chemicals, called neurotransmitters, to communicate between neurons within and across these stations in the pain pathway. These chemicals are released by neurons in tiny packets (vesicles) into the space between two cells. When they reach their target cell, they bind to special proteins on the surface of the cells called receptors. The transmitter then activates the receptor, which functions much like a gate. The gate will either close to block (inhibitory receptor) the signal or open to send (excitatory receptor) the signal along to the next station.

There are many different neurotransmitters in the human body and they play a role in normal function as well as in disease. In the case of nociception and pain, they act in various combinations at all levels of the nervous system to transmit and modify signals generated by noxious stimuli.

One excitatory neurotransmitter of special interest to pain research-ers is glutamate, which plays a major role in nervous system function and in pain pathophysiology. The modulation of glutamate neurotrans-mission is complex, but it plays a key role in heightening the sensitivity to pain through increased responsiveness of excitatory receptors in the spinal cord dorsal horn and in the brain. This is part of a process called central sensitization and contributes to making pain persist. A great deal of attention has been given to developing molecules/drugs that block certain receptors for glutamate for their potential in reducing pain.

Unlike glutamate, GABA (or gamma-aminobutyric acid) is predom-inately an inhibitory neurotransmitter in that it generally decreases or blocks the activity of neurons. Most of what we know of its role in pain is related to its function in inhibiting spinal cord neurons from transmitting pain signals and therefore dampening pain. Chemicals that are similar to GABA have been explored as possible analgesics, but because GABA is so widespread in the nervous system it is difficult to make a GABA-like drug without affecting other nervous system functions. As we learn more about the specific roles of GABA receptors, drug development may be accelerated.

Norepinephrine and serotonin are neurotransmitters used by the descending pain pathways from the brain stem to dampen the incom-ing signals from painful stimuli from the site of the injury or inflam-mation. Drugs that modulate the activity of these transmitters, such as some antidepressants, are effective in treating some chronic pain conditions, likely by enhancing the availability of the transmitters through a recycling and reuse process. Serotonin receptors also are present on the nerves that supply the surface of the brain involved in migraines, and their modulation by a class of drugs called "triptans" is effective in acutely treating migraine.

The opioids are another important class of neurotransmitters that are involved in pain control, as well as pleasure and addiction. Their receptors are found throughout the body and can be activated by endog-enous (produced by our bodies) opioid peptides that are released by neurons in the brain. The enkephalins, dynorphins, and endorphins are some of the body's own natural painkillers. They may be more familiar for the role of endorphins in the feeling of well-being during exercise—the runner's high. Opioid receptors also can be activated by morphine, which mimics the effect of our endogenous opioids. Mor-phine is a natural product and like similar synthetic opioids, is a very potent, but potentially addictive painkiller that is used broadly for severe acute and chronic pain management. Together the opioids provide effective pain relief for many people with pain. Other peptides also transmit neuronal signals and play a role in pain responses. Scientists have shown that mice bred experimentally to lack a gene for two peptides, called tachykinins-neurokinin A and substance P, have a reduced response to severe pain. When exposed to mild pain, these mice react in the same way as mice that carry the missing gene. But when exposed to more severe pain, the mice exhibit a reduced pain response. This suggests that the two peptides are involved in the perception of pain sensations, especially moderate-to-severe pain.

Genetics of Pain

Differences in our genes highlight how different we are in respect to pain. Scientists believe that genetic variations can determine our risk for developing chronic pain, how sensitive we are to painful stimuli, whether or not certain therapies will ease our pain, and how we respond to acute or chronic pain. Many genes contribute to pain perception, and mutations in one or more pain-related genes account for some of the variability of each individual's pain experiences. Some people born genetically insensate to pain—meaning they cannot feel pain—have a mutation in part of a gene that plays a role in electrical activity of nerve cells. A different mutation in that same gene can cause a severe and disabling pain condition. Scientists have identified many genes involved in pain by screening large numbers of people with pain conditions for shared gene mutations. While genes play a role in determining our sensitivity to pain, they only account for a portion of this variability. Ultimately, our individual sensitivity to pain is governed by a complex interaction of genes, cognitions, mood, our environment and early life experiences.

Inflammation and Pain

The link between the nervous and immune systems also is important. Cytokines, a group of proteins found in the nervous system, are also part of the immune system—the body's shield for fighting off disease and responding to tissue injury. Cytokines can trigger pain by promoting inflammation, even in the absence of injury or damage. After trauma, cytokine levels rise in the brain and spinal cord and at the site where the injury occurred. Improvements in our understanding of the precise role of cytokines in producing pain may lead to new classes of drugs that can block the action of these substances to produce analgesia.

Neural Circuits and Chronic Pain

The pain that we perceive when we have an injury or infection alerts us to the potential for tissue damage. Sometimes this protective pain persists after the healing occurs or may even appear when there was no apparent cause. This persistent pain is linked to changes in our nervous system, which responds to internal and external change by reorganizing and adapting throughout life. This phenomenon is known as neuronal plasticity, a process that allows us to learn, remember, and recover from brain injury. Following an injury or disease process, sometimes the nervous system undergoes a structural and functional reorganization that is not a healthy form of plasticity. Long-term, maladaptive changes in both the peripheral and central nervous system can make us hypersensitive to pain and can make pain persist after injuries have healed. For example, sensory neurons in the peripheral nervous system, which normally detect noxious/painful stimuli, may alter the electrical or molecular signals that they send to the spinal cord. This in turn triggers genes to alter production of receptors and chemical transmitters in spinal cord neurons setting up a chronic pain state. Scientists have methods to identify which genes' activities change with injury and chronic pain. Knowledge of the proteins that ultimately are synthesized by these genes are providing new targets for therapy development. Increased physiological excitation of neurons in the spinal cord, in turn enhance pain signaling pathways to the brainstem and in the brain. This hypersensitivity of the central nervous system is called central sensitization. It is difficult to reverse and makes pain persist beyond its protective role.

How Is Pain Diagnosed?

There is no way to tell accurately how much pain a person has. Tools to measure pain intensity, to show pain through imaging technology, to locate pain precisely, and to assess the effect of pain on someone's life, offer some insight into how much pain a person has. They do not, however, provide objective measures of pain. Sometimes, as in the case of headaches, physicians find that the best aid to diagnosis is the person's own description of the type, duration, and location of pain. Defining pain as sharp or dull, constant or intermittent, burning or aching may give the best clues to the cause of pain. These descriptions are part of what is called the pain history, taken by the physician during the preliminary examination of a person with pain. Developing a test for assessing pain would be a very useful tool in diagnosing and treating pain.

Physicians, however, do have a number of approaches and technologies they use to find the cause of pain. Primarily these include:

- A musculoskeletal and neurological examination
- Laboratory tests (e.g., blood, urine, cerebrospinal fluid)
- Electrodiagnostic procedures include electromyography (EMG), nerve conduction studies, evoked potential (EP) studies, and quantitative sensory testing
- Imaging, especially magnetic resonance imaging or MRI
- X-rays

How Is Pain Treated?

The goal of pain management is to improve function, enabling individuals to work, attend school, and participate in day-to-day activities. People with pain and their physicians have a number of options for treatment; some are more effective than others. Sometimes, relaxation and the use of imagery as a distraction provide relief. These methods may be powerful and effective, according to those who advocate their use. Whatever the treatment regime, it is important to remember that, while not all pain is curable, all pain is treatable. The following treatments are among the most common.

Treatment varies depending on the duration and type of pain. For the most part, the medications listed below have been shown in clinical trials to relieve or prevent pain associated with a specific condition(s), but none have been proven fully effective in relieving all types of pain. A healthcare professional should be consulted to determine which medication is effective for a given pain condition and what to expect for pain relief and side effects. Evidence for the procedures listed below is variable in its quality. In some cases, evidence suggesting that some treatments are effective is anecdotal—or based on personal experience—and in other cases it is collected from well-designed clinical trials.

- Acetaminophen
- Acupuncture
- Analgesic
- Anticonvulsants
- Antidepressants
- Beta-blockers

- Biofeedback
- Capsaicin
- Chiropractic care
- Cognitive-behavioral therapy
- Counseling
- Electrical stimulation
  - TENS
  - Peripheral nerve stimulation
  - Spinal cord stimulation
  - Deep brain stimulation
- Exercise
- Hypnosis
- Low-power lasers
- Magnets
- Marijuana (cannabis)
- Nerve blocks
  - Sympathectomy or sympathetic blockade
  - Neurolytic blocks
  - Surgical blocks
    - Spinal dorsal rhizotomy
- Nonsteroidal anti-inflammatory drugs (NSAIDs)
  - Aspirin
  - COX-2 inhibitors
  - Ibuprofen
- Opioids
- Physical therapy and rehabilitation
- R.I.C.E. (Rest, Ice, Compression, and Elevation)
- Serotonergic agonists
- Surgery

Gender and Pain

It is widely believed that pain affects men and women differently. In fact, according to the Institute of Medicine's report: *Relieving Pain in America,* women often report a higher prevalence of chronic pain than men and are at a greater risk for many pain conditions. Women are likely to have more pain from certain diseases, such as cancer. Also, a number of chronic pain disorders occur only in women and others occur predominantly in women. These include chronic fatigue syndrome, endometriosis, fibromyalgia, interstitial cystitis, vulvodynia, and temporomandibular disorders.

The IOM report mentions at least three theories that may explain the differences in pain experience by gender:

- A gender-role theory that assumes it is more socially acceptable for women to report pain;

- An exposure theory that suggests women are exposed to more pain risk factors; and

- A vulnerability theory proposing that women are more vulnerable to developing certain types of pain, such as musculoskeletal pain.

Of these, the vulnerability theory is best supported by scientific evidence.

A greater understanding of gender differences in pain may lead to better avenues of pain management.

Pain in the Elderly and Children

Pain is the number one complaint of older Americans, and one in five older Americans takes a painkiller regularly. Pain management in older people differs from than in younger people. For example, older persons are much more likely to experience medication-related side effects than younger ones. In 1998, the American Geriatrics Society (AGS) issued guidelines for improving the management of pain and quality of life in older people. The guidelines contained several non-drug approaches to treatment, including exercise, and recommended that, whenever possible, people use alternatives to aspirin, ibuprofen, and other NSAIDs because of the drugs' side effects, including stomach irritation and gastrointestinal bleeding.

In the updated guidelines, the AGS recommends that NSAIDs and COX-2s be considered rarely, and with extreme caution, in highly selected individuals due to possible increased cardiovascular risk and gastrointestinal bleeding.

For older adults, acetaminophen is the first-line treatment for mild to moderate pain, according to the guidelines.

Pain in children also requires special attention, particularly because young children are not always able to describe the degree of pain they are experiencing. Although treating pain in children poses a special challenge to physicians and parents alike, children should never be undertreated. Special tools for measuring pain in children have been developed that, when combined with cues used by parents, help physicians select the most effective treatments.

Nonsteroidal agents, and especially acetaminophen, are most often prescribed for control of pain in children. In the case of severe pain or pain following surgery, acetaminophen may be combined with codeine.

Chapter 2

Facts and Figures on Pain

An analysis of data from the National Health Interview Survey (NHIS) has found that most American adults have experienced some level of pain, from brief to more lasting (chronic) pain, and from relatively minor to more severe pain. The analysis helps to unravel the complexities of a Nation in pain. It found that an estimated 25.3 million adults (11.2 percent) experience chronic pain—that is, they had pain every day for the preceding 3 months. Nearly 40 million adults (17.6 percent) experience severe levels of pain. Those with severe pain are also likely to have worse health status.

"The number of people who suffer from severe and chronic pain is striking," said Josephine P. Briggs, M.D., director of National Center for Complementary and Integrative Health (NCCIH). "This analysis adds valuable new scope to our understanding of pain and could inform the National Pain Strategy in the areas of population research and disparities. It may help shape future research, development, and targeting of effective pain interventions, including complementary health approaches."

Pain is one of the leading reasons Americans turn to complementary health approaches such as yoga, massage, and meditation—which may help manage pain and other symptoms that are not consistently addressed by prescription drugs and other conventional treatments.

This chapter contains text excerpted from the following sources: Text in this chapter begins with excerpts from "NIH Analysis Shows Americans Are in Pain," National Center for Complementary and Integrative Health (NCCIH), August 11, 2015; Text beginning with the heading "What Is Chronic Pain?" is excerpted from "Pain in America Infographic," National Institutes of Health (NIH), September 10, 2014.

The NHIS is an annual study in which tens of thousands of Americans are interviewed about their health—and illness-related experiences. The NHIS asked participants about the frequency and intensity of pain experienced in the prior 3 months. The survey results are based on combined data from 8,781 American adults from a subsection of the larger NHIS.

Researchers assigned pain severity using an approach developed by the Washington Group on Disability Statistics, which provides four categories of pain. Among the findings of the analysis:

- An estimated 23.4 million adults (10.3 percent) experience a lot of pain.

- An estimated 126 million adults (55.7 percent) reported some type of pain in the 3 months prior to the survey.

- Adults in the two most severe pain groups were likely to have worse health status, use more healthcare, and suffer from more disability than those with less severe pain. However, approximately half of individuals with the most severe pain still rated their overall health as good or better.

- There were associations between pain severity and race, ethnicity, language preference, gender, and age. Women, older individuals, and non-Hispanics were more likely to report any pain, while Asians were less likely.

- Minorities who did not choose to be interviewed in English are markedly less likely to report pain.

- The impact of gender on pain varies by race and ethnicity.

"This report begins to answer calls for better national data on the nature and extent of the pain problem," said Richard L. Nahin, Ph.D., M.P.H., lead epidemiologist for NCCIH and author of the analysis. "The experience of pain is subjective. It's not surprising then that the data show varied responses to pain even in those with similar levels of pain. Continuing analyses of these data may help identify subpopulations that would benefit from additional pain treatment options."

What Is Chronic Pain?

Chronic pain is considered a disease itself. It can be influenced by environmental and psychological factors and is resistant to most medical treatments.

Acute pain often results from disease, inflammation, or injury to tissues. It generally comes on suddenly.

100 million adults suffer from chronic pain in the United States.

- About 1/2 have daily pain

- Up to 1/3 have mild pain

- 1/3 or more have moderate pain

- Less than 1/3 have severe pain

These are three of the most common types of pain:

- Low back pain

- Severe headache or migraine

- Neck pain

Many people suffer from more than one kind of chronic pain. Chronic pain affects emotional state:

- Depression

- Anger

- Anxiety

- Fear

Who Suffers the Most?

- **Women** experience pain differently from men. Women feel pain more intensely and are at greater risk of developing chronic pain conditions than men.

- **African Americans and Hispanics** are less likely than whites to receive adequate pain relief despite comparable severity.

- **African Americans** with chronic pain report lower quality pain management, more disabling pain severity, and lower quality of life because of pain, than whites.

- **30 percent of adults 65 years and older** report low back pain compared to 23 percent of adults ages 18–44.

- **Approximately 50 percent of older adults and nursing home residents** experience debilitating pain or suffer from pain on a daily basis.

Challenges

- A majority of clinicians, especially primary healthcare professionals, have not been well trained in pain and pain management.

- The estimated economic impact of pain from direct medical costs to loss of productive time ranges from $560–$635 billion every year.

Chapter 3

Pain Perception

Chapter Contents

Section 3.1

Theory of Pain

This section includes text excerpted from "The Gate
Control Theory of Pain," U.S. Department of Veterans
Affairs (VA), July 2013. Reviewed June 2017.

The Gate Control Theory

The way in which we experience pain is very complex. All sorts of factors influence our experience, including our thoughts and feelings.

For example, you will probably be aware that there are times when, even though you have pain, you are only dimly aware of it. This can happen, for example, when you are really engrossed in doing something interesting or having to face a situation which demands all your attention. A very good example of this are the stories you might have heard about wounded soldiers, who despite being seriously injured will continue in battle and not really be aware of much pain until after the danger has passed.

On the other hand, you will probably be aware of how in some circumstances your pain can feel much worse. Indeed, you may find that the more you think about your pain, the worse it can feel.

Nerves from all over the body run to the spinal cord, which is the first main meeting point for the nervous system. In the spinal cord, you might imagine a series of gates into which messages about pain arrive from all over the body.

These gates can sometimes be much more open than at other times. This is important because it is through these gates that messages from your body pass towards your brain. If the gates are more open, then a lot of pain messages pass through to the brain and you are likely to experience a high level of pain. If the gates are more closed, then fewer messages get through and you are likely to experience less pain. So, what are the factors that make a difference to how open or closed the gates are?

Factors That Open the Gate

There are three main ways in which the gates to pain can be made more open, so that the pain feels worse. These are to do with how we feel about things, how we think about things, and what we are doing.

1. **Stress and Tension.** All sorts of emotional states can lead to the gates to pain being more open. These include being anxious, worried, angry, and depressed. Having a lot of tension in the body is a common way of opening the pain gates.

2. **Mental Factors.** One of the most effective ways of opening the gates and increasing your pain is to focus all your attention on it. Boredom can also lead to the pain gates opening.

3. **Lack of Activity.** Another factor that seems to open the gates to pain is to not move around, to have stiff joints and to lack fitness.

Factors That Close the Gate

In the same way as above, the way we feel, the way we think and what we do can all have a part to play in helping to close the gates to pain.

1. **Relaxation and Contentment.** Feeling generally happy and optimistic has been found to help to close the gates to pain. Also, feeling relaxed in yourself seems to be a particularly useful way of closing the gates.

2. **Mental Factors.** Being involved and taking an interest in life helps to close the gates. Also if you concentrate intensely on something other than the pain (e.g., work, T.V., book), then this can distract you from any pain, helping to close the gates.

3. **Activity.** Taking the right amount of exercise, so that you develop your fitness, can help to close the gates.

4. **Other Physical Factors.** You may also find that for you certain types of medication can help to close the gates, as might certain types of counter-stimulation (e.g., heat, massage, tens, acupuncture).

Putting Theory into Practice

So, how can you apply the gate control theory of pain to you? The best way is to experiment with some of the ideas that are described above. How might you be able to use the fact that emotional factors can make a difference? Are there ways of becoming more relaxed, for example? And what about mental factors? Are there ways that you can get more involved in life? Can you use distraction more than you have been doing? And what about physical factors? Could you increase your fitness and activity levels (provided that you don't over do it)? And might you be able to make more use of counter-stimulation?

Knowing about the gate control theory of pain can give you the opportunity to experiment with what opens and what closes the gates for you. Keep a record of your experiments. For example, you might have two headings "factors that open the gate" and "factors that close the gate." And put what you find into practice. You might not be able to remove your pain, but you might well find that, for at least some of the time, you can influence just how much the gates are open or closed to your pain.

Section 3.2

Types and Ways People Experience Pain

This section includes text excerpted from "Pain: You Can Get Help," National Institute on Aging (NIA), National Institutes of Health (NIH), May 2015.

You've probably been in pain at one time or another. Maybe you've had a headache or bruise—pain that doesn't last too long. But, many older people have ongoing pain from health problems like arthritis, cancer, diabetes, or shingles. They may even have many different kinds of pain.

Pain can be your body's way of warning you that something is wrong. Always tell the doctor where you hurt and exactly how it feels.

Acute Pain and Chronic Pain

There are two kinds of pain. Acute pain begins suddenly, lasts for a short time, and goes away as your body heals. You might feel acute pain after surgery or if you have a broken bone, infected tooth, or kidney stone.

Pain that lasts for several months or years is called chronic (or persistent) pain. This pain often affects older people. Examples include rheumatoid arthritis (RA) and sciatica. In some cases, chronic pain follows after acute pain from an injury or other health issue has gone away, like postherpetic neuralgia after shingles.

Living with any type of pain can be very hard. It can cause many other problems. For instance, pain can:

- Get in the way of your daily activities

- Disturb your sleep and eating habits

- Make it difficult to continue working

- Cause depression or anxiety

Describing Pain

Many people have a hard time describing pain. Think about these questions when you explain how the pain feels:

- Where does it hurt?

- When did it start? Does the pain come and go?

- What does it feel like? Is the pain sharp, dull, or burning? Would you use some other word to describe it?

- Do you have other symptoms?

- When do you feel the pain? In the morning? In the evening? After eating?

- Is there anything you do that makes the pain feel better or worse? For example, does using a heating pad or ice pack help? Does changing your position from lying down to sitting up make it better? Have you tried any over-the-counter medications for it?

Your doctor or nurse may ask you to rate your pain on a scale of 0 to 10, with 0 being no pain and 10 being the worst pain you can imagine. Or, your doctor may ask if the pain is mild, moderate, or severe. Some doctors or nurses have pictures of faces that show different expressions of pain. You point to the face that shows how you feel.

Attitudes about Pain

Everyone reacts to pain differently. Many older people have been told not to talk about their aches and pains. Some people feel they should be brave and not complain when they hurt. Other people are quick to report pain and ask for help.

Worrying about pain is a common problem. This worry can make you afraid to stay active, and it can separate you from your friends and family. Working with your doctor, you can find ways to continue to take part in physical and social activities despite being in pain.

Some people put off going to the doctor because they think pain is just part of aging and nothing can help. This is not true! It is important to see a doctor if you have a new pain. Finding a way to manage your pain is often easier if it is addressed early.

Some Facts about Pain

- Most people don't have to live with pain. There are pain treatments. While not all pain can be cured, most pain can be managed. If your doctor has not been able to help you, ask to see a pain specialist.

- Most people who properly take doctor-prescribed narcotic drugs for pain relief do not become addicted. If you take your medicine exactly the way your doctor tells you, then you are not likely to develop an addiction problem. Let your doctor know if you have a personal or family history of substance abuse.

- The side effects from pain medicine usually are not worse than the pain. Side effects from pain medicine like constipation, dry mouth, and drowsiness may be a problem when you first begin taking the medicine. These problems can often be treated and may go away as your body gets used to the medicine.

- Your doctor will not think you're a whiner or a sissy if you talk about your pain. If you are in pain, tell your doctor so you can get the help you need.

- If you use pain medicine now, it will still work when you need it later. Using medicine at the first sign of pain may help control your pain later.

- Pain is not "all in your head." No one but you knows how your pain feels. If you're in pain, talk with your doctor.

Chapter 4

Chronic Pain Affects Mental Health and Sleep

Chapter Contents

Section 4.1

Understanding Chronic Pain

This section includes text excerpted from "Chronic Pain Primer," U.S. Department of Veterans Affairs (VA), June 17, 2015.

Chronic pain (noncancer pain) generally refers to intractable pain that exists for three or more months and does not resolve in response to treatment. There is some variation in terms of the required pain duration, in that some conditions may become chronic in as little as one month, while some pain specialists adhere to the six-month pain duration criteria employed in the past.

Chronic Pain versus Psychogenic Pain

Perhaps no other issue has done as much damage to individuals with chronic pain as this one. Many healthcare professionals fail to recognize the complexity of pain and believe that it can be dichotomized based on the presence or absence of physical findings, secondary gain, or prior emotional problems. As a result, countless individuals have been informed that "The pain is all in your head." And if these same individuals react with anger and hurt, healthcare staff are ready to compound the problem by labeling the individual as hostile, demanding, or aggressive.

In actuality, the correspondence between physical findings (e.g., Magnetic resonance imaging (MRI), computerized tomography (CT), or X-ray results) and pain complaints is fairly low (generally, 40% to 60%). Individuals may have abnormal tests (e.g., MRI shows a "bulging disk" or a herniation) with no pain, or substantial pain with negative results. This is because chronic pain can develop in the absence of the gross skeletal changes healthcare professionals are able to detect with current technology. Muscle strain and inflammation are common causes of chronic pain, yet may be extremely difficult to detect. Other conditions may be due to systemic problems (e.g., human immunodeficiency virus (HIV)-related pain or sickle cell pain), trauma to nerves (e.g., postthoracotomy pain), circulatory difficulties (e.g., diabetic neuropathy), central nervous system (CNS) dysfunction (e.g., central pain syndromes), or many others. Yet, in each of these cases they may be unable to "see" the cause of the problem. Instead, they have to rely on the person's report of their pain, coupled with behavioral observations and indirect medical data. This does not mean that the pain is psychogenic. Rather, it means that they are less able to detect or understand its cause.

In actuality, healthy individuals feigning pain for secondary gain purposes are relatively rare. And in most cases, clear monetary motives will be evident. Additionally, the presence of secondary gain does not at all indicate that an individual's pain is less "real." In this country most individuals with chronic pain receive at least some type of benefit (not necessarily monetary) for pain complaints. Therefore, exaggeration of pain or related problems is to be expected. Unfortunately, many less aware practitioners use the presence of secondary gain or pain amplification as an indication that the person's pain is not "real."

Factors Influencing the Experience of Pain

Pain is a complex response by the organism to a number of factors.

Physiological/Biological factors

- Site of injury or source of painful stimuli
- Intensity of stimulation/degree of tissue damage
- Type and density of receptors present
- Biologically-based individual differences in pain threshold and sensitivity
- Amount of competing sensory (large fiber) activity

Psychological factors

- Emotional status of the individual (in general, negative emotions increase pain; positive emotions reduce pain)
- Attentional effects
- Individual beliefs and expectations regarding the experience of pain (pain can be experienced with no noxious stimulation if it is expected)
- The individual's belief regarding their ability to establish control over the pain

- The individual's history of pain experiences and pain sensations (cultural and learning effects)

- General physical health of the person with pain

As pain duration increases, more of these factors begin to influence the experience of pain. Thus, successful chronic pain treatment often involves multiple specialties delivering a range of interventions for a variety of related problems.

Section 4.2

Chronic Pain Syndromes

This section includes text excerpted from "Chronic Pain Primer," U.S. Department of Veterans Affairs (VA), June 17, 2015.

In deciding how to treat chronic pain, it is important to distinguish between **chronic pain** and a **chronic pain syndrome**. A chronic pain syndrome differs from chronic pain in that people with a chronic pain syndrome, over time, develop a number of related life problems beyond the sensation of pain itself. It is important to distinguish between the two because they respond to different types of treatment.

Most individuals with chronic pain (estimates are about 75% nationally) do not develop the more complicated and distressful chronic pain syndrome. Although they may experience the pain for the remainder of their lives, little change in their daily regimen of activities, family relationships, work, or other life components occurs. Many of these individuals may never seek treatment for pain. Those that do often require less intensive, single-modality interventions.

The 25 percent who do develop chronic pain syndromes tend to experience increasing physical, emotional, and social deterioration over time. They may abuse pain medications (usually narcotics and/or muscle relaxants), and typically require more intensive, multimodal treatment to stop the cycle of increasing dysfunction.

Symptoms of Chronic Pain Syndromes

- Reduced activity
- Impaired sleep
- Depression
- Suicidal ideation
- Social withdrawal
- Irritability
- Fatigue
- Memory and cognitive impairment
- Poor self-esteem
- Less interest in sex
- Relationship problems
- Pain behaviors
- Kinesiophobia, or the avoidance of certain movements or activities due to fear of reinjury or re-experiencing the pain.
- Helplessness
- Hopelessness
- Alcohol abuse
- Medication abuse
- Guilt
- Anxiety
- Misbehavior by children in the home
- Loss of employment

There are at present no empirical methods of determining whether or not a chronic pain syndrome is present. Distinctions between the two are based on clinical judgments. Generally, the more of the above symptoms the individual reports or the more severe the symptoms are, the more severe the chronic pain syndrome is. However, the above are symptoms of a chronic pain syndrome only when they are primarily or mostly due to the pain itself. For example, individuals with a history of substance abuse or depression which preceded their chronic pain would not meet the requirement that their symptoms be primarily due to their pain.

How Do Chronic Pain Syndromes Develop?

As individuals try to cope with chronic pain, they adopt predictable patterns of behavior which appear to provide short-term relief. Unfortunately, the long-term effects of these patterns tends to be increased pain and more daily impairment. Typically this results from the chronic pain cycle:

pain > less activity > weaker muscles > more pain > less activity > weaker muscles

The deterioration is exacerbated by **Kinesiophobia**, or avoidance of certain movements or activities due to fear of reinjury or re-experiencing the pain. Kinesiophobia leads to more protective behaviors, or changes in posture, gait, or movement that reduce the pain for the short term. Unfortunately, over time they may lead to increased muscle weakness, reduced circulation, muscle spasms and inflammation, reduced flexibility, and, in some cases, muscle atrophy.

Models of Treatment

There are four primary models of chronic pain service delivery, which are based on the results of the International Association for the Study of Pain (IASP) Task Force on Guidelines for Desirable Characteristics for Pain Treatment Facilities. These models are represented both in the private sector and in the VA.

Single service clinics or modality-oriented clinics are outpatient clinics that provide a specific type of treatment for pain but do not provide comprehensive assessment or management. Most often they are staffed by individuals from a single discipline with some expertise in a range of pain interventions falling within their areas of specialty training. Examples include a nerve block clinic, a transcutaneous nerve stimulation (TENS) clinic, or a biofeedback clinic. In general, these approaches are best suited for individuals with chronic pain, but without a chronic pain syndrome. The goal of treatment is pain reduction.

The next level of intervention occurs within a **pain clinic**. These outpatient clinics specifically focus on the diagnosis and management of individuals with chronic pain. They are staffed by individuals from one or more disciplines with specialized training in chronic pain. They may focus only on selected pain problems (e.g., a "headache clinic" or a "back pain clinic"), or on more general pain conditions. They may refer to outside consultants or staff for services not available within the clinic. They are most appropriate for individuals with more severe pain but without a chronic pain syndrome. However, those with mild chronic pain syndromes also may be appropriate.

As healthcare professionals increase in treatment intensity and complexity, they next come to the **multidisciplinary (or interdisciplinary) pain clinic**. This level of intervention includes a specific outpatient or inpatient program of treatment which typically includes at a minimum physical restoration, medical, educational, and psychological services delivered by an identifiable team of individuals from a range of disciplines with extensive training and experience in chronic pain interventions. These pain programs are most suited for those with mild to moderate chronic pain syndromes who require more global and intensive treatment of their pain and their related areas of dysfunction. Goals include improvement in pain, activity level, flexibility, strength, endurance, and psychosocial functioning.

The final type of treatment delivery is provided through a **multidisciplinary (or interdisciplinary) pain center**. The pain center is the largest and most complex type of pain treatment model, and typically is associated with a medical school or teaching hospital. Such centers offer treatment of both acute and chronic pain using a dedicated, interdisciplinary staff working in a team setting. Staff specialize in pain treatment. Unlike the multidisciplinary pain clinic, pain centers also must engage in active pain-related research and staff education. Pain centers are most appropriate for individuals with moderate to severe chronic pain syndromes, and for those with less severe pain syndromes but very complex and refractory pain problems. They also are most appropriate for individuals with chronic pain whose rehabilitation is complicated by concurrent medical or emotional problems that require closer monitoring and the immediate availability of emergent and supportive services. The Chronic Pain Rehabilitation Program at James A. Haley Veterans Hospital is the only program in the VA that currently meets the pain center criteria and is CARF-accredited.

Section 4.3

Depression and Chronic Pain

This section includes text excerpted from "Depression and Chronic Pain," U.S. Department of Health and Human Services (HHS), June 6, 2013. Reviewed June 2017.

What Is Depression?

Major depressive disorder, or depression, is a serious mental illness. Depression interferes with your daily life and routine and reduces your quality of life. About 6.7 percent of U.S. adults ages 18 and older have depression.

Signs and Symptoms of Depression

- Ongoing sad, anxious, or empty feelings
- Feeling hopeless
- Feeling guilty, worthless, or helpless
- Feeling irritable or restless
- Loss of interest in activities or hobbies once enjoyable, including sex
- Feeling tired all the time
- Difficulty concentrating, remembering details, or making decisions
- Difficulty falling asleep or staying asleep, a condition called insomnia, or sleeping all the time
- Overeating or loss of appetite
- Thoughts of death and suicide or suicide attempts
- Ongoing aches and pains, headaches, cramps, or digestive
- Problems that do not ease with treatment.

What Is Chronic Pain?

Chronic pain is pain that lasts for weeks, months, or even years. It often does not ease with regular pain medication. Chronic pain can have a distinct cause, such as a temporary injury or infection or a long-term disease. But some chronic pain has no obvious cause. Like depression, chronic pain can cause problems with sleep and daily activities, reducing your quality of life.

How Are Depression and Chronic Pain Linked?

Scientists don't yet know how depression and chronic pain are linked, but the illnesses are known to occur together. Chronic pain can worsen depression symptoms and is a risk factor for suicide in people who are depressed.

Bodily aches and pains are a common symptom of depression. Studies show that people with more severe depression feel more intense pain. According to recent research, people with depression have higher than normal levels of proteins called cytokines. Cytokines send messages to cells that affect how the immune system responds to infection and disease, including the strength and length of the response. In this way, cytokines can trigger pain by promoting inflammation, which is the body's response to infection or injury. Inflammation helps protect the body by destroying, removing, or isolating the infected or injured area. In addition to pain, signs of inflammation include swelling, redness, heat, and sometimes loss of function.

Many studies are finding that inflammation may be a link between depression and illnesses that often occur with depression. Further research may help doctors and scientists better understand this connection and find better ways to diagnose and treat depression and other illnesses. One disorder that has been shown to occur with depression is fibromyalgia. Fibromyalgia causes chronic, widespread muscle pain, tiredness, and multiple tender points—places on the body that hurt in response to light pressure. People with fibromyalgia are more likely to have depression and other mental illnesses than the general population. Studies have shown that depression and fibromyalgia share risk factors and treatments.

How Is Depression Treated in People Who Have Chronic Pain?

Depression is diagnosed and treated by a healthcare provider. Treating depression can help you manage your chronic pain and improve your overall health. Recovery from depression takes time but treatments are effective. At present, the most common treatments for depression include:

- Cognitive behavioral therapy (CBT)

- Selective serotonin reuptake inhibitor (SSRI)

- Serotonin and norepinephrine reuptake inhibitor (SNRI)

While currently available depression treatments are generally well tolerated and safe, talk with your healthcare provider about side effects, possible drug interactions, and other treatment options.

Not everyone responds to treatment the same way. Medications can take several weeks to work, may need to be combined with ongoing talk therapy, or may need to be changed or adjusted to minimize side effects and achieve the best results. People living with chronic pain may be able to manage their symptoms through lifestyle changes. For example, regular aerobic exercise may help reduce some symptoms of chronic pain. Exercise may also boost your mood and help treat your depression. Talk therapy may also be helpful in treating your chronic pain.

Section 4.4

Pain and Posttraumatic Stress Disorder (PTSD)

This section includes text excerpted from "The Experience of Chronic Pain and PTSD: A Guide for Healthcare Providers," U.S. Department of Veterans Affairs (VA), February 23, 2016.

About Chronic Pain

According to the International Association for the Study of Pain (IASP), chronic pain involves suffering from pain in a particular area of the body (e.g., in the back or the neck) for at least three to six months. Chronic pain may be as severe as, if not more severe than, acute pain but the individual's experience is "modulated and compounded by the prolonged or recurrent nature of the chronic state, and further complicated by a multitude of economic and psycho-social factors." In stark contrast to acute pain, chronic pain persists beyond the amount of time that is normal for an injury to heal.

Chronic pain can have a variety of sources including disease processes or injuries. Some chronic pain stems from a traumatic event, such as a physical or sexual assault, a motor vehicle accident, or some type of disaster. Under these circumstances the person may experience both chronic pain and posttraumatic stress disorder (PTSD).

How Common Is Chronic Pain?

Approximately one in three Americans (more than twelve million people) suffer from some kind of recurring pain in their lifetimes, and three million of these individuals are seriously disabled from their chronic pain conditions. Eighty to ninety percent of Americans experience chronic cervical or lower back problems.

Evaluating Chronic Pain

Medical providers have a difficult time ascertaining the accuracy of patients' pain severity. Care providers generally assess chronic pain by administering physical examinations and having patients perform various tasks, such as exercises that help the provider evaluate the patient's strength, flexibility, and reflexes. At times, patients are asked to rate their pain on a scale from "no pain at all to "completely unbearable." Yet, because every person is different and perceives and experiences pain in different ways, it is difficult for medical providers to determine how much pain an individual is experiencing.

In addition, healthcare providers usually base their determination of pain severity on their own perceptions of how much pain seems appropriate for a given injury or pain condition. There is often very little consistency between providers regarding the measurement of their patients' pain. This creates obvious frustration for providers, but this can be even more exasperating for the individual who is suffering from chronic pain. It is common for patients to be disbelieved, or to have the level of their pain or disability minimized. Many times, this frustration causes patients to go from provider to provider in search of answers and relief from their pain. Additionally, this kind of experience often contributes to an increased sense of helplessness and despair, which can subsequently increase tension and pain, as well as emotional distress.

What Is the Experience of Chronic Pain Like Physically?

There are many forms of chronic pain, and each type of condition results in different experiences of pain and disability. As an example, chronic low back pain (CLBP), the most pervasive or common type of pain, is known to result in severe disability and limitation of movement.

Most patients with chronic pain resort to invasive assessment or treatment procedures, including surgery, to help ameliorate the pain. Individuals with chronic pain are less able to function in daily life than those who do not suffer from chronic pain. Patients with severe chronic pain and limited mobility oftentimes are unable to perform activities of daily living, such as walking, standing, sitting, lifting light objects, doing paperwork, standing in line at a grocery store, going shopping, or working. Many patients with chronic pain cannot work because of their pain or physical limitations.

What Is the Experience of Chronic Pain Like Psychologically?

Chronic pain and the disability that often comes with it can lead to a cognitive reevaluation and reintegration of one's belief systems, values, emotions, and feelings of self-worth. Numerous studies have indicated that many patients who experience chronic pain (up to 100%) tend also to be clinically depressed. In fact, depression is the most common psychiatric diagnosis in patients with chronic pain. The experience of progressive, consistent chronic pain and disability also translates for many individuals into having thoughts of suicide as a means of ending their pain and frustration.

Posttraumatic Stress Disorder (PTSD) and Chronic Pain

The prevalence of PTSD is substantially elevated in patients with chronic pain. A current PTSD prevalence of 35 percent was seen in a sample of chronic pain patients, compared to 3.5 percent in the general population. In a study of patients with chronic low back pain, 51 percent of the patients evidenced significant PTSD symptoms. In another study of patients who experienced chronic pain following a motor vehicle accident, researchers found that 50 percent of the patients developed PTSD.

One symptom of PTSD is that the person becomes emotionally or physically upset when reminded of the traumatic event. For people with chronic pain, the pain may actually serve as a reminder of the traumatic event, which will tend to exacerbate the PTSD.

Past Experiences, Present Pain

It is important to recognize that certain types of chronic pain are more common in individuals who have experienced specific traumas. For example, adult survivors of physical, psychological, or sexual abuse tend to be more at risk for developing certain types of chronic pain later in their lives. The most common forms of chronic pain for survivors of these kinds of trauma involve:

- pain in the pelvis, lower back, face, and bladder;
- fibromyalgia;
- interstitial cystitis; and
- nonremitting whiplash syndromes.

Some of the theories as to why this relationship occurs relate to personality development, neurobiology or neurophysiology, memory, behavior, and personal coping styles. In order to increase our understanding of the relationships between certain traumas and specific kinds of chronic pain, it is essential that healthcare providers ask both male and female patients with chronic pain about their childhood experiences. It is particularly important to gather this information for those patients where the source or basis for their pain conditions is unknown.

Treating Individuals Who Have Chronic Pain and PTSD

Cognitive-behavioral therapy (CBT) is a psychotherapeutic intervention that helps patients manage chronic pain. Other types of treatment that help patients with chronic pain include: stress inoculation training, behavior modification/operant conditioning, self-directed treatments, and adjunctive treatments such as biofeedback and relaxation training. There are also manualized treatments that specifically address avoidance behaviors and hypervigilance, because these behaviors tend to reinforce fear reactions.

Research suggests that providing CBT treatments to address PTSD symptoms in patients with chronic pain may lead to improvements in pain-related functioning. This has been seen even when the pain was not addressed specifically in the intervention. When treating patients with chronic pain, it is vital that healthcare providers address patients' symptoms of PTSD and depression. In so doing, they increase the likelihood that patients will have improvements in their levels of pain as well as in their physical and emotional functioning.

Recommendations for Healthcare Providers

When patients are coping with a chronic pain condition, it is difficult for them to hear from a healthcare provider that they will need to "live with it" and "manage the pain" for the rest of their lives. Being faced with the news of impending health problems, ongoing severe pain, and disability is extremely difficult. These individuals may have lost their physical abilities, and they have lost the assurance that they can fully control whatever is going on in their lives. Much like losing a loved one, these individuals will need to grieve their losses. This may take some time and will vary from person to person. Here are some suggestions for assisting these individuals:

- **Gather a thorough biopsychosocial history and assess the individual for medical and psychiatric problems**. Do a risk assessment for suicidal and homicidal ideation. Also ask about misuse of substances, such as drugs or alcohol, including over-the-counter and prescription drugs or narcotics. Taking appropriate steps to ensure someone is clean and sober and not using medications or other substances to self-medicate is a necessary component of treatment.

- **Assess for PTSD symptoms**. A quick screen is the Primary Care PTSD Screen (PC-PTSD) that has been designed for use in primary care and other medical settings.

- **Make appropriate referrals for PTSD, depression, other psychiatric disorders, or significant spiritual issues**. Likewise, help build up or stabilize the patient's social support network, as this will act as a buffer against the stress they are experiencing.

Understand that prior to patients being able to come to an acceptance about the permanence of their condition, they will be feeling very much out of control and helpless. Their lives essentially revolve around trying to regain their sense of control. This can sometimes be difficult, particularly when treatments don't seem to help or the patient's support system is weak. There may be times when they become outwardly angry or depressed. Restoring some sense of control and empowering the patient is a fundamental part of the treatment process.

Section 4.5

Pain and Sleep

Pain is the leading cause of insomnia. People who experience chronic pain—which includes about 15 percent of the overall U.S. population and half of all elderly people—often have trouble falling asleep and staying asleep. In fact, about 65 percent of people with chronic pain report having disrupted sleep or nonrestorative sleep, resulting in an average deficit of 42 minutes between the amount of sleep they need and the amount they actually get. Shorter sleep duration and poorer sleep quality, in turn, exacerbate chronic pain and interfere with activities, work, mood, relationships, and other aspects of daily life.

About Chronic Pain

People who experience chronic pain often have trouble falling asleep. Most people prepare for sleep by eliminating distractions and trying to relax. This process may include preparing the covers and pillows, turning off the lights, quieting noises in the bedroom, and making themselves comfortable. For people with chronic pain, however, distractions may serve as a pain management tool. As long as they are able to focus on working, socializing, preparing meals, performing household tasks, reading, watching television, or engaging in recreational activities, their perception of pain tends to decrease. When they eliminate distractions and try to fall asleep, however, their brain tends to focus on the pain. Their level of stress and experience of pain may increase with the amount of time it takes them to fall asleep.

People dealing with pain also tend to have trouble sleeping through the night. Research has shown, for instance, that people with chronic back pain experience a number of microarousals—or changes from a deeper to a lighter stage of sleep—per hour each night. Such disruptions to the normal stages of sleep lead to frequent awakenings during the night and less restorative sleep. The poor quality of sleep means that people with chronic pain do not feel rested and refreshed in the morning. As a result, they often experience drowsiness, diminished energy, depressed mood, and increased pain throughout the day.

In some cases, people with pain also have other medical problems that disrupt sleep, such as restless leg syndrome or nocturnal leg cramps. People with restless leg syndrome experience an uncomfortable tingling or tickling sensation in their legs at night. This sensation creates an uncontrollable urge to move the legs, which can result in involuntary kicking or jerking motions during sleep. The symptoms of restless leg syndrome can contribute to problems falling asleep or staying asleep. They are sometimes relieved through massage, hot baths before bedtime, daily exercise, or eliminating caffeine or nicotine. They can also be treated with prescription medications.

Nocturnal leg cramps are sudden, painful muscle spasms that tend to occur during sleep or during the process of falling asleep. They may affect the feet, calves, or thighs and last between a few seconds and several minutes. Dehydration is the most common cause of muscle cramps, so staying well hydrated during the day can help prevent them from occurring. Overuse of the leg muscles is another factor that sometimes contributes to nocturnal cramping. Stretching before bedtime often helps with this problem. Deficiencies in calcium, magnesium, or potassium may also cause muscle cramps, so supplementing intake of these minerals in the diet may also prove helpful.

Improving Pain and Sleep

When pain impacts sleep, it is important to treat both problems together with a multidisciplinary approach. Since chronic pain and insomnia reinforce each other in a vicious cycle, treatments aimed at improving pain may also help improve sleep, while treatments aimed at improving sleep may also help improve pain. Many behavioral and psychological approaches are available to treat both pain and sleep issues.

Practices and habits that can lead to better quality sleep are known as "sleep hygiene." In many cases, people who experience chronic pain develop bad habits and poor sleep hygiene over time. Some of the practices that have proven safe and effective in improving sleep include the following:

- Develop a regular routine to help the body get into a consistent, healthy sleep-wake cycle. Try to go to bed at the same time every night and wake up at the same time each morning. Chronic pain sufferers sometimes try to compensate for having trouble falling asleep by sleeping late the next morning, but this practice disrupts the sleep-wake pattern.

- Avoid taking naps during the day, which can make insomnia worse in the long run by disrupting the sleep-wake cycle.

- Do not go to bed unless sleepy. Instead, spend some time engaging in relaxing activities like listening to music, reading a book, or meditating.

- Get out of bed if sleep does not come within 30 minutes. Trying to fall asleep for hours on end only increases anxiety levels and turns the bedroom into a stressful place. Instead, get up and return to a relaxing activity until a feeling of drowsiness occurs.

- Develop bedtime rituals to aid in relaxation and train the body to fall asleep. Suggestions include taking a warm bath or shower, listening to music, reading a book, or having a light snack.

- Avoid caffeine, nicotine, and alcohol before bedtime. Research has shown that these substances can be disruptive to a good night's sleep.

- Exercise at least four to six hours before bedtime. Although regular exercise can help ease chronic pain and promote good sleep, vigorous exercise within a few hours of bedtime can disrupt sleep.

- Create a comfortable, pleasant, relaxing sleep environment. People with chronic pain tend to be highly sensitive to environmental factors, such as light, noise, temperature, mattresses, and bedding. As a result, choosing comfortable bedding, making sure the temperature is neither too hot nor too cold, and eliminating sources of distracting noise or light can make a big difference in helping them get a good night's sleep.

- Try alternative techniques such as meditation, yoga, deep breathing, deep muscle relaxation, or hypnosis to aid in chronic pain management and relaxation. These techniques can help people reduce stress, decrease the perception of pain, and improve sleep.

If these approaches are not effective in improving sleep, chronic pain sufferers should consult a doctor. A variety of medications are available to help address sleep problems. Before taking any sleep medication, however, patients must be sure to tell the doctor about any other medications they may be taking for chronic pain or other medical conditions.

References

1. "Chronic Pain and Insomnia: Breaking the Cycle," Drugs and Usage, December 23, 2015.

2. "Pain and Sleep," National Sleep Foundation, 2016.

3. Silberman, Stephanie. "What's Really Causing Your Sleepless Nights?" Huffington Post, July 21, 2011.

Chapter 5

Substance Use and Pain

Chapter Contents

Section 5.1

The Effects of Cigarette Smoke on Pain

"The Effects of Cigarette Smoke on Pain,"
© 2017 Omnigraphics. Reviewed June 2017.

Many of smoking's harmful effects are well known, including its link to heart disease, respiratory disease, and cancer. Smoking is a factor in one among five deaths in the United States and is the greatest preventable cause of disease and death. However, what is less well known is its link to chronic pain. Many recent research studies have found that smoking makes pain worse and can interfere with effective pain management. Paradoxically, individuals with chronic pain tend to smoke more than the general public at large. While the overall smoking rate in the United States is 22 percent, more than half of patients who opt for pain management are found to be smokers.

What Is the Effect of Smoking on Pain?

Nicotine, the addictive ingredient in cigarettes, is a proven pain killer, but it is generally effective only in the short term. Despite this short-term effect, smokers have overall lower thresholds of pain compared to nonsmokers. The reasons are not fully understood, but scientists believe that contributing factors may include the effect of smoking on how the body regulates inflammation and perceives pain as well as the role smoking plays in the development of chronic, painful conditions. Smokers with chronic pain often fall into a cycle of smoking to cope with pain, which in turn interferes with pain management, leading the patient to smoke more when their pain threshold has invariably changed.

How Does Smoking Interfere with Pain Management?

Smoking affects the body and chronic pain in a number of different ways:

Aches and Pains: Smokers experience pain in the neck, arm, back, and legs and existing pain becomes worse with smoking.

Bones: Smoking affects the musculoskeletal system, which includes the muscles, bones, tendons, and ligaments. Smoking acts on osteoblasts, the cells that develop into bone. It also interferes with the absorption of calcium from food and can lead to osteoporosis. Weakening of bones increases the incidence of fractures, which in turn produces acute and ongoing pain.

Decrease in oxygen supply to the body: Smoking decreases the level of oxygen in the blood and also affects blood circulation. Healing of wounds takes longer in such conditions and can also have an effect on how the body regulates inflammation. Lack of enough oxygen in blood also affects the production of osteoblasts and increases healing time for fractures.

Chronic disease: Multiple sclerosis, lupus, fibromyalgia, and arthritis are chronic and painful conditions than can be made worse by smoking.

Degenerative disc disease: Smoking hardens arterial walls which impede blood flow in areas like bones and discs in the spinal cord that are fed by smaller vessels. The spine is starved of oxygen as a result so that after an injury or collapse, the spine becomes less capable of repairing itself and degenerates.

Increased perception of pain: Research indicates that smoking affects brain circuits associated with pain. The nervous system becomes more sensitive to pain and perceives pain more acutely.

Effect on Pain Medication: Smokers often require higher dosages of analgesics or narcotics for effective pain management according to research.

What Can Smokers Do?

Simply put, the most effective way for patients who smoke to overcome chronic pain is to quit. Smoking cessation has been repeatedly linked to the reduction of chronic pain and to an overall improvement in health. Smokers should be well prepared and armed with techniques to aid their decision to quit and succeed. Some strategies include:

- Designate a day for not smoking.

- Enlist the support of friends and relatives to help you quit.

- Find ways of becoming physically active.

- Stop stocking up on cigarettes and throw away ashtrays, matches and lighters.

- Join a smoking cessation program.

- Change your daily routine and break associations linked to smoking.

- Use nicotine substitute products like inhalers, patches, and gum to reduce dependence.

- Take it slow by handling it one day at a time.

Patients can also consult a pain management specialist to determine how quitting smoking can work as part of an overall program to address their chronic pain.

References

1.   Thompson, Dennis Jr. "Chronic Pain and Smoking,"Everyday Health Media, LLC, 2017.

2.   Ingraham, Paul. "Smoking and Chronic Pain," PainScience. com, Nov 18, 2016.

3.   "Smokers Have More Aches and Pains," WebMD, LLC, Jan 8, 2003.

4.   Whiteman, Honor. "Smoking Linked to Increased Risk of Chronic Back Pain," MedicalNewsToday, Nov 4, 2014.

5.   "Smoking & Joint Pain—Why Smokers Have More Aches and Pains?" ConsumerHealthDigest, Jun 15, 2017.

6.   "The Shocking Truth behind Smoking and Pain," Advanced Pain Management, Jan 17, 2017.

7.   Macadaeg., Dr. "What You Don't Know about Smoking and Your Spine," Indiana Spine Group, n.d.

Section 5.2

Alcohol and Chronic Pain

This section includes text excerpted from "Using Alcohol to
Relieve Your Pain: What Are the Risks?" National Institute on
Alcohol Abuse and Alcoholism (NIAAA), July 2013.
Reviewed June 2017.

People have used alcohol to relieve pain since ancient times.
Laboratory studies confirm that alcohol does indeed reduce pain in
humans and in animals. Moreover, recent research suggests that
as many as 28 percent of people experiencing chronic pain turn to
alcohol to alleviate their suffering. Despite this, using alcohol to
alleviate pain places people at risk for a number of harmful health
consequences.

What Are the Risks?

Mixing alcohol and pain medicines can be harmful.

- Mixing alcohol and acetaminophen can cause acute liver failure

- Mixing alcohol and aspirin increases risk for gastric bleeding

- Alcohol increases analgesic, reinforcing, and sedative effects of
  opiates, elevating risk for combined misuse of alcohol and opiates as well as overdose

If you're taking medications to manage your pain, talk to your doctor or pharmacist about any reactions that may result from mixing
them with alcohol.

Analgesic doses of alcohol exceed moderate drinking guidelines.

- The greatest pain-reducing effects occur when alcohol is administered at doses exceeding guidelines for moderate daily alcohol
  use.*

According to the Dietary Guidelines for Americans, *drinking in mod-
eration is defined as having no more than 1 drink per day for women
and no more than 2 drinks per day for men.*

- Tolerance develops to alcohol's analgesic effects so that it takes more alcohol to produce the same effects. Increasing alcohol use to stay ahead of tolerance can lead to other problems, including the development of alcohol dependence.

  Chronic alcohol drinking makes pain worse.

- Withdrawal from chronic alcohol use often increases pain sensitivity which could motivate some people to continue drinking or even increase their drinking to reverse withdrawal-related increases in pain.

- Prolonged, excessive alcohol exposure generates a painful small fiber peripheral neuropathy, the most common neurologic complication associated with alcoholism.

If you use alcohol to relieve your pain, it is important to learn about possible adverse health effects. Ask your healthcare provider if any alcohol use is safe for you.

Section 5.3

Opioid Abuse and Chronic Pain

This chapter contains text excerpted from the following sources: Text under the heading "Opioids as Prescribed Medication" is excerpted from "Opioids and Chronic Pain," U.S. National Library of Medicine (NLM), National Institutes of Health (NIH), 2011. Reviewed June 2017; Text under the heading "Opioid Crisis and Chronic Pain" is excerpted from "Responsibly and Sensitively Addressing Chronic Pain amid an Opioid Crisis," National Institute on Drug Abuse (NIDA), September 2, 2016.

Opioids as Prescribed Medication

Opioids are commonly prescribed because they are effective in relieving many types of pain. These medications are classified as narcotics and can be dangerous when abused. When used properly, opioids such as morphine have long been known to help the severe pain that follows surgery and to alleviate the suffering of people with advanced cancer. Recently, morphine and similar drugs have been used to treat chronic pain not caused by cancer. For many people, they have been remarkably helpful; for others, it either hasn't worked or has created problems over time.

Taken as directed, opioids can manage pain effectively when used for a short amount of time. With long-term use, people need to be screened and monitored because a fraction of those treated will develop an addiction disorder, abuse the drugs, or give them to others. Long-term daily use of opioids leads to physical dependence, which is not to be confused with addiction disorder. An addiction disorder occurs in about 5 percent of people who take these pain relievers as directed over the period of a year. An addiction disorder can be treated, but like those who misuse or illegally distribute prescription drugs, the prescriber needs to be vigilant to identify and address these problems. That is why everyone who uses prescription opioids needs to be screened and closely monitored.

Opioid Crisis and Chronic Pain

Medicine is not perfect. Guidelines and practices that make sense at one point in time, often based on the best available evidence and theory, are frequently reversed when better data emerge—and sometimes only after patients have been harmed. An analysis of articles in the New England Journal of Medicine from 2001 to 2010 identified 146 reversals of recommended medical practice during that decade alone. The increased aggressiveness in treating moderate acute and chronic forms of pain using opioids during the 1990s, abetted by heavy marketing of these drugs, will undoubtedly go down in history as another of those failed strategies, whose reversal we are now seeing in revised pain management guidelines such as those released by the CDC this past March.

Although the exact numbers are not known, the majority of people with opioid use disorders are not pain patients and did not start that way. However, overprescribing of opioids in clinical settings made these drugs available in large quantities for diversion and misuse; and there is growing evidence that treating certain kinds of pain (both acute and chronic) with opioids can have the unintended effect of worsening it for some patients. Recent studies are shedding new light on why using opioids to kill pain in the short term can have the paradoxical effect of actually intensifying and prolonging pain—an effect known as opioid-induced hyperalgesia. For example, a recent study using a rat model of chronic nerve pain found that morphine significantly

47

enhanced sensitivity to pain following injury and prolonged the pain of the injury well beyond the point at which the tissues had healed; the priming of glial cells in the spine by inflammation may be why. The risk of hyperalgesia is another reason, besides addiction risk, that the CDC is now counseling less reliance on opioids for management of chronic pain except in cancer pain and palliative care.

It is particularly tragic that these lessons about opioids—both their addictiveness and their ability to actually increase pain—were learned as much as a century and a half ago but were forgotten or ignored. In the late 19th and early 20th century, widespread sale and medicinal use of opioids like morphine, heroin, and opium (as well as other widely misused pharmaceuticals like cocaine) led to increased misuse and addiction. Early drug policies in America, like the Harrison Narcotics Tax Act of 1914, were designed to address this problem by restricting and regulating the sale and prescribing of habit-forming substances. What is not as widely known is that increased pain sensitivity as a result of opioid dependency, then called "morphia," was also described in the medical literature as early as 1870.

Given what we are now learning about opioids' paradoxical effects, one has to wonder whether overtreatment with opioids might have contributed to the rise in chronic pain in America instead of just treating it. Without better epidemiological data on pain trends over time, it is only possible to speculate. The United States consumes the vast majority of the world's opioid medications, and pain prevalence in the United States is higher than in most other developed countries. The rise in opioid prescribing, especially since pain was declared the "fifth vital sign" in 1996 (the same year OxyContin was approved), paralleled a rise in diagnoses for common forms of pain including chronic low back pain. But it is hard to disentangle these trends from other contributing variables like increased obesity in the U.S. population, which can also increase pain, as well as the increased survival from chronic diseases that produce pain. Future research will need to closely examine these questions.

In any case, people with chronic pain are real victims of these shifting tides of medical practice, and we cannot forget about these patients in our haste to end the opioid misuse crisis. Health organizations are now taking steps to revise how to diagnose and manage pain in this country, but as yet, medicine has little to offer chronic pain patients in place of opioids. Many patients with chronic pain are understandably concerned that the only medications that give them some relief are less and less available to them, and they complain of being stigmatized as "addicts" because of the almost inevitable physical dependence that comes with long-term opioid treatment, which is frequently confused with addiction. Physicians must understand that dependence on opioids is not the same as addiction; and the potential dangers of restricting opioid medications on which patients are physically dependent could be devastating in the current drug landscape, where counterfeit pain pills made with the very potent opioid medication fentanyl are causing overdoses and claiming many lives.

The Surgeon General's letter is a call for physicians to assume greater responsibility in addressing the opioid crisis. Responsibly addressing pain includes treating existing pain patients with sensitivity and care, understanding the difficult nuances of opioid tolerance and physical dependence and their distinctness from opioid use disorders including addiction, and following appropriate strategies for addressing hyperalgesia. It is also incumbent on researchers in their field to redouble their efforts to search for new pain medications (and non-drug treatments) that have less misuse and dependence liability. Similarly, insurance and healthcare providers need to cover and offer evidence-based alternatives to the management of chronic pain even when they are more costly than opioid medications. Safe and effective pain management needs to be a top priority for researchers and for the healthcare system.

Chapter 6

Coping with Chronic Pain

Chapter Contents

Section 6.1

Learning to Control Pain

This section includes text excerpted from "Halt the
Hurt!" NIH News in Health, National Institutes of
Health (NIH), March 2012. Reviewed June 2017.

Pain—it's something we've all experienced. From our first skinned
knee to the headaches, back pain, and creaky joints as we age, pain
is something we encounter many times. Most pain is acute and goes
away quickly. But in some cases, when pain develops slowly or persists
for months or even years, then it's called chronic pain, and it can be
tricky to treat.

Chronic pain is a huge problem. Over 115 million people nation-
wide—about 1 in 3 Americans—suffer from some kind of long-term
pain. It's the leading reason that people miss work.

National Institutes of Health (NIH)-funded scientists are working
to better understand and treat chronic pain. They're uncovering the
intricate pathways that lead to long-term pain. And they're looking for
approaches beyond medication that might help you control your pain.

Chronic pain differs in many ways from acute pain. Acute pain is
part of the body's response to an injury or short-term illness. Acute
pain can help prevent more serious injury. For instance, it can make
you quickly pull your finger away from a hot stove or keep your weight
off a broken ankle. The causes of acute pain can usually be diagnosed
and treated, and the pain eventually ends.

But the causes of chronic pain aren't always clear. "It's a complex problem that involves more than just the physical aspects of
where the hurt seems to be," says Dr. John Killen, deputy director
of NIH's National Center for Complementary and Alternative Medicine (NCCAM). "There's a lot of accumulating scientific evidence that
chronic pain is partly a problem of how the brain processes pain."

Chronic pain can come in many forms, and it accompanies several conditions including low-back pain, arthritis, cancer, migraine,
fibromyalgia, endometriosis, and inflammatory bowel disease. These
persistent pains can severely limit your ability to move around and
perform day-to-day tasks. Chronic pain can lead to depression and

anxiety. It's hard to look on the bright side when pain just won't go away. Some experts say that chronic pain is a disease itself.

The complexities of chronic pain can make it difficult to treat. Many of today's medications for chronic pain target inflammation. These drugs include aspirin, ibuprofen and COX-2 inhibitors. But if taken at high doses for a long time, these drugs can irritate your stomach and digestive system and possibly harm your kidneys. And they don't work for everyone.

"With hard-to-treat pain, the opioids are also used, sometimes in combination with the other drugs," says Dr. Raymond Dionne, who oversees some of NIH's clinical pain research. Opioids include prescription painkillers such as codeine and morphine and brand-name drugs such as Vicodin, Oxycontin and Percocet. Opioids affect the processes by which the brain perceives pain. If used improperly, though, opioids can be addictive, and increasingly high doses may be needed to keep pain in check.

"As with all drugs, you have to find a balance between effectiveness and side effects," says Dionne. He and other researchers have studied potential new pain medications to learn more about how they work in the body. But for the most part, pain medications are similar to those used 5 or more decades ago. That's why some researchers are looking for approaches beyond medications.

"One thing we know is that currently available drug therapies don't provide all the answers. Many people find that medications don't fully relieve their chronic pain, and they can experience unpleasant side effects," Killen says. "Evidence on a number of fronts, for several conditions, suggests that mind and body approaches can be helpful additions to conventional medicine for managing chronic pain."

Research has shown that patients with chronic low-back pain might benefit from acupuncture, massage therapy, yoga or cognitive-behavioral therapy (a type of talk therapy).

NIH-funded scientists have also found that people with fibromyalgia pain might find relief through tai chi. This mind-body technique combines meditation, slow movements, deep breathing and relaxation.

But how much these approaches truly help is still an open question. Studies of pain relief can be difficult to interpret. Researchers must rely on patients to complete questionnaires and rate their own levels of pain.

One puzzler is that the exposure to the exact same pain-causing thing, or stimulus, can lead to completely different responses in different people. For example, when an identical heat stimulus is applied to different people's arms, one may report feeling uncomfortable, while another might say that the pain is extreme.

"How do we account for these differences? We've now learned that genes play a role," says Dr. Sean Mackey, who heads Stanford University's neuroscience and pain lab. "Some differences involve our personality and mood states, including anxiety."

Mackey and his team are using brain scans to gain insights into how we process and feel pain. One study found that a painful stimulus can activate different brain regions in people who are anxious than in those who are fearful of pain.

In another study, volunteers were taught strategies that could turn on specific brain regions. One technique involved mentally changing the meaning of the pain and thinking about it in a non-threatening way.

"We found that with repeated training, people can learn how to build up this brain area, almost like a muscle, and make its activity much stronger," says Mackey. "That led to a significant improvement overall in their pain perception." The researchers also found that different types of mental strategies, such as distraction, engaged different brain regions.

Another study found that intense feelings of passionate love can provide surprisingly effective pain relief. "It turns out that the areas of the brain activated by intense love are the same areas that drugs use to reduce pain," says Mackay.

"We can't write a prescription for patients to go home and have a passionate love affair," says Mackey. "But we can suggest that you go out and do things that are rewarding, that are emotionally meaningful. Go for a walk on a moonlit beach. Go listen to some music you never listened to before. Do something that's novel and exciting."

That's a prescription that should be painless to try.

Tips for Pain Relief

- **Keep your weight in check**. Extra weight can slow healing and make some pain worse, especially in the back, knees, hips and feet.

- **Exercise.** Pain may make you inactive, which can lead to a cycle of more pain and loss of function. Ask your doctor if exercise might help.

- **Get enough sleep.** It will improve healing and your mood.

- **Avoid tobacco, caffeine, and alcohol.** They can set back your treatment and increase pain.

- **Get the right medical help.** If your regular doctor hasn't found a helpful approach for pain relief, ask to see a pain specialist.

- **Join a pain support group.** Talk with others about how they deal with pain. Share your ideas and thoughts while learning from those in the group.

Section 6.2

Managing Chronic Pain

This section includes text excerpted from "You Can
Manage Your Chronic Pain to Live a Good Life,"
Substance Abuse and Mental Health Services
Administration (SAMIISA), 2013. Reviewed June 2017.

Chronic Pain Doesn't Mean You Always Have to Suffer

The word chronic means constant, lasting a long time, or coming back again and again. When you have pain that has bothered you for more than 3 months and doesn't seem to get better with time, you may be experiencing chronic pain. Major causes of chronic pain include lower back problems, nerve damage, and migraine headaches. Pain also can be a part of many diseases, such as sickle cell anemia, arthritis, pancreatitis, fibromyalgia, and HIV/AIDS. There are many other causes of pain, and sometimes the cause is unknown.

Chronic pain can be difficult to bear, even awful. It can lead you to lose sleep, to become anxious and depressed, to have a hard time keeping up on the job, and to stop doing things you did before. These changes can add stress, produce more pain, and trigger new health problems. If unmanaged, pain can become the center of your life. In many cases, chronic pain is a lifelong condition. However, by managing your pain, you can usually continue to enjoy the activities that matter to you. One of the most important things you can do to manage your pain is to safeguard your recovery from mental illness or addiction. A clear mind helps you think better, so that you take the right steps to manage your pain.

Work with Healthcare Providers to Manage Pain

If you have chronic pain, talk to your healthcare providers about it at your next scheduled appointment, or set up a new appointment just for this purpose. Don't put off talking to your care providers in hope that the pain will go away. Medical professionals may be able to determine what's causing the pain and help you deal with that problem. Even if the source of pain remains a mystery, care providers can work with you to try different strategies until you find a combination that reduces your suffering.

If you have a history with drugs or alcohol, you may hesitate to seek medical care for your pain. If you have a history of mental illness, you may be equally reluctant. You may be afraid that care providers will judge you or think you are being dishonest. Or, you may be afraid that you will be persuaded to take medications that could trigger your addiction. If you don't know what's causing the pain, you might be afraid that others will think it's all in your head. But for your own sake, you should contact a care provider. Chances are good that the professionals you meet with will treat you respect fully, help you maintain your recovery, and work with you to find ways to reduce your pain. If this isn't true for the first care providers you contact, then you may want to meet with others who are more responsive to your concerns. Many different types of care providers can work with you to manage pain. These include primary care doctors or specialists, nurses, and other members of a doctor's team including physician assistants and nurse practitioners. Psychologists, addiction treatment counselors, and other types of counselors also may be able to help. Several professionals may become involved in your pain care. If this is the case, it's important that they coordinate your care with each other. You can help make sure this happens by asking, "Who is serving as the point person for my pain care?"

Help your care providers understand how much pain you have. When you meet with care providers about your pain, they will try to learn where the pain is coming from and what it is like. They will ask questions about your general health and your exercise habits. They also will ask specific questions about the pain. Pain usually increases and decreases across time, so it is important for your care providers to know the most pain, the least pain, and the typical pain you feel in a given day. Since pain treatment often does not make all pain go away, care providers also will need to know what level of pain you can live with. This can be different from person to person. You may be asked to rate episodes of pain on a numerical scale of 0 to 10, or on a picture scale, such as a set of frowning and smiling faces. You also may be asked to use a scale to rate your quality of life on such factors as sleep, stress, and ability to perform daily activities. Having high scores doesn't mean your pain is impossible to treat, and having low scores doesn't mean you should try to ignore your pain. Pain scores are just one of many tools that care providers use to understand your pain. Every time you see your care providers about pain, you may be asked to give pain scores. These will be compared with your past pain scores to see if treatment is helping to reduce your pain.

Be as specific as you can about your level of pain. Sometimes your pain can feel like an 11 on a scale of 0 to 10. Chronic pain affects more than your body—it can affect your mood, your relationships, and your ability to be independent. It can also challenge your recovery from mental illness or addiction. When you are asked to rate your pain level, try to separate the feeling of pain from the suffering and disruption it is causing. Name a level that is only about your pain. Try not to underreport or overreport your pain. If you are worried that your care providers will prescribe medications that could put your recovery at risk, you may be tempted to report less pain than you feel. On the other hand, if you are worried that your care providers won't give you pain relief medications unless your pain is unbearable, you may be tempted to report more pain than you feel. In general, your pain level is only one factor that is considered when prescribing pain medications. Be straightforward about your pain level, and speak up about your concerns about pain medications. Help your care providers understand how the pain affects you. Try not to answer questions about pain with one word, such as "yes," "no," or "fine." Instead, give some details. Help your care providers understand what activities are important to you, but that are hard to do now because of your pain.

Be ready to share information about your mental and emotional health. Some conditions can make your chronic pain worse. For example, if you were in an accident or terrible incident, you may have flashbacks or other symptoms of posttraumatic stress disorder (PTSD). These can make pain more intense. Being depressed, anxious, or under a lot of stress can make pain feel worse, too. Your care providers will ask questions about your state of mind, because the way you feel mentally and emotionally has a bearing on the best way to treat your pain while minimizing risk to your recovery.

Disclose to care providers your addiction and recovery history. It's very important that your care providers know your history of drug and alcohol use and about your progress in recovery. If they don't ask about this, you should volunteer the information, so that they can develop a pain management plan that fits with your recovery plan. Be sure to mention if you are in recovery with the help of medications, such as methadone, buprenorphine, or naltrexone. These medications can affect how pain medications work for you. Your doctor is required by law to keep this information confidential and not share it with others (such as employers) who are not involved in your healthcare.

Work with care providers to create a pain management plan. Chronic pain differs from person to person and from one moment to the next. That's why you need to have a pain management plan that's designed for you. This plan may include both action steps and medications for overall management of pain, plus guidance on what to do when you have episodes of acute pain. It's important to note that pain management is a process. You and your care providers will need to monitor your plan on an ongoing basis and make adjustments as needed, so that it continues to help you manage your pain.

Go back for checkups. Your care providers will want to see you again after you start a pain management plan. This is so they can find out how the plan is working for you and make adjustments as needed. These meetings are opportunities for you to ask any questions you might have. Checkups also can help you avoid addiction risk behaviors. Care providers can look for signs that show unusual drug use on your part, such as borrowing somebody else's medications or increasing doses of the medication you take without prior approval. Your care providers will try to determine whether such behavior indicates your pain is not being treated effectively or whether you are having a relapse. In either case, your care providers will work with you to make sure your pain is managed in the best way possible while protecting your recovery.

Pain Can Be Treated in Many Ways

Your care providers may advise you to do a number of things to reduce your pain. If you are already taking steps on your own to manage your chronic pain, tell your care providers. If they don't ask about this, volunteer the information, so that it is part of the management plan you build together. Each piece of your plan may help to some degree. All of the pieces together may do quite a bit to ease the pain.

Some of them will require a significant commitment and active involvement, but they can be the keys to effective management of pain.

Pain Management Begins with You

It's understandable that you want to get rid of your pain completely, but that is often not possible. Although you may always have some pain to manage, you can still improve your quality of life. You can manage your chronic pain. You can have a good life.

Section 6.3

Dealing with Chronic Pain

This section includes text excerpted from "Dealing with Chronic Pain," U.S. Department of Veterans Affairs (VA), January 2015.

Pain is called "chronic" when its lasts over a long period of time. This includes pain that you feel regularly, even if it comes and goes. Chronic pain can affect a particular part of the body, such as the back, shoulders, or knee, or be experienced as general all-over body pain. Living with pain can interfere with your life because of the negative impact it has on how you are feeling and functioning day to day. However, by managing pain effectively (often referred to as pain management) you can feel better and live better.

Work with an Understanding and Knowledgeable Doctor to Evaluate Treatment Options

While primary care providers (PCPs) can often help you deal effectively with painful symptoms, depending on the severity and duration of those symptoms it may be important to talk to your PCP about a referral to a doctor who specializes in pain medicine. Most Department of Veterans Affairs (VA) Medical Centers have a pain management clinic, where Veterans can be referred. Developing an open and trusting relationship with this doctor is important in treating your pain. Communicate with your doctor about where the pain is, how bad it is, and how often it occurs. Also talk about what makes the pain better or worse.

Since pain symptoms vary from person to person, pain management treatment strategies and treatments also need to be individualized. Medication alone is often not sufficient to treat pain and sometimes too many medications or taking them for prolonged periods of time can cause other problems. Additional treatments for you might include interventions for your specific type of pain or non-traditional treatments. As time passes, it is important for you and your doctor to reevaluate what's working for you and what can be done differently to accommodate any changes in your symptoms. Finding the right combination is the key.

Take Care of the Things You Can Control

Getting enough sleep, eating healthy, and exercising is essential to maintaining function and health and even more so when you are dealing with chronic pain. The good news is these are things you can control and do for yourself. It may seem that trying to exercise does not make sense- you have pain so you do not want to move, or are afraid to cause more pain. Studies show that low-impact graded aerobic exercise (such as walking, swimming, or biking) can actually help reduce the pain.

Ask your doctor which exercises are safe for you. He or she may even recommend you work with a physical therapist that will tailor an exercise program to best meet your needs. Other things you can do yourself are: therapies for the mind and body such as meditation and yoga (non-traditional treatments often referred to as Complementary and Integrative medicine practices).

These may help reduce stress, improve mood, and make you less aware of pain which will help you feel better. Again, your doctor can help you decide which techniques may be beneficial for you.

Care for Your Emotional Health

Chronic pain is often accompanied by undesired changes in your personal routine. These changes might include: loss of function, inability to work, and deterioration of personal relationships. Because of negative life changes, people in chronic pain have an increased risk for emotional health issues such as depression and anxiety. Your emotions may range from: fear, anger, and denial to hope and optimism.

Every person feels different emotions at different times, and some-times emotions can make controlling pain more difficult. Taking care of the emotional aspects of chronic pain is a necessary part of treating your overall pain. Your doctor may want to prescribe medication for depression, anxiety, and sleep disturbances and, may also suggest cognitive behavioral therapy (CBT).

CBT is based on the idea that emotions and behavior are influenced by our thoughts about a situation (e.g., "this is awful" vs. "this is uncomfortable"). By learning to modify the way we think about difficult situations, we can cope better and avoid acting in ways that make the situation worse. This is part of your doctor's approach to treating pain as a "whole" not just the part that physically hurts. Some things you can do to help yourself deal with the emotional aspects of pain are to: keep a journal of your emotions, talk to loved ones about how you feel, or join a local support group.

Section 6.4

Seniors and Chronic Pain

This section includes text excerpted from "Seniors and
Chronic Pain," U.S. National Library of Medicine (NLM), National
Institutes of Health (NIH),October 4, 2011. Reviewed June 2017.

Chronic pain is a growing problem among older Americans. Under-standing the causes of this pain, the special medical needs of the elderly, and the role of pain self-management can help seniors reduce or eliminate this condition.

As the United States evolves into a nation with an older population, greater attention is being paid to healthcare problems more common among the elderly. Research has shown that 50 percent of older adults who live on their own and 75–85 percent of the elderly in care facili-ties suffer from chronic pain. Yet, pain among older adults is largely undertreated, with serious health consequences, such as depression, anxiety, decreased mobility, social isolation, poor sleep, and related health risks.

There are natural changes that occur with aging that affect pain—sleep patterns change, muscles and joints gradually become more rigid, and energy decreases. Frequently, older people don't report their pain, because they don't know that it can be treated or they believe it will lead to expensive tests or more medications. And there can be conditions, such as vision or hearing loss or dementia that can limit communication about pain.

To help overcome these barriers, treatment of chronic pain may involve a team of different pain management specialists—including a physician, nurse practitioner, physician assistant, pharmacist, and others who specialize in pain management.

"It takes a team to take care of a patient," says Ann M. Berger, M.D., chief of the National Institutes of Health (NIH) Clinical Center's Pain and Palliative Care Service. The service brings together people from a variety of disciplines to help patients manage their symptoms and relieve their physical, emotional, and spiritual suffering.

"We're the quality-of-life team; that's how I introduce ourselves to our patients," says Dr. Berger. "This is the first truly integrative approach to pain management."

Since pain, especially chronic, long-term pain, is prevalent across so many different diseases and conditions, the NIH also created a Pain Consortium to help study all aspects of pain prevention and treatment. This interdisciplinary Consortium is composed of 18 different Institutes and Centers and helps coordinate planning for key research opportunities in every aspect of pain.

Treating pain in older adults requires special care because nutritional problems or multiple medical problems—diabetes, heart disease, arthritis—are common. Helping seniors self-manage their pain is an important part of reducing or eliminating that pain.

Questions to Ask Your Healthcare Provider

Communication with your caregiver or care team is the best way to help you manage or end your chronic pain.

- What is causing my pain? What can I do about it?
- What is the name of the pain medicine I will be taking?
- How long will it take for the medicine to work?
- What side effects should I expect?
- If I forget to take the pain medicine, what should I do?

- When should I take the pain medicine—on a regular schedule? Before, with, or after meals? At bedtime?

- Are there any dangers to taking this pain medicine I should know about?

- Will this pain medicine cause problems with any other prescription drugs or over-the-counter medicines I am taking?

Chapter 7

Relaxation Techniques for People with Chronic Pain

What Are Relaxation Techniques?

Relaxation techniques include a number of practices such as progressive relaxation, guided imagery, biofeedback, self-hypnosis, and deep breathing exercises. The goal is similar in all: to produce the body's natural relaxation response, characterized by slower breathing, lower blood pressure, and a feeling of increased well-being.

Meditation and practices that include meditation with movement, such as yoga and tai chi, can also promote relaxation. You can find information about these practices elsewhere on the National Center for Complementary and Integrative Health (NCCIH) Website www. nccih.nih.gov.

Stress management programs commonly include relaxation techniques. Relaxation techniques have also been studied to see whether they might be of value in managing various health problems.

The Importance of Practice

Relaxation techniques are skills, and like other skills, they need practice. People who use relaxation techniques frequently are more

---

This chapter includes text excerpted from "Relaxation Techniques for Health," National Center for Complementary and Integrative Health (NCCIH), May 2016.

likely to benefit from them. Regular, frequent practice is particularly important if you're using relaxation techniques to help manage a chronic health problem. Continuing use of relaxation techniques is more effective than short-term use.

Relaxation techniques include the following:

Autogenic Training

In autogenic training, you learn to concentrate on the physical sensations of warmth, heaviness, and relaxation in different parts of your body.

Biofeedback-Assisted Relaxation

Biofeedback techniques measure body functions and give you information about them so that you can learn to control them. Biofeedback-assisted relaxation uses electronic devices to teach you to produce changes in your body that are associated with relaxation, such as reduced muscle tension.

Deep Breathing or Breathing Exercises

This technique involves focusing on taking slow, deep, even breaths.

Guided Imagery

For this technique, people are taught to focus on pleasant images to replace negative or stressful feelings. Guided imagery may be self-directed or led by a practitioner or a recording.

Progressive Relaxation

This technique, also called Jacobson relaxation or progressive muscle relaxation, involves tightening and relaxing various muscle groups. Progressive relaxation is often combined with guided imagery and breathing exercises.

Self-Hypnosis

In self-hypnosis programs, people are taught to produce the relaxation response when prompted by a phrase or nonverbal cue (called a "suggestion").

What the Science Says about the Effectiveness of Relaxation Techniques for Pain

Researchers have evaluated relaxation techniques to see whether they could play a role in managing a variety of conditions, including the following:

Childbirth

Relaxation techniques such as guided imagery, progressive muscle relaxation, and breathing techniques may be useful in managing labor pain. Studies have shown that women who were taught self-hypnosis have a decreased need for pain medicine during labor. Biofeedback hasn't been shown to relieve labor pain.

Fibromyalgia

Studies of guided imagery for fibromyalgia have had inconsistent results. An evaluation of the research concluded that electromyographic (EMG) biofeedback, in which people are taught to control and reduce muscle tension, helped to reduce fibromyalgia pain, at least for short periods of time. However, EMG biofeedback didn't affect sleep problems, depression, fatigue, or health-related quality of life in people with fibromyalgia, and its long-term effects haven't been established.

Headache

- **Biofeedback.** Biofeedback has been studied for both tension headaches and migraines.

  - An evaluation of high-quality studies concluded that there's conflicting evidence about whether biofeedback can relieve tension headaches.

  - Studies have shown decreases in the frequency of migraines in people who were using biofeedback. However, it's unclear whether biofeedback is better than a placebo.

- **Other Relaxation Techniques.** Relaxation techniques other than biofeedback have been studied for tension headaches. An evaluation of high-quality studies found conflicting evidence on whether relaxation techniques are better than no treatment or a placebo. Some studies suggest that other relaxation techniques are less effective than biofeedback.

Pain

Evaluations of the research evidence have found promising but not conclusive evidence that guided imagery may help relieve some musculoskeletal pain (pain involving the bones or muscles) and other types of pain.

An analysis of data on hospitalized cancer patients showed that those who received integrative medicine therapies, such as guided imagery and relaxation response training, during their hospitalization had reductions in both pain and anxiety.

Pain in Children and Adolescents

An evaluation of the scientific evidence found that psychological therapies, which may include relaxation techniques as well as other approaches such as cognitive-behavioral therapy, can reduce pain in children and adolescents with chronic headaches or other types of chronic pain. The evidence is particularly promising for headaches: the effect on pain may last for several months after treatment, and the therapies also help to reduce anxiety.

Temporomandibular Joint Dysfunction

Problems with the temporomandibular joint (the joint that connects the jaw to the side of the head) can cause pain and difficulty moving the jaw. A few studies have shown that programs that include relaxation techniques may help relieve symptoms of temporomandibular joint dysfunction.

What the Science Says about the Safety and Side Effects of Relaxation Techniques

- Relaxation techniques are generally considered safe for healthy people. However, occasionally, people report negative experiences such as increased anxiety, intrusive thoughts, or fear of losing control.

- There have been rare reports that certain relaxation techniques might cause or worsen symptoms in people with epilepsy or certain psychiatric conditions, or with a history of abuse or trauma. People with heart disease should talk to their healthcare provider before doing progressive muscle relaxation.

Who Teaches Relaxation Techniques?

A variety of professionals, including physicians, psychologists, social workers, nurses, and complementary health practitioners, may teach relaxation techniques. Also, people sometimes learn the simpler relaxation techniques on their own.

Chapter 8

Physical Activity Helps Relieve Arthritis Pain

The Benefits of Physical Activity for Adults with Arthritis

Regular physical activity has many benefits for people with arthritis. Participating in arthritis-friendly physical activity improves pain, function, mood, and quality of life without making symptoms worse. Being physically active can also delay the onset of disability and help people with arthritis manage other chronic conditions such as diabetes, heart disease, and obesity.

Safe, enjoyable physical activity is possible for most adults with arthritis. Most people with arthritis can safely exercise on their own or join one of many proven programs available in communities across the country.

Types of Arthritis-Friendly Activity

Adults with arthritis should follow either the Active Adult or Active Older Adult Guidelines from the *Physical Activity Guidelines for Americans*, whichever meets your personal health goals and matches your abilities. Remember to start slow and pay attention to how your body

This chapter includes text excerpted from "Physical Activity for Arthritis," Centers for Disease Control and Prevention (CDC), April 18, 2017.

tolerates activity. The most important thing to remember is to find out what works best for you.

Aerobic activities. Aerobic activity is also called "cardio," endurance, or conditioning exercise. It is any activity that makes your heart beat faster and makes you breathe a little harder than when you are sitting, standing or lying. You want to do activity that is moderate or vigorous intensity and that does not twist or "pound" your joints too much. Some people with arthritis can do vigorous activities such as running and can even tolerate some activities that are harder on the joints like basketball or tennis. You should choose the activities that are right for you and that are enjoyable. Remember, each person is different, but there are a wide variety of activities that you can do to meet the Guidelines.

Table 8.1. Examples of Moderate and Vigorous Intensity Aerobic Activities

Moderate Intensity	Vigorous Intensity
• Brisk Walking.	• Jogging/running.
• Bicycling.	• Singles tennis.
• Swimming.	• Swimming.
• Mowing the grass, heavy yard work.	• Jumping rope.
• Doubles tennis.	• Conditioning Machines (e.g., stair climbers, elliptical, stationary bike).
• Social dancing.	• Sports (e.g., soccer, basketball, football, racquetball).
• Conditioning Machines (e.g., stair climbers, elliptical, stationary bike).	• Aerobic dance or spinning classes.
• Tai Chi, yoga.	
• Sports (e.g., softball, baseball, volleyball).	
• Skiing, roller and ice skating.	

Muscle strengthening activities. You should do activities that strengthen your muscles at least 2 days per week in addition to your aerobic activities. Muscle strengthening activities are especially important for people with arthritis because having strong muscles takes some of the pressure off the joints.

You can do muscle strengthening exercises in your home, at a gym, or at a community center. You should do exercises that work all the major muscle groups of the body (e.g., legs, hips, back, abdomen, chest, shoulders, and arms). You should do at least 1 set of 8–12 repetitions for each muscle group. There are many ways you can do muscle strengthening activities:

- Lifting weights using machines, dumbbells, or weight cuffs.
- Working with resistance bands.
- Using your own bodyweight as resistance (e.g., push-ups, sit ups).
- Heavy gardening (e.g., digging, shoveling).
- Some group exercise classes.
- Muscle strengthening exercise videos.

Balance activities. Many older adults and some adults with arthritis and other chronic diseases may be prone to falling. If you are worried about falling or are at risk of falling, you should include activities that improve balance at least 3 days per week as part of your activity plan. Balance activities can be part of your aerobic or your muscle strengthening activities. Examples of activities that improve balance include the following:

- Tai Chi.
- Backward walking, side stepping, heel and toe walking.
- Standing on 1 foot.
- Some group exercise classes.

Additional Recommendations for People with Arthritis

Stay flexible. In addition to the activities recommended above, flexibility exercises are also important. Many people with arthritis have joint stiffness that makes daily tasks such as bathing and fixing meals difficult. Doing daily flexibility exercises for all upper (e.g., neck, shoulder, elbow, wrist, and finger) and lower (e.g., low back, hip, knee, ankle, and toes) joints of the body helps maintain essential range of motion.

More Information for Older Adults

If you have arthritis, you should follow either the Active Adult or Active Older Adult recommendations, whichever meets your personal health goals and matches your abilities. You should do this activity in addition to your usual daily activity. You may notice that the recommended amount and type of activity are the same for the Active Adult and Active Older Adult except for the additional recommendation to include activities that promote balance. Read some additional details for the Active Older Adult below:

Prevent falls. Have you fallen in the past? Do you have trouble walking? If so, you may be at high risk of falling. Activities that improve or maintain balance should be included in your physical activity plan. Examples of activities that have been proven to help balance include walking backwards, standing on one leg, and Tai Chi. Some exercise classes offered in many local communities include exercises that are good for balance.

Stay active. Any physical activity is better than none. If you cannot do 150 minutes of moderate intensity activity every week, it is important to be as active as your health allows. People with arthritis often have symptoms that come and go. This may mean that one week you can do 150 minutes of moderate intensity activity and the next week you can't. You may have to change your activity level depending on your arthritis symptoms, but try to stay as active as your symptoms allow. Learn how to modify your activity with tips for S.M.A.R.T. activity, below.

Adjust the level of effort. Some activities take more effort for older adults and those with low fitness or poor function. For example, walking at a brisk pace for a 23-year-old healthy male is moderate intensity, but the same activity may be vigorous activity for a 77-year-old male with diabetes. You should adjust the level of effort during activity so that it is comfortable for you. Find out how to measure your level of effort.

Talk to your doctor. If you have arthritis or another chronic health condition, you should already be under the care of a doctor or other healthcare provider. Healthcare providers and certified exercise professionals can answer your questions about how much and what types of activity are right for you.

How Hard Are You Working?

Moderate intensity activity makes your heart beat a little faster and you breathe a little harder. You can talk easily while doing moderate intensity activity, but you may not be able to sing comfortably.

Vigorous intensity activity makes your heart beat much faster and you may not be able to talk comfortably without stopping to catch your breath.

Relative intensity can be estimated using a scale of 0 to 10 where sitting is 0 and 10 is the highest level of effort possible. Moderate intensity activity is a 5 or 6 and vigorous intensity activity is a 7 or 8.

The **talk test** is a simple way to measure relative intensity. In general, if you're doing moderate-intensity activity you can talk, but not sing, during the activity. If you are doing vigorous-intensity activity, you will not be able to say more than a few words without pausing for a breath.

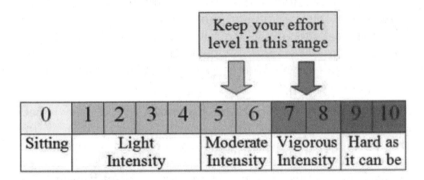

Figure 8.1. *Talk Test*

Tips for Starting and Maintaining a Physical Activity Program

Safe, enjoyable physical activity is possible for most every adult with arthritis. The most important thing to remember is to find out what works best for you. At first glance, 150 minutes of activity per week sounds like a lot, but if you pay attention to the following tips you will be well on your way to getting the recommended amount of activity in no time!

Studies show that some increase in pain, stiffness, and swelling is normal when starting an activity program. If you have increased swelling or pain that does not get better with rest then talk to your healthcare provider. It may take 6–8 weeks for your joints to accommodate to your increased activity level, but sticking with your activity program will result in long-term pain relief.

Here is an easy way to remember these tips: Make **S.M.A.R.T** choices!

- **Start low, and go slow.** Many adults with arthritis are inactive, even though their doctor may have told them being active will help their arthritis. You may want to be more active but just don't know where to start or how much to do. You may be worried that using your joints and muscles may make your arthritis worse. The good news is that the opposite is true, physical activity will help your arthritis! The first key to starting activity safely is to **start low.** This may mean you can only walk 5 minutes at a time every other day. The second key is to **go slow**. People with arthritis may take more time for their body to adjust to a new level of activity. For example, healthy children can usually increase the amount of activity a little each week, while older adults and those with chronic conditions may take 3–4 weeks to adjust to a new activity level. You should add activity in small amounts, at least 10 minutes at a time, and allow enough time for your body to adjust to the new level before adding more activity.

- **Modify activity as needed.** Remember, any activity is better than none. Your arthritis symptoms, such as pain, stiffness and fatigue, may come and go and you may have good days and bad days. You may want to stop activity completely when your arthritis symptoms increase, but it is important that you first try to modify your activity to stay as active as possible without making your symptoms worse.

If you currently do some activity or feel confident that you can safely plan your own activity program, you should look for safe places to be physically active. For example, if you walk in your neighborhood or a local park make sure the sidewalks or pathways are level and free of obstructions, are well-lighted, and are separated from heavy traffic.

- **Activities should be "joint friendly."** Choose activities that are easy on the joints like walking, bicycling, water aerobics, or dancing. These activities have a low risk of injury and do not twist or "pound" the joints too much.

- **Recognize safe places and ways to be active.** Safety is important for starting and maintaining an activity plan. If you are currently inactive or you do not have the confidence to start your own physical activity program, an exercise class designed for people with arthritis may be a good option. If you plan and direct your own activity, find safe places to be active. For example, while walking in your neighborhood or at a local park, make sure the sidewalks or pathways are level and free of obstructions, are well-lighted, and are separated from heavy traffic.

- **Talk to a health professional.** You should already be under the care of a healthcare professional for your arthritis, who is a good source of information about physical activity. Healthcare professionals and certified exercise professionals can answer your questions about how much and what types of activity match your abilities and health goals.

Chapter 9

Ergonomics to Avoid Workplace Pain

Ergonomics looks at what kind of work you do, what tools you use and your whole job environment. The aim is to find the best fit between you and your job conditions. Examples of ergonomic changes to your work might include:

- Adjusting the position of your computer keyboard to prevent carpal tunnel syndrome

- Being sure that the height of your desk chair allows your feet to rest flat on floor

- Learning the right way to lift heavy objects to prevent back injuries

- Using handle coatings or special gloves to suppress vibrations from power tools

No matter what the job is, the goal is to make sure that you are safe, comfortable, and less prone to work-related injuries.

This chapter contains text excerpted from the following sources: Text in this chapter begins with excerpts from "Ergonomics," U.S. National Library of Medicine (NLM), National Institutes of Health (NIH), December 31, 2016; Text beginning with the heading "Computers" is excerpted from "Ergonomics—Prevention," Division of Occupational Health and Safety (DOHS), National Institutes of Health (NIH), September 2, 2016.

Computers

Monitor Placement

You should consider how the placement and maintenance of the monitor can affect both the eyes and the musculoskeletal system. The following suggestions can help prevent the development of eye strain, neck pain, and shoulder fatigue while using your computer workstation:

- Make sure the surface of the viewing screen is clean.

- Adjust brightness and contrast to optimum comfort.

- Position the monitor directly in front of you to avoid excessive twisting of the neck.

- Position the monitor approximately 20–26 inches (arm's length) from you.

- Tilt top of the monitor back 10 to 20 degrees.

- Position monitors at right angles from windows to reduce glare.

- Position monitors away from direct lighting which creates excessive glare or use a glare filter over the monitor to reduce glare.

- The top of the viewing screen should be at eye level when the user is sitting in an upright position.

Note: Bifocal wearers may need to lower monitor a couple of inches.

Adjusting Your Chair

Contrary to popular belief, sitting, which most people believe is relaxing, is hard on the back. Sitting for long periods of time can cause increased pressure on the intervertebral discs, the springy, shock-absorbing part of the spine. Sitting is hard on the feet and lungs. Gravity tends to pool blood in the legs and feet and create a sluggish return to the heart. The following recommendations can help increase comfort when using a computer:

- Don't stay in one static position for extended periods of time.

- When performing daily tasks, alternate between sitting and standing.

- Adjust height of backrest to support the natural inward curvature of the lower back.

- It may be useful to use a rolled towel or lumbar pad to support the lower back.

- The backrest angle is set so that your hip-torso angle is 90 degrees or greater.

- Adjust height of chair so feet rest flat on floor (use footrest if necessary).

  - Sit upright in the chair with the low back against the backrest and the shoulders touching the backrest.

  - Thighs should be parallel to the floor and knees at about the same level as the hips.

  - Back of knees should not come in direct contact with the edge of the seat pan (there should be 2–3 inches between the edge of the seat and the back of the knee).

- Don't use armrests to slouch.

- Adjust height and/or width of armrests so they allow the user to rest arms at their sides and relax/drop their shoulders while keyboarding.

- When armrests are used, elbows and lower arms should rest lightly so as not to cause circulatory or nerve problems.

Desktop Placement

If you are like many computer users, your computer, keyboard, and mouse are resting on your desk or a portable computer workstation. There is no specific height recommended for your desktop; however, the working height of your desk should be approximately elbow height for light duty desk work.

To allow for proper alignment of your arms your keyboard should be approximately 1 inch to 2 inches above your thighs. Most times this requires a desk which is 25 inches to 29 inches in height (depending upon size of individual) or the use of an articulating keyboard tray. The area underneath the desk should always be clean to accommodate the user's legs and allow for stretching.

The desktop should be organized so frequently used objects are close to the user to avoid excessive extended reaching. If a document holder is used, it should be placed at approximately the same height as the monitor and at the same distance from the eyes to prevent frequent eye shifts between the screen and reference materials.

Keyboard and Mouse Placement

Many ergonomic problems associated with computer workstations occur in the forearm, wrist, and hand. Continuous work on the computer exposes soft tissues in these areas to repetition, awkward postures, and forceful exertions.

The following adjustments should be made to your workstation to help prevent the development of an ergonomic problem in the upper extremities:

- Adjust keyboard height so shoulders can relax and allow arms to rest at sides (an articulating keyboard tray is often necessary to accommodate proper height and distance).

- Keyboard should be close to the user to avoid excessive extended reaching.

- Forearms parallel to the floor (approximately 90 degree angle at elbow).

- Mouse should be placed adjacent to keyboard and at the same height as the keyboard (use articulating keyboard tray if necessary).

- Avoid extended and elevated reaching for keyboard and mouse. Wrist should be in neutral position (not excessively flexed or extended).

- Do not rest the hand on the mouse when you are not using it. Rest hands in your lap when not entering data.

Lighting

Lighting not suited to working with a Video Display Terminal (VDT) is a major contributing factor in visual discomforts including eyestrain, burning or itching eyes, and blurred or double vision. Typical office environments have illumination levels of 75 to 100 foot-candles, but according to the American National Standards Institute (ANSI), computer workstations require only 18 to 46 foot-candles. Use the following recommendations to reduce eyestrain and eye fatigue:

- Close drapes/blinds to reduce glare. Adjust lighting to avoid glare on screen (light source should come at a 90 degree angle, with low watt lights rather than high.) Place monitor at 90 degree angle to windows (where possible). Reduce overhead lighting (where possible). Use indirect or shielded lighting where possible. Walls should be painted medium or dark color and not have reflective finish.

- Use a glare screen to reduce glare (alternatively, place a large manila folder on top of the monitor and let it hang over the monitor 2 inches to 3 inches to reduce glare from overhead lighting).

Industrial and Shops

Whole-Body Vibration

Whole-body vibration is experienced in any work condition that involves sitting, standing, or lying on a vibrating surface. Excessive levels and durations of exposure to whole-body vibrations may contribute to back pain and performance problems. If you spend a considerable amount of your work day on a vibrating seat or floor and experience any of the following signs or symptoms contact your Safety and Health Specialist.

- Blurred vision.

- Decrease in manual coordination.

- Drowsiness (even with proper rest).

- Lower back pain.

- Insomnia.

- Headaches.

- Upset stomach.

Hand-Arm Vibration

Vibrating hand tools or workpieces transmit vibrations to the holder, and depending on the vibration level and duration factors, may contribute to Raynaud syndrome or vibration-induced white finger disorders. These disorders show a progression of symptoms beginning with occasional or intermittent numbness or blanching of the tips of a few finger to more persistent attacks, affecting greater parts of most fingers and reducing tactile discrimination and manual dexterity. If you notice the onset of any of these symptoms, contact your Safety and Health Specialist.

The following recommendations can help reduce the likelihood of developing hand-arm vibration syndromes:

- Select power tools with anti-vibration properties.

- Use handle coatings that suppress vibrations. Increase coefficient of friction on handles to reduce force requirements.

- Keep power tools balanced and lubricated to minimize vibration.

- Incorporate job rotation. Have more than one person perform tasks that involve exposure to hand-arm vibration.

- Use vibration attenuation gloves.

Hand Tool Use and Selection Principles

Implementing the following suggestions for proper selection and usage of hand tools will help reduce the likelihood of developing work-related musculoskeletal disorders (WMSDs) in the hands, wrists, and arms:

- **Maintain straight wrists**. Avoid bending or rotating the wrists; a variety of bent-handle tools are commercially available.

- **Avoid static muscle loading**. Reduce both the weight and size of the tool. Do not raise or extend elbows when working with heavy tools. Provide counter balance support devices for larger, heavier tools.

- **Avoid stress on soft tissues**. Stress concentrations result from poorly designed tools that exert pressure on the palms or fingers. Examples include short-handled pliers and tools with finger grooves that do not fit the worker's hand.

- **Reduce grip force requirements**. The greater the effort to maintain control of a hand tool, the higher the potential for injury. A compressible gripping surface rather than hard plastic should be used.

- **Whenever possible, select tools that use a full-hand power grip rather than a precision finger grip**.

- **Avoid sharp edges and pinch points**. Select tools that will not cut or pinch the hands even when gloves are not worn.

- **Avoid repetitive trigger-finger actions**. Select tools with large switches that can be operated with all four fingers.

- **Wear gloves that fit**. Tight-fitting gloves can put pressure on the hands, while loose-fitting gloves reduce grip strength and pose other safety hazards.

If your job involves the frequent use of hand-tools and you frequently experience numbing, blanching, pins-and-needles, or dull pain in the hands or forearms, contact your Safety and Health Specialist.

Laboratories

Repetitive Pipetting

The following are recommended for control of ergonomic hazards associated with repetitive pipetting:

- Use pipettes with newer trigger mechanisms requiring less force to activate, and use the pointer finger to aspirate and the thumb to dispense (e.g., Rainin-Latch Mode Pipette).
- Use pipettes that fit comfortably in the user's hand.
- For tasks such as mixing or aliquoting, use an electronic pipette with mixing functions.

Additional Recommendations

- Use a multichannel pipette for large aliquoting tasks.
- Take micro-breaks of 2 minutes for every 20 minutes of pipetting. Mild hand exercises and stretches are beneficial.
- Clean pipettes on scheduled basis (this reduces "sticking" and improves quality of work).
- Adjust the workstation so the individual doesn't have to work with their arms in an elevated position. Work with arms close to the body.
- Rotate pipetting activities between laboratory tasks, hands, and people.
- Use thin-wall pipette tips that fit correctly and are easy to eject.
- Use minimal force when applying pipette tips.
- Keep samples and instruments within easy reach.
- Use an adjustable stool or chair when sitting at a lab bench

- If it is necessary to stand for long periods of time during pipetting, use an anti-fatigue matting.

Microscopy

The following are recommended to control hazards associated with microscopy:

- Try pulling the microscope toward the edge of the work surface to position the operator in a more upright posture.

- Try elevating the microscope. This can help position the operator in a more upright posture and reduce rounding of the shoulders and neck.

- Maintain neutral spine.

- Use an ergonomically designed chair that provides adequate back support, adjustable height, and adjustable seat angle.

- Use armrests to support the operator's forearms while using adjustment knobs on the microscope.

Proper Workstation Setup for Microscopy

- Make sure there is adequate room under the work surface so the operator can pull the chair up to the ocular(s).

- Provide footrests and discourage the use of foot rings on stools.

- Provide sit-stand seats for areas where there is restricted legroom.

- Encourage frequent breaks from microscopy work as well as stretching exercises

- Use television systems where possible to eliminate the use of binocular eyepieces.

Biosafety Cabinets and Laboratory Workbenches

The following are recommended for control of ergonomic hazards associated with biosafety cabinets and laboratory workbenches:

- Use an ergonomically designed chair that provides adequate back support, adjustable seat angle, and height adjustability between 28 inches to 33 inches.

- Use footrests for individuals whose feet do not rest comfortably on the floor.

- Apply closed-cell foam padding to the front edge of the biosafety cabinet (away from the downdraft) or workbench. This reduces contact forces by increasing the surface area that comes into contact with the forearm and therefore reduces the chances of impinging nerves, tendons, or blood vessels. If applying closed-cell padding to front edge of biosafety cabinet, make sure the material can be properly decontaminated.

- Remove drawers, supplies, refrigerators, etc. from under the workbenches and cabinet doors from under biosafety cabinets (provides legroom).

- Use a turntable to store equipment near the worker. This reduces excessive reaching and twisting, which places an increased load on the low back.

- Use anti-fatigue matting for laboratory personnel who must stand for extended periods of time.

- Take frequent micro-breaks to perform stretching exercises.

New biosafety cabinets may be purchased that incorporate the features below. Desirable features for the new biosafety cabinets include:

- A perforated front grill reduced by 1 inch to 2 inches to bring the work platform closer to the laboratory worker-adjustable height (hand-crank or hydraulic lift). Nonglare glass on the sash window and/or adjustable Plexiglas barriers.

- A platform configuration with "wells" for placement of tall containers.

Microtome or Cryostat

The following are recommended for control of ergonomic hazards associated with microtome or cryostat use:

- Lower the workstation to keep arms closer to body.

- Apply padding to the front edge of work surface to eliminate sharp edges and increase the amount of blood flow to the hands.

- Retrofit the existing handle with an adapter that will allow the operator to use the handwheel in a pistol grip position. This will alleviate repetitive wrist flexion and extension.

- Consider use of an automatic foot operated cryostat when frequent cryo-sectioning is performed.

- Avoid placing utensils such as forceps inside the cryostat.

- Use an ergonomically designed chair.

- Take frequent "micro-breaks." These breaks should be used to perform stretching exercises, especially the hands.

Flow Cytometer

The use of a flow cytometer requires frequent lateral bending, neck and back flexion, and extended arm reaching. This is due to the receiving port being located on the bottom of the flow cytometer. The operator must sit in awkward positions in order to see the controls. The following are recommended for control of ergonomic hazards associated with using a flow cytometer:

- Raise the flow cytometer by placing a block between the flow cytometer and the workbench.

- Use an electric or hydraulic adjustable table. Each individual will be able to adjust the flow cytometer to a height which is most comfortable.

- Use an ergonomically designed chair.

- Place the top of the monitor so the top of the screen is approximately at eye level.

Glove Boxes or Anaerobic Chambers

Working in glove boxes or anaerobic chambers requires extended static loading on the shoulders. Extending the arms for more than a couple of minutes can become very exhausting. In addition to static loading and frequent side reaching, the thick gloves also make the user over compensate on grip strength. The following are recommended for control of ergonomic hazards associated with using a glove box:

- Move all needed materials for the experiment from the side chamber to the main chamber at one time to reduce the amount of side reaching.

- Use highly absorbent hand powder for glove comfort.

- Utilize job enlargement to avoid long continuous use of glove boxes.

- Provide anti-fatigue matting for extended use of the glove box.

- If necessary, use a sit-stand seat to alleviate stress on the low back.

- Take frequent breaks to perform stretching exercises and relieve static loading from the shoulders.

Manipulating Centrifuge Rotors

Centrifuge rotors present a unique lifting hazard in the laboratory. The following are recommended for control of ergonomic hazards associated with lifting centrifuge rotors:

- Use a second person to assist with the lift.

- Use a cart to transport rotors.

- Look for manufacturers' which produces lighter weight rotors.

- Implement a pulley system, which would attach to the ceiling directly above the centrifuge.

Micro-Manipulation and Fine Motor Skills

The following are recommended for control or ergonomic hazards associated with micro-manipulation techniques:

- Use plastic vials with fewer threads. This will reduce twisting motions during capping and uncapping lids.

- Use small pieces of foam similar to the type used on pencils and pens, to prevent soreness on the fingertips, where fingers and forceps articulate. This will distribute the force over a greater surface area, thus reducing the compressive forces on the soft tissue.

- Practice using the forceps between the 1st and 2nd digits instead of using the thumb and 1st digit. Then try alternating between the two positions to reduce the use of the thumb. The thumb is used repetitively with almost every job task performed in the laboratory.

- Tilt storage bins toward the worker to reduce wrist flexion while reaching for supplies.

- Encourage micro-breaks and hand exercises.

Patient Care

Assisting another individual in a change of position requires proper body mechanics on your part. Proper body mechanics (positioning) will make your job easier to perform and reduce the risk of injury. Proper body mechanics requires that the natural curves of the spine are maintained in proper alignment. Look at the natural curves of your back and understand how to successfully maintain these curves:

- Bend your knees to get up and down.

- Keep the object close to the body in order to minimize forces on your body.

- Pivot and don't twist.

- Don't try to do more than you can handle. Respect your limits.

Part Two

Musculoskeletal Pain

Chapter 10

Arthritis and Rheumatic Diseases

Chapter Contents

Section 10.1

Basic Information about Arthritis and Rheumatic Diseases

This section includes text excerpted from "Arthritis and Rheumatic Diseases," National Institute of Arthritis and Musculoskeletal and Skin Diseases (NIAMS), October 2014.

Arthritis and Rheumatic Diseases

"Arthritis" literally means joint inflammation. Although joint inflammation is a symptom or sign rather than a specific diagnosis, the term arthritis is often used to refer to any disorder that affects the joints. These disorders fall within the broader category of rheumatic diseases. These are diseases characterized by inflammation (signs include redness or heat, swelling, and symptoms such as pain) and loss of function of one or more connecting or supporting structures of the body. They especially affect joints, tendons, ligaments, bones, and muscles. Common signs and symptoms are pain, swelling, and stiffness. Some rheumatic diseases also can involve internal organs.

There are more than 100 rheumatic diseases that collectively affect more than 46 million Americans. This section provides brief descriptions of some of the more common forms of arthritis and rheumatic diseases as well information about their causes, diagnosis, and treatments.

Examples of Rheumatic Diseases

The most common type of arthritis, osteoarthritis, damages both the cartilage, which is the tissue that cushions the ends of bones within the joint and the underlying bone. **Osteoarthritis** can cause joint pain and stiffness. Disability results most often when the disease affects the spine and the weight-bearing joints (the knees and hips). **Rheumatoid arthritis**, which is less common, is an inflammatory disease of the immune system that attacks the lining of the joint, called the "synovium," resulting in pain and swelling and loss of function in the joints. The most commonly affected joints are those in the hands and feet.

94

Causes of Rheumatic Diseases

There are likely many genes and combinations of genes that predispose people to rheumatic diseases. Some have been identified. In rheumatoid arthritis, juvenile arthritis, and lupus, for example, patients may have a variation in a gene that codes for an enzyme called protein tyrosine phosphatase nonreceptor 22 (PTPN22). In osteoarthritis, inherited cartilage weakness may play a role.

In people who are genetically susceptible, factors in the environment may trigger the disease. For example, scientists have found a connection between *Epstein-Barr* virus and lupus. Excessive stress on a joint from repeated injury may lead to osteoarthritis. Hormone or other male-female differences may also play a role. For example, lupus, rheumatoid arthritis, scleroderma, and fibromyalgia are more common among women.

Other Rheumatic Diseases

- **Bursitis.** A condition involving inflammation of the bursae (small, fluid-filled sacs that help reduce friction between bones and other moving structures in the joints) that produces pain and tenderness and may limit the movement of nearby joints.

- **Fibromyalgia.** A chronic disorder characterized by the presence of tender points—points on the body that are painful upon the application of pressure—and widespread muscle pain. Many people also experience fatigue and sleep disturbances.

- **Gout.** A type of arthritis resulting from deposits of needle-like crystals of uric acid in the joints, usually beginning in the big toe. The crystals cause episodic inflammation, swelling, and pain in the affected joint(s).

- **Infectious arthritis.** A general term used to describe forms of arthritis that are caused by infectious agents such as bacteria or viruses. Parvovirus arthritis and gonococcal arthritis are examples of infectious arthritis, as is the arthritis that occurs with Lyme disease, a bacterial infection following the bite of certain infected ticks.

- **Juvenile idiopathic arthritis.** The most common form of arthritis in childhood, causes pain, stiffness, swelling, and loss of function of the joints. It may be associated with rashes or fevers and may affect various parts of the body.

- **Polymyalgia rheumatica.** A condition involving tendons, muscles, ligaments, and tissues around the joint that causes pain, aching, and morning stiffness in the shoulders, hips, neck, and lower back. It is sometimes the first sign of giant cell arteritis, a disease of the arteries characterized by headaches, inflammation, weakness, weight loss, and fever.

- **Polymyositis.** A rheumatic disease that causes inflammation and weakness in the muscles. The disease may affect the whole body and cause disability.

- **Scleroderma** (also known as systemic sclerosis). A condition in which an excessive production of collagen (a fiber-like protein) leads to thickening of and damage to the skin, blood vessels, joints, and sometimes internal organs such as the lungs and kidneys.

- **Spondyloarthropathies.** A group of rheumatic diseases that principally affects the spine. One common form—ankylosing spondylitis—also may affect the hips, shoulders, and knees. Another spondyloarthropathy, reactive arthritis, develops after an infection involving the lower urinary tract, bowel, or other organ and is commonly associated with eye problems, skin rashes, and mouth sores. Psoriatic arthritis, which is a form of arthritis that occurs in some patients with the skin disorder psoriasis, is also considered a spondlyoarthropathy. Psoriatic arthritis often affects the joints at the ends of the fingers and toes and is accompanied by changes in the fingernails and toenails. Back pain may occur if the spine is involved.

- **Systemic lupus erythematosus** (also known as "lupus" or SLE). An autoimmune disease in which the immune system attacks the body's own healthy cells and tissues. This can result in inflammation of and damage to the joints, skin, kidneys, heart, lungs, blood vessels, and brain.

- **Tendinitis.** Inflammation of tendons (tough cords of tissue that connect muscle to bone) that is caused by overuse, injury, or a rheumatic condition and may restrict movement of nearby joints.

Who Is Affected?

Rheumatic diseases affect an estimated 46 million people in the United States of all races and ages, including an estimated 294,000 children. Some rheumatic diseases are more common among certain populations. For example, as noted above, rheumatoid arthritis, scleroderma, fibromyalgia, and lupus predominantly affect women. The spondyloarthropathies and gout are more common in men. However, after menopause, the incidence of gout in women begins to rise. Lupus is more common in and tends to be more severe in African Americans and Hispanics than Caucasians.

Signs and Symptoms of Arthritis and Rheumatic Diseases

Different types of arthritis and rheumatic diseases have different signs and symptoms. In general, people who have arthritis feel pain and stiffness in one or more joints. Pain and stiffness may be accompanied by tenderness, warmth, redness in a joint, and/or difficulty using or moving a joint normally.

Diagnosis of Arthritis and Rheumatic Diseases

The diagnosis of a rheumatic disease may be made by a general practitioner or a rheumatologist, a doctor who specializes in diagnosing and treating arthritis and other rheumatic diseases.

Based on the findings of the history and physical exam, the doctor may order laboratory tests and X-rays or other imaging tests to help confirm a diagnosis. Samples of blood, urine, or synovial fluid (lubricating fluid found in the joint) may be needed for the lab tests. Many of these same tests may be useful later for monitoring the disease or the effectiveness of treatments.

The doctor may need to see the patient more than once and possibly a number of times to make an accurate diagnosis.

Treatment of Arthritis and Rheumatic Diseases

Treatments for arthritis and rheumatic diseases vary depending on the specific disease or condition; however, treatment generally includes the following:

- Exercise

- Diet

- Medications

  - Oral analgesics

- Topical analgesics

- Nonsteroidal anti-inflammatory drugs (NSAIDs)

- Disease-modifying antirheumatic drugs (DMARDs)

- Biologic response modifiers

- Janus kinase inhibitors

- Corticosteroids

- Heat and cold therapies

- Relaxation therapy

- Splints and braces

- Assistive devices

- Surgery

Section 10.2

Rheumatoid Arthritis

This section includes text excerpted from "Handout on
Health: Rheumatoid Arthritis," National Institute of Arthritis and
Musculoskeletal and Skin Diseases (NIAMS), February 2016.

Rheumatoid arthritis (RA) is an inflammatory disease that causes
pain, swelling, stiffness, and loss of function in the joints. It occurs when
the immune system, which normally defends the body from invading
organisms, turns its attack against the membrane lining the joints.

Rheumatoid arthritis has several features that make it different from other kinds of arthritis. For example, rheumatoid arthritis
generally occurs in a symmetrical pattern, meaning that if one knee
or hand is involved, the other one also is. The disease often affects
the wrist joints and the finger joints closest to the hand. It can also
affect other parts of the body besides the joints. In addition, people
with rheumatoid arthritis may have fatigue, occasional fevers, and
a loss of energy.

The course of rheumatoid arthritis can range from mild to severe. In most cases it is chronic, meaning it lasts a long time—often a lifetime. For many people, periods of relatively mild disease activity are punctuated by flares, or times of heightened disease activity. In others, symptoms are constant.

Features of rheumatoid arthritis:

- Tender, warm, swollen joints

- Symmetrical pattern of affected joints

- Joint inflammation often affecting the wrist and finger joints closest to the hand

- Joint inflammation sometimes affecting other joints, including the neck, shoulders, elbows, hips, knees, ankles, and feet

- Fatigue, occasional fevers, a loss of energy

- Pain and stiffness lasting for more than 30 minutes in the morning or after a long rest

- Symptoms that last for many years

- Variability of symptoms among people with the disease.

Who Has Rheumatoid Arthritis?

Scientists estimate that about 1.5 million people, or about 0.6 percent of the U.S. adult population, have rheumatoid arthritis. Interestingly, some recent studies have suggested that although the number of new cases of rheumatoid arthritis for older people is increasing, the overall number of new cases may actually be going down.

Rheumatoid arthritis occurs in all races and ethnic groups. Although the disease often begins in middle age and occurs with increased frequency in older people, older teenagers and young adults may also be diagnosed with the disease. (Children and younger teenagers may be diagnosed with juvenile idiopathic arthritis, a condition related to rheumatoid arthritis.) Like some other forms of arthritis, rheumatoid arthritis occurs much more frequently in women than in men. About two to three times as many women as men have the disease.

What Happens in Rheumatoid Arthritis?

Rheumatoid arthritis is primarily a disease of the joints. A joint is the point where two or more bones come together. With a few exceptions (in

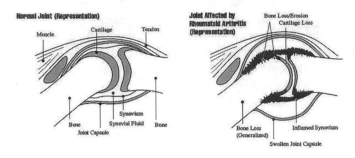

Figure 10.1. *Joint Rheumatoid Arthritis*

A joint (the place where two bones meet) is surrounded by a capsule that protects and supports it. The joint capsule is lined with a type of tissue called synovium, which produces synovial fluid that lubricates and nourishes joint tissues. In rheumatoid arthritis, the synovium becomes inflamed, causing warmth, redness, swelling, and pain. As the disease progresses, the inflamed synovium invades and damages the cartilage and bone of the joint. Surrounding muscles, ligaments, and tendons become weakened. Rheumatoid arthritis also can cause more generalized bone loss that may lead to osteoporosis (fragile bones that are prone to fracture).

the skull and pelvis, for example), joints are designed to allow movement between the bones and to absorb shock from movements like walking or repetitive motions. The ends of the bones are covered by a tough, elastic tissue called cartilage. The joint is surrounded by a capsule that protects and supports it. The joint capsule is lined with a type of tissue called synovium, which produces synovial fluid, a clear substance that lubricates and nourishes the cartilage and bones inside the joint capsule.

Like many other rheumatic diseases, rheumatoid arthritis is an autoimmune disease (auto means self), so called because a person's immune system, which normally helps protect the body from infection and disease, attacks joint tissues for unknown reasons. White blood cells, the agents of the immune system, travel to the synovium and cause inflammation (synovitis), characterized by warmth, redness, swelling, and pain—typical symptoms of rheumatoid arthritis. During the inflammation process, the normally thin synovium becomes thick and makes the joint swollen, puffy, and sometimes warm to the touch.

As rheumatoid arthritis progresses, the inflamed synovium invades and destroys the cartilage and bone within the joint. The surrounding muscles, ligaments, and tendons that support and stabilize the joint become weak and unable to work normally. These effects lead to the pain and joint damage often seen in rheumatoid arthritis. Researchers studying rheumatoid arthritis now believe that it begins to damage bones during the first year or two that a person has the disease, which is one reason why early diagnosis and treatment are so important.

Some people with rheumatoid arthritis also have symptoms in places other than their joints. Many people with rheumatoid arthritis develop anemia, or a decrease in the production of red blood cells. Other effects that occur less often include neck pain and dry eyes and mouth. Very rarely, people may have inflammation of the blood vessels (vasculitis), the lining of the lungs (pleurisy), or the sac enclosing the heart (pericarditis).

How Does Rheumatoid Arthritis Affect People's Lives?

Rheumatoid arthritis affects people differently. Some people have mild or moderate forms of the disease, with periods of worsening symptoms, called flares, and periods in which they feel better, called remissions. Others have a severe form of the disease that is active most of the time, lasts for many years or a lifetime, and leads to serious joint damage and disability.

Although rheumatoid arthritis is primarily a disease of the joints, its effects are not just physical. Many people with rheumatoid arthritis also experience issues related to:

- depression, anxiety
- feelings of helplessness
- low self-esteem

Rheumatoid arthritis can affect virtually every area of a person's life from work life to family life. It can also interfere with the joys and responsibilities of family life and may affect the decision to have children.

Fortunately, current treatment strategies allow most people with the disease to lead active and productive lives. These strategies include pain-relieving drugs and medications that slow joint damage, a balance between rest and exercise, and patient education and support programs. In recent years, research has led to a new understanding of rheumatoid arthritis and has increased the likelihood that, in time, researchers will find even better ways to treat the disease.

What Causes Rheumatoid Arthritis?

Scientists still do not know exactly what causes the immune system to turn against the body's own tissues in rheumatoid arthritis, but research over the last few years has begun to piece together the factors involved.

Genetic (inherited) factors. Scientists have discovered that certain genes known to play a role in the immune system are associated with a tendency to develop rheumatoid arthritis. For the genes that have been linked to rheumatoid arthritis, the frequency of the risky gene is only modestly higher in those with rheumatoid arthritis compared with healthy controls. In other words, individual genes by themselves confer only a small relative risk of disease. Some people who have these particular genes never develop the disease. These observations suggest that although a person's genetic makeup plays an important role in determining if he or she will develop rheumatoid arthritis, it is not the only factor. What is clear, however, is that more than one gene is involved in determining whether a person develops rheumatoid arthritis and how severe the disease will become.

Environmental factors. Many scientists think that something must occur to trigger the disease process in people whose genetic makeup makes them susceptible to rheumatoid arthritis. A variety of factors have been suggested, but a specific agent has not been identified.

Other factors. Some scientists also think that a variety of hormonal factors may be involved. Women are more likely to develop rheumatoid arthritis than men. The disease may improve during pregnancy and flare after pregnancy. Breastfeeding may also aggravate the disease. Contraceptive use may increase a person's likelihood of developing rheumatoid arthritis. This suggests hormones, or possibly deficiencies or changes in certain hormones, may promote the development of rheumatoid arthritis in a genetically susceptible person who has been exposed to a triggering agent from the environment.

Even though all the answers are not known, one thing is certain; rheumatoid arthritis develops as a result of an interaction of many factors. Researchers are trying to understand these factors and how they work together.

How Is Rheumatoid Arthritis Diagnosed?

Rheumatoid arthritis can be difficult to diagnose in its early stages for several reasons. First, there is no single test for the disease. In addition, symptoms differ from person to person and can be more severe in some people than in others. Also, symptoms can be similar to those of other types of arthritis and joint conditions, and it may take some time for other conditions to be ruled out. Finally, the full range of symptoms develops over time, and only a few symptoms may be present in the early stages. As a result, doctors use a variety of the following tools to diagnose the disease and to rule out other conditions:

- Medical history
- Physical examination
- Laboratory tests
  - Rheumatoid factor (RF)
  - Anti-CCP antibodies
  - Others
- X-rays

How Is Rheumatoid Arthritis Treated?

Doctors use a variety of approaches to treat rheumatoid arthritis. These are used in different combinations and at different times during the course of the disease and are chosen according to the patient's individual situation. No matter what treatment the doctor and patient choose, however, the goals are the same: to relieve pain, reduce inflammation, slow down or stop joint damage, and improve the person's sense of well-being and ability to function.

Good communication between the patient and doctor is necessary for effective treatment. Talking to the doctor can help ensure that exercise and pain management programs are provided as needed, and that drugs are prescribed appropriately. Talking to the doctor can also help people who are making decisions about surgery.

Goals of treatment:

- Relieve pain
- Reduce inflammation
- Slow down or stop joint damage
- Improve a person's sense of well-being and ability to function

Current treatment approaches:

- Lifestyle

- Medications

- Surgery

- Routine monitoring and ongoing care

- Health behavior changes

  - Rest and exercise

  - Joint care

  - Stress reduction

  - Healthful diet

  - Climate

- Medications

- Routine monitoring and ongoing care

- Alternative and complementary therapies

Who Treats Rheumatoid Arthritis?

Diagnosing and treating rheumatoid arthritis requires a team effort involving the patient and several types of healthcare professionals.

The primary doctor to treat arthritis may be an **internist,** a doctor who specializes in the diagnosis and medical treatment of adults, or a **rheumatologist**, a doctor who specializes in arthritis and other diseases of the bones, joints, and muscles.

As treatment progresses, other professionals often help. These may include the following:

- Orthopaedists

- Physical therapists

- Occupational therapists

- Dietitians

- Nurse educators

- Psychologists

What You Can Do: The Importance of Self-Care

Although healthcare professionals can prescribe or recommend treatments to help patients manage their rheumatoid arthritis, the real key to living well with the disease lies with the patients themselves. Research shows that people who take part in their own care report less pain and make fewer doctor visits. They also enjoy a better quality of life.

Self-management programs teach about rheumatoid arthritis and its treatments, exercise and relaxation approaches, communication between patients and healthcare providers, and problem solving. Research on these programs has shown that they help people:

- understand the disease.

- reduce their pain while remaining active.

- cope physically, emotionally, and mentally.

- feel greater control over the disease and build a sense of confidence in the ability to function and lead full, active, and independent lives.

Section 10.3

Osteoarthritis

This section includes text excerpted from "Handout on Health: Osteoarthritis," National Institute of Arthritis and Musculoskeletal and Skin Diseases (NIAMS), May 2016.

Osteoarthritis is the most common type of arthritis and is seen especially among older people. Sometimes it is called degenerative joint disease. Osteoarthritis mostly affects cartilage, the hard but slippery tissue that covers the ends of bones where they meet to form a joint. Healthy cartilage allows bones to glide over one another. It also absorbs energy from the shock of physical movement. In osteoarthritis, the surface layer of cartilage breaks and wears away. This allows bones under the cartilage to rub together, causing pain, swelling, and loss of motion of the joint. Over time, the joint may lose its normal shape. Also, small deposits of bone—called osteophytes or bone spurs—may grow on the edges of the joint. Bits of bone or cartilage can break off and float inside the joint space. This causes more pain and damage.

People with osteoarthritis usually have joint pain and stiffness. Unlike some other forms of arthritis, such as rheumatoid arthritis, osteoarthritis affects only joint function. It does not affect skin tissue, the lungs, the eyes, or the blood vessels.

In rheumatoid arthritis, another common form of arthritis, the immune system attacks the tissues of the joints, leading to pain, inflammation, and eventually joint damage and malformation. It typically begins at a younger age than osteoarthritis, causes swelling and redness in joints, and may make people feel sick, tired, and feverish. Also, the joint involvement of rheumatoid arthritis is symmetrical; that is, if one joint is affected, the same joint on the opposite side of the body is usually similarly affected. Osteoarthritis, on the other hand, can occur in a single joint or can affect a joint on one side of the body much more severely.

Who Has Osteoarthritis?

Osteoarthritis is by far the most common type of arthritis, and the percentage of people who have it grows higher with age. An estimated 27 million Americans age 25 and older have osteoarthritis.

Although osteoarthritis becomes more common with age, younger people can develop it, usually as the result of a joint injury, a joint malformation, or a genetic defect in joint cartilage. Both men and women have the disease. Before age 45, more men than women have osteoarthritis; after age 45, it is more common in women. It is also more likely to occur in people who are overweight and in those with jobs that stress particular joints.

How Does Osteoarthritis Affect People?

People with osteoarthritis usually experience joint pain and stiffness. The most commonly affected joints are those at the ends of the fingers (closest to the nail), thumbs, neck, lower back, knees, and hips.

Osteoarthritis affects different people differently. It may progress quickly, but for most people, joint damage develops gradually over years. In some people, osteoarthritis is relatively mild and interferes little with day-to-day life; in others, it causes significant pain and disability.

Osteoarthritis Basics: The Joint and Its Parts

A joint is the point where two or more bones are connected. With a few exceptions (in the skull and pelvis, for example), joints are designed to allow movement between the bones and to absorb shock from movements like walking or repetitive motions. These movable joints are made up of the following parts:

- **Cartilage.** A hard but slippery coating on the end of each bone. Cartilage breaks down and wears away in osteoarthritis.

- **Joint capsule.** A tough membrane sac that encloses all the bones and other joint parts.

- **Synovium.** A thin membrane inside the joint capsule that secretes synovial fluid.

- **Synovial fluid.** A fluid that lubricates the joint and keeps the cartilage smooth and healthy.

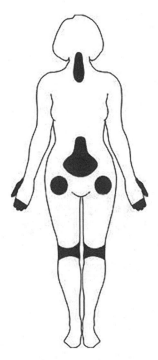

Figure 10.2. *Areas That Affect Osteoarthritis*

Osteoarthritis most often occurs in the hands (at the ends of the fingers and thumbs), spine (neck and lower back), knees, and hips.

- **Ligaments, tendons, and muscles.** Tissues that surround the bones and joints, and allow the joints to bend and move. Ligaments are tough, cord-like tissues that connect one bone to another.

- **Tendons.** Tough, fibrous cords that connect muscles to bones. Muscles are bundles of specialized cells that, when stimulated by nerves, either relax or contract to produce movement.

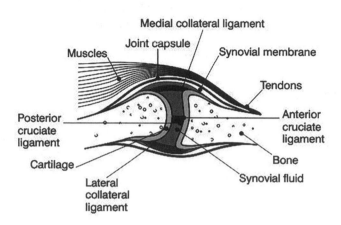

Figure 10.3. *A Healthy Joint (Representation)*

In a healthy joint, the ends of bones are encased in smooth cartilage. Together, they are protected by a joint capsule lined with a synovial membrane that produces synovial fluid. The capsule and fluid protect the cartilage, muscles, and connective tissues.

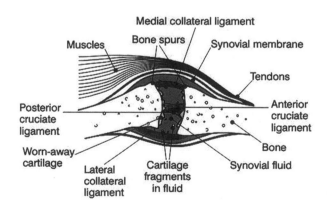

Figure 10.4. *A Joint with Severe Osteoarthritis (Representation)*

With osteoarthritis, the cartilage becomes worn away. Spurs grow out from the edge of the bone, and synovial fluid increases. Altogether, the joint feels stiff and sore.

How Do You Know If You Have Osteoarthritis?

Usually, osteoarthritis comes on slowly. Early in the disease, your joints may ache after physical work or exercise. Later on, joint pain may become more persistent. You may also experience joint stiffness, particularly when you first wake up in the morning or have been in one position for a long time.

Although osteoarthritis can occur in any joint, most often it affects the hands, knees, hips, and spine (either at the neck or lower back). Different characteristics of the disease can depend on the specific joint(s) affected. The joints that are most often affected by osteoarthritis includes:

- **Hands.** Osteoarthritis of the hands seems to have some hereditary characteristics; that is, it runs in families. If your mother or grandmother has or had osteoarthritis in their hands, you're at greater-than-average risk of having it too. Women are more likely than men to have osteoarthritis in the hands. For most women, it develops after menopause.

- **Knees.** The knees are among the joints most commonly affected by osteoarthritis. Symptoms of knee osteoarthritis include stiffness, swelling, and pain, which make it hard to walk, climb, and get in and out of chairs and bathtubs. Osteoarthritis in the knees can lead to disability.

- **Hips.** The hips are also common sites of osteoarthritis. As with knee osteoarthritis, symptoms of hip osteoarthritis include pain and stiffness of the joint itself. But sometimes pain is felt in the groin, inner thigh, buttocks, or even the knees. Osteoarthritis of the hip may limit moving and bending, making daily activities such as dressing and putting on shoes a challenge.

- **Spine.** Osteoarthritis of the spine may show up as stiffness and pain in the neck or lower back. In some cases, arthritis-related changes in the spine can cause pressure on the nerves where they exit the spinal column, resulting in weakness, tingling, or numbness of the arms and legs. In severe cases, this can even affect bladder and bowel function.

How Do Doctors Diagnose Osteoarthritis?

No single test can diagnose osteoarthritis; however, sometimes doctors use tests to help confirm a diagnosis or rule out other conditions that could be causing your symptoms. Most doctors use a combination of the following methods:

- Clinical History
- Physical Examination
- X-Rays
- Magnetic Resonance Imaging (MRI)
- Other Tests
  - Blood tests
  - Joint aspiration

How Is Osteoarthritis Treated?

Most successful treatment programs involve a combination of approaches tailored to the patient's needs, lifestyle, and health. Most programs include ways to manage pain and improve function. These approaches are described below.

Four goals of osteoarthritis treatment include:

1. to control pain
2. to improve joint function
3. to maintain normal body weight
4. to achieve a healthy lifestyle

Treatment approaches to osteoarthritis include:

- exercise
  - Strengthening exercises
  - Aerobic activities
  - Range-of-motion activities
  - Balance and agility exercises
- weight control
- nondrug pain relief techniques and alternative therapies
  - Heat and cold
  - Transcutaneous electrical nerve stimulation (TENS)
  - Massage

- Acupuncture
- Nutritional supplements
- medications to control pain
  - Over-the-counter pain relievers
  - NSAIDs (nonsteroidal anti-inflammatory drugs)
  - Narcotic or central acting agents
  - Corticosteroids
  - Hyaluronic acid substitutes
  - Other medications such as pain-relieving creams, rubs, and sprays
- surgery
  - Removal of loose pieces of bone and cartilage from the joint if they are causing symptoms of buckling or locking (arthroscopic debridement).
  - Repositioning of bones (osteotomy).
  - Resurfacing (smoothing out) bones (joint resurfacing).

Who Provides Care for People with Osteoarthritis?

Treating arthritis often requires a multidisciplinary or team approach. Many types of health professionals care for people with arthritis. You may choose a few or more of the following professionals to be part of your healthcare team:

- Primary care physicians
- Rheumatologists
- Orthopaedists
- Physical therapists
- Occupational therapists
- Dietitians
- Nurse educators
- Physiatrists (rehabilitation specialists)
- Licensed acupuncture therapists
- Psychologists

- Social workers

- Chiropractors

- Massage therapists

Section 10.4

Reactive Arthritis

This section includes text excerpted from "Questions and Answers
about Reactive Arthritis," National Institute of Arthritis and
Musculoskeletal and Skin Diseases (NIAMS), October 2016.

Reactive arthritis is a form of arthritis, or joint inflammation, that
occurs as a "reaction" to an infection elsewhere in the body. Inflammation is a characteristic reaction of tissues to injury or disease and is
marked by swelling, redness, heat, and pain. Besides this joint inflammation, reactive arthritis is associated with two other symptoms: redness and inflammation of the eyes (conjunctivitis) and inflammation
of the urinary tract (urethritis). These symptoms may occur alone,
together, or not at all.

Reactive arthritis is a type of "spondyloarthritis" a group of disorders that can cause inflammation throughout the body, especially in
the spine. (Examples of other disorders in this group include psoriatic
arthritis, ankylosing spondylitis, and the kind of arthritis that sometimes accompanies inflammatory bowel disease.)

In many patients, reactive arthritis is triggered by an infection
in the bladder, the urethra, or, in women, the vagina (the urogenital
tract) that is often transmitted through sexual contact. This form of
the disorder is sometimes called genitourinary or urogenital reactive
arthritis. Another form of reactive arthritis is caused by an infection
in the intestinal tract from eating food or handling substances that
are contaminated with bacteria. This form of arthritis is sometimes
called enteric or gastrointestinal reactive arthritis.

The symptoms of reactive arthritis usually last several months,
although symptoms can return or develop into a long-term disease in
a small percentage of people.

What Causes Reactive Arthritis?

Reactive arthritis typically begins within 2 to 4 weeks after infection. The bacterium most often associated with reactive arthritis is *Chlamydia trachomatis*, commonly known as chlamydia. It is usually acquired through sexual contact. Some evidence also shows that respiratory infections with *Chlamydia pneumoniae* may trigger reactive arthritis.

Infections in the digestive tract that may trigger reactive arthritis include *Salmonella, Shigella, Yersinia,* and *Campylobacter*. People may become infected with these bacteria after eating or handling improperly prepared food, such as meats that are not stored at the proper temperature.

Doctors do not know exactly why some people exposed to these bacteria develop reactive arthritis and others do not, but they have identified a genetic factor, human leukocyte antigen (HLA) B27, that increases a person's chance of developing reactive arthritis. However, inheriting the HLA *B27* gene does not necessarily mean you will get reactive arthritis.

Is Reactive Arthritis Contagious?

Reactive arthritis is not contagious; that is, a person with the disorder cannot pass the arthritis on to someone else. However, the bacteria that can trigger reactive arthritis can be passed from person to person.

Who Gets Reactive Arthritis?

Overall, young adult men are most likely to develop reactive arthritis. However, evidence shows that although men are nine times more likely than women to develop reactive arthritis caused by sexually acquired infections, women and men are equally likely to develop reactive arthritis as a result of food-borne infections. Women with reactive arthritis often have milder symptoms than men.

What Are the Symptoms of Reactive Arthritis?

Reactive arthritis most typically results in inflammation of the urogenital tract, the joints, and the eyes. Less common symptoms are mouth ulcers and skin rashes. Any of these symptoms may be so mild that patients do not notice them. They usually come and go over a period of several weeks to several months.

Joint Symptoms

Reactive arthritis typically involves pain and swelling in the knees, ankles, and feet. Wrists, fingers, and other joints are affected less often. People with reactive arthritis commonly develop inflammation of the tendons (tendinitis) or at places where tendons attach to the bone (enthesitis). In many people with reactive arthritis, this results in heel pain or irritation of the Achilles tendon at the back of the ankle. Some people with reactive arthritis also develop heel spurs, which are bony growths in the heel that may cause chronic (long-lasting) foot pain. Approximately half of people with reactive arthritis report low-back and buttock pain.

Reactive arthritis also can cause spondylitis (inflammation of the vertebrae in the spinal column) or sacroiliitis (inflammation of the joints in the lower back that connect the spine to the pelvis). People with reactive arthritis who have the HLA *B27* gene are even more likely to develop spondylitis and/or sacroiliitis.

Eye Involvement

Conjunctivitis, an inflammation of the mucous membrane that covers the eyeball and eyelid, develops in approximately half of people with reactive arthritis. Some people may develop uveitis, which is an inflammation of the inner eye. Conjunctivitis and uveitis can cause redness of the eyes, eye pain and irritation, and blurred vision. Eye involvement typically occurs early in the course of reactive arthritis, and symptoms may come and go.

How Is Reactive Arthritis Diagnosed?

Doctors sometimes find it difficult to diagnose reactive arthritis because there is no specific laboratory test to confirm that a person has it. A doctor may order a blood test to detect the genetic factor HLA *B27*, but even if the result is positive, the presence of HLA *B27* does not always mean that a person has the disorder.

At the beginning of an examination, the doctor will probably take a complete medical history and note current symptoms as well as any previous medical problems or infections. Before and after seeing the doctor, it is sometimes useful for the patient to keep a record of the symptoms that occur, when they occur, and how long they last. It is especially important to report any flu-like symptoms, such as fever, vomiting, or diarrhea, because they may be evidence of a bacterial infection.

The doctor may use various blood tests besides the HLA *B27* test to help rule out other conditions and confirm a suspected diagnosis of reactive arthritis. For example, the doctor may order rheumatoid factor or antinuclear antibody tests. Most people who have reactive arthritis will have negative results on these tests. If a patient's test results are positive, he or she may have some other form of arthritis (such as rheumatoid arthritis) or another rheumatic disease (such as lupus). Doctors also may order a blood test to determine the erythrocyte sedimentation rate (sed rate), which is the rate at which red blood cells settle to the bottom of a test tube of blood. A high sed rate often indicates inflammation somewhere in the body. Typically, people with rheumatic diseases, including reactive arthritis, have an elevated sed rate.

The doctor also is likely to perform tests for infections that might be associated with reactive arthritis. Patients generally are tested for a *Chlamydia* infection because studies have shown that early treatment of *Chlamydia*-induced reactive arthritis may reduce the progression of the disease. The doctor may look for bacterial infections by testing cell samples taken from the patient's throat as well as the urethra in men or cervix in women. Urine and stool samples also may be tested. A sample of synovial fluid (the fluid that lubricates the joints) may be removed from the arthritic joint. Studies of synovial fluid can help the doctor rule out infection in the joint.

Doctors sometimes use X-rays to help diagnose reactive arthritis and to rule out other causes of arthritis. X-rays can detect some of the symptoms of reactive arthritis, including spondylitis, sacroiliitis, swelling of soft tissues, damage to cartilage or bone margins of the joint, and calcium deposits where the tendon attaches to the bone.

What Type of Doctor Treats Reactive Arthritis?

A person with reactive arthritis probably will need to see several different types of doctors because reactive arthritis affects different parts of the body. However, it may be helpful to the doctors and the patient for one doctor, usually a rheumatologist (a doctor specializing in arthritis), to manage the complete treatment plan. This doctor can coordinate treatments and monitor the side effects from the various medicines the patient may take. The following specialists treat other features that affect different parts of the body.

- Ophthalmologist
- Gynecologist

- Urologist
- Dermatologist
- Orthopaedist
- Physiatrist

How Is Reactive Arthritis Treated?

Although there is no cure for reactive arthritis, some treatments relieve symptoms of the disorder. The doctor is likely to use one or more of the following treatments:

- Nonsteroidal Anti-Inflammatory Drugs (NSAIDs)
- Corticosteroid Injections
- Topical Corticosteroids
- Antibiotics
- Immunosuppressive Medicines
- Exercise

What Is the Prognosis for People Who Have Reactive Arthritis?

Most people with reactive arthritis recover fully from the initial flare of symptoms and are able to return to regular activities a few months after the first symptoms appear. In such cases, the symptoms of arthritis may last up to a year, although these are usually very mild and do not interfere with daily activities. Some people with reactive arthritis will have chronic (long-term) arthritis, which usually is mild. Studies show that between 15 and 50 percent of patients will develop symptoms again sometime after the initial flare has disappeared. It is possible that such relapses may be caused by reinfection. Back pain and arthritis are the symptoms that most commonly reappear. A few patients will have chronic, severe arthritis that is difficult to control with treatment and may cause joint damage.

Section 10.5

Gout

This section includes text excerpted from "Questions and Answers about Gout," National Institute of Arthritis and Musculoskeletal and Skin Diseases (NIAMS), April 2016.

Gout is a painful condition that occurs when the bodily waste product uric acid is deposited as needle-like crystals in the joints and/or soft tissues. In the joints, these uric acid crystals cause inflammatory arthritis, which in turn leads to intermittent swelling, redness, heat, pain, and stiffness in the joints.

In many people, gout initially affects the joints of the big toe. But many other joints and areas around the joints can be affected in addition to or instead of the big toe. These include the insteps, ankles, heels, knees, wrists, fingers, and elbows. Chalky deposits of uric acid, also known as tophi, can appear as lumps under the skin that surrounds the joints and covers the rim of the ear. Uric acid crystals can also collect in the kidneys and cause kidney stones.

What Is Uric Acid?

Uric acid is a substance that results from the breakdown of purines. A normal part of all human tissue, purines are found in many foods. Normally, uric acid is dissolved in the blood and passed through the kidneys into the urine, where it is eliminated.

If there is an increase in the production of uric acid or if the kidneys do not eliminate enough uric acid from the body, levels of it build up in the blood (a condition called hyperuricemia). Hyperuricemia also may result when a person eats too many high-purine foods, such as liver, dried beans and peas, anchovies, and gravies. Hyperuricemia is not a disease, and by itself it is not dangerous. However, if excess uric acid crystals form as a result of hyperuricemia, gout can develop. The crystals form and accumulate in the joint, causing inflammation.

What Are the Four Stages of Gout?

Gout can progress through four stages:

1. **Asymptomatic (without symptoms) hyperuricemia.** In this stage, a person has elevated levels of uric acid in the blood (hyperuricemia), but no other symptoms. Treatment is usually not required.

2. **Acute gout or acute gouty arthritis.** In this stage, hyperuricemia has caused the deposit of uric acid crystals in joint spaces. This leads to a sudden onset of intense pain and swelling in the joints, which also may be warm and very tender. An acute attack commonly occurs at night and can be triggered by stressful events, alcohol or drugs, or the presence of another illness. Attacks usually subside within 3 to 10 days, even without treatment, and the next attack may not occur for months or even years. Over time, however, attacks can last longer and occur more frequently.

3. **Interval or intercritical gout.** This is the period between acute attacks. In this stage, a person does not have any symptoms.

4. **Chronic tophaceous gout.** This is the most disabling stage of gout. It usually develops over a long period, such as 10 years. In this stage, the disease may have caused permanent damage to the affected joints and sometimes to the kidneys. With proper treatment, most people with gout do not progress to this advanced stage.

When It's Not Gout, It May Be Pseudogout

Gout is sometimes confused with other forms of arthritis because the symptoms—acute and episodic attacks of joint warmth, pain, swelling, and stiffness—can be similar. One form of arthritis often confused with gout is called pseudogout or calcium pyrophosphate deposition (CPPD). The pain, swelling, and redness of pseudogout can also come on suddenly and may be severe, closely resembling the symptoms of gout. However, the crystals that irritate the joint are calcium phosphate crystals, not uric acid.

What Causes Gout?

A number of risk factors are associated with hyperuricemia and gout. They include:

- **Genetics.** Many people with gout have a family history of the disease. Estimates range from 20 to 80 percent.

- **Gender and age.** It is more common in men than in women and more common in adults than in children.

- **Weight.** Being overweight increases the risk of developing hyperuricemia and gout because there is more tissue available for turnover or breakdown, which leads to excess uric acid production.

- **Alcohol consumption.** Drinking too much alcohol can lead to hyperuricemia, because alcohol interferes with the removal of uric acid from the body.

- **Diet.** Eating too many foods that are rich in purines can cause or aggravate gout in some people.

- **Lead exposure.** In some cases, exposure to lead in the environment can cause gout.

- **Other health problems.** Renal insufficiency, or the inability of the kidneys to eliminate waste products, is a common cause of gout in older people. Other medical problems that contribute to high blood levels of uric acid include:

  - high blood pressure

  - hypothyroidism (underactive thyroid gland)

  - conditions that cause an excessively rapid turnover of cells, such as psoriasis, hemolytic anemia, or some cancers

  - Kelley-Seegmiller syndrome or Lesch-Nyhan syndrome, two rare conditions in which the enzyme that helps control uric acid levels either is not present or is found in insufficient quantities.

- **Medications.** A number of medications may put people at risk for developing hyperuricemia and gout. They include:

- **Diuretics,** which are taken to eliminate excess fluid from the body in conditions like hypertension, edema, and heart disease, and which decrease the amount of uric acid passed in the urine

- **Salicylate-containing drugs**, such as aspirin

- **Niacin**, a vitamin also known as nicotinic acid

- **Cyclosporine**, a medication that suppresses the body's immune system (the system that protects the body from infection and disease). This medication is used in the treatment of some auto-immune diseases, and to prevent the body's rejection of trans-planted organs

- **Levodopa**, a medicine used to support communication along nerve pathways in the treatment of Parkinson disease

Who Is Likely to Develop Gout?

Scientists estimate that 6 million adults age 20 and older report having had gout at some time in their lives. It is rare in children and young adults. Men, particularly those between the ages of 40 and 50, are more likely to develop gout than women, who rarely develop the disorder before menopause. People who have had an organ transplant are more susceptible to gout.

How Is Gout Diagnosed?

Gout may be difficult for doctors to diagnose because the symptoms can be vague, and gout often mimics other conditions. Although most people with gout have hyperuricemia at some time during the course of their disease, it may not be present during an acute attack. In addition, having hyperuricemia alone does not mean that a person will get gout. In fact, most people with hyperuricemia do not develop the disease.

To confirm a diagnosis of gout, a doctor may insert a needle into an inflamed joint and draw a sample of synovial fluid, the substance that lubricates a joint. The joint fluid is placed on a slide and examined under a microscope for uric acid crystals. Their absence, however, does not completely rule out the diagnosis.

The doctor also may find it helpful to look for uric acid crystals around joints to diagnose gout. Gout attacks may mimic joint infections, and a doctor who suspects a joint infection (rather than gout) may also culture the joint fluid to see whether bacteria are present.

Signs and symptoms of gout:

- hyperuricemia
- presence of uric acid crystals in joint fluid
- more than one attack of acute arthritis
- arthritis that develops in a day, producing a swollen, red, and warm joint
- attack of arthritis in only one joint, often the toe, ankle, or knee.

How Is Gout Treated?

With proper treatment, most people who have gout are able to control their symptoms and live productive lives. Gout can be treated with one or a combination of therapies. The goals of treatment are to ease the pain associated with acute attacks, to prevent future attacks, and to avoid the formation of tophi and kidney stones. Successful treatment can reduce discomfort caused by the symptoms of gout, as well as long-term damage to the affected joints. Treatment will help to prevent disability due to gout.

The most common treatments for an acute attack of gout are nonsteroidal anti-inflammatory drugs (NSAIDs) taken orally (by mouth), or corticosteroids, which are taken orally or injected into the affected joint. NSAIDs reduce the inflammation caused by deposits of uric acid crystals, but have no effect on the amount of uric acid in the body.

Corticosteroids are strong anti-inflammatory hormones. The most commonly prescribed corticosteroid is prednisone. Patients often begin to improve within a few hours of treatment with a corticosteroid, and the attack usually goes away completely within a week or so. When NSAIDs or corticosteroids do not control symptoms, the doctor may consider using colchicine. The doctor also may consider prescribing other medicines to treat hyperuricemia and reduce the frequency of sudden attacks and the development of tophi. People who have other medical problems, such as high blood pressure or high blood triglycerides (fats), may find that the drugs they take for those conditions can also be useful for gout. The doctor may also recommend losing weight, for those who are overweight; limiting alcohol consumption; and avoiding or limiting high-purine foods, which can increase uric acid levels.

What Can People with Gout Do to Stay Healthy?

Fortunately, gout can be controlled. People with gout can decrease the severity of attacks and reduce their risk of future attacks by taking their medications as prescribed. Acute gout is best controlled if medications are taken at the first sign of pain or inflammation. Other steps you can take to stay healthy and minimize gout's effect on your life include the following:

- Tell your doctor about all the medicines and vitamins you take. He or she can tell you if any of them increase your risk of hyperuricemia.

- Plan follow-up visits with your doctor to evaluate your progress.

- Drink plenty of nonalcoholic fluids, especially water. Nonalcoholic fluids help remove uric acid from the body. Alcohol, on the other hand, can raise the levels of uric acid in your blood.

- Exercise regularly and maintain a healthy body weight. Lose weight if you are overweight, but avoid low-carbohydrate diets that are designed for quick weight loss. When carbohydrate intake is insufficient, your body can't completely burn its own fat. As a consequence, substances called ketones form and are released into the bloodstream, resulting in a condition called ketosis. After a short time, ketosis can increase the level of uric acid in your blood.

- Avoid foods that are high in purines. High-purine foods include:

  - anchovies

  - asparagus

  - beef kidneys

  - brains

  - dried beans and peas

  - game meats

  - gravy

  - herring

  - liver

  - mackerel

  - mushrooms

  - sardines

  - scallops

  - sweetbreads

Section 10.6

Polymyalgia Rheumatica

This section includes text excerpted from "Questions and
Answers about Polymyalgia Rheumatica and Giant Cell
Arteritis," National Institute of Arthritis and Musculoskeletal
and Skin Diseases (NIAMS), May 2016.

What Is Polymyalgia Rheumatica?

Polymyalgia rheumatica is a rheumatic disorder associated with
moderate-to-severe musculoskeletal pain and stiffness in the neck,
shoulder, and hip area. Stiffness is most noticeable in the morning or
after a period of inactivity. This disorder may develop rapidly; in some
people it comes on literally overnight. But for most people, polymyalgia
rheumatica develops more gradually.

The cause of polymyalgia rheumatica is not known. But it is associated with immune system problems, genetic factors, and an event, such
as an infection, that triggers symptoms. The fact that polymyalgia rheumatica is rare in people under the age of 50 and becomes more common
as age increases, suggests that it may be linked to the aging process.

Polymyalgia rheumatica usually resolves within 1 to several years.
The symptoms of polymyalgia rheumatica are quickly controlled by
treatment with corticosteroids, but symptoms return if treatment is
stopped too early. Corticosteroid treatment does not appear to influence the length of the disease.

What Is Giant Cell Arteritis?

Giant cell arteritis is a form of vasculitis, a group of disorders that
results in inflammation of blood vessels. This inflammation causes
the arteries to narrow, impeding adequate blood flow. In giant cell
arteritis, the vessels most involved are those of the head, especially the
temporal arteries (located on each side of the head). For this reason,
the disorder is sometimes called temporal arteritis. However, other
blood vessels can also become inflamed in giant cell arteritis. For a good
prognosis, it is critical to receive early treatment, before irreversible
tissue damage occurs.

How Are Polymyalgia Rheumatica and Giant Cell Arteritis Related?

It is unclear how or why polymyalgia rheumatica and giant cell arteritis frequently occur together. But some people with polymyalgia rheumatica also develop giant cell arteritis either simultaneously, or after the musculoskeletal symptoms have disappeared. Other people with giant cell arteritis also have polymyalgia rheumatica at some time while the arteries are inflamed.

When undiagnosed or untreated, giant cell arteritis can cause potentially serious problems, including permanent vision loss and stroke. So regardless of why giant cell arteritis might occur along with polymyalgia rheumatica, it is important that doctors look for symptoms of the arteritis in anyone diagnosed with polymyalgia rheumatica.

Patients, too, must learn and watch for symptoms of giant cell arteritis, because early detection and proper treatment are key to preventing complications. Any symptoms should be reported to your doctor immediately.

What Are the Symptoms of Polymyalgia Rheumatica?

In addition to the musculoskeletal stiffness mentioned earlier, people with polymyalgia rheumatica also may have flu-like symptoms, including fever, weakness, and weight loss.

What Are the Symptoms of Giant Cell Arteritis?

Early symptoms of giant cell arteritis may resemble flu symptoms such as fatigue, loss of appetite, and fever. Symptoms specifically related to the inflamed arteries of the head include headaches, pain and tenderness over the temples, double vision or visual loss, dizziness or problems with coordination, and balance. Pain may also affect the jaw and tongue, especially when eating, and opening the mouth wide may become difficult. In rare cases, giant cell arteritis causes ulceration of the scalp.

Who Is at Risk for These Conditions?

Caucasian women over the age of 50 have the highest risk of developing polymyalgia rheumatica and giant cell arteritis. Although women are more likely than men to develop the conditions, research suggests that men with giant cell arteritis are more likely to suffer potentially blinding eye involvement. Both conditions almost exclusively affect people over the age of 50. The incidence of both peaks between 70 and 80 years of age.

Polymyalgia rheumatica and giant cell arteritis are both quite common. It is estimated that 711,000 Americans have polymyalgia rheumatica and 228,000 have giant cell arteritis.

How Are Polymyalgia Rheumatica and Giant Cell Arteritis Diagnosed?

A diagnosis of polymyalgia rheumatica is based primarily on the patient's medical history and symptoms, and on a physical examination. No single test is available to definitively diagnose polymyalgia rheumatica. However, doctors often use lab tests to confirm a diagnosis or rule out other diagnoses or possible reasons for the patient's symptoms.

The most typical laboratory finding in people with polymyalgia rheumatica is an elevated erythrocyte sedimentation rate, commonly referred to as the sed rate. This test measures inflammation by determining how quickly red blood cells fall to the bottom of a test tube of unclotted blood. Rapidly descending cells (an elevated sed rate) indicate inflammation in the body. Although the sed rate measurement is a helpful diagnostic tool, it alone does not confirm polymyalgia rheumatica. An abnormal result indicates only that tissue is inflamed, but this is also a symptom of many forms of arthritis and other rheumatic diseases.

Before making a diagnosis of polymyalgia rheumatica, the doctor may order additional tests. For example, the C-reactive protein test is another common means of measuring inflammation. There is also a common test for rheumatoid factor, an antibody (a protein made by the immune system) that is sometimes found in the blood of people with rheumatoid arthritis. Although polymyalgia rheumatica and rheumatoid arthritis share many symptoms, those with polymyalgia rheumatica rarely test positive for rheumatoid factor. Therefore, a positive rheumatoid factor might suggest a diagnosis of rheumatoid arthritis instead of polymyalgia rheumatica.

As with polymyalgia rheumatica, a diagnosis of giant cell arteritis is based largely on symptoms and a physical examination. The exam may reveal that the temporal artery is inflamed and tender to the touch, and that it has a reduced pulse.

When a doctor suspects giant cell arteritis a temporal artery biopsy is typically ordered. In this procedure, a small section of the artery is removed through an incision in the skin over the temple area and examined under a microscope. A biopsy that is positive for giant cell arteritis will show abnormal cells in the artery walls. Some patients showing symptoms of giant cell arteritis will have negative biopsy results. In such cases, the doctor may suggest a second biopsy.

How Are They Treated?

The treatment of choice for both polymyalgia rheumatica and giant cell arteritis is corticosteroid medication, such as prednisone.[1]

Polymyalgia rheumatica responds to a low daily dose of corticosteroids that is increased as needed until symptoms disappear. At this point, the doctor may gradually reduce the dosage to determine the lowest amount needed to alleviate symptoms. Most patients can discontinue medication after 6 months to 2 years. If symptoms recur, corticosteroid treatment is required again.

Nonsteroidal anti-inflammatory drugs (NSAIDs), such as aspirin and ibuprofen, also may be used to treat polymyalgia rheumatica. The medication must be taken daily, and long-term use may cause stomach irritation. For most patients, NSAIDs alone are not enough to relieve symptoms.[2]

Even without treatment, polymyalgia rheumatica usually disappears in 1 to several years. With treatment, however, symptoms disappear quickly, usually in 24 to 48 hours. If corticosteroids don't bring improvement, the doctor is likely to consider other possible diagnoses.

Giant cell arteritis is treated with high doses of corticosteroids. If not treated promptly, the condition carries a small but definite risk of blindness, so corticosteroids should be started as soon as possible, perhaps

---

[2] *All medicines can have side effects. Some medicines and side effects are mentioned in this section. Some side effects may be more severe than others. You should review the package insert that comes with your medicine and ask your healthcare provider or pharmacist if you have any questions about the possible side effects.*

[3] *Warning: Side effects of NSAIDs include stomach problems; skin rashes; high blood pressure; fluid retention; and liver, kidney, and heart problems. The longer a person uses NSAIDs, the more likely he or she is to have side effects, ranging from mild to serious. Many other drugs cannot be taken when a patient is being treated with NSAIDs, because NSAIDs alter the way the body uses or eliminates these other drugs. Check with your healthcare provider or pharmacist before you take NSAIDs. NSAIDs should only be used at the lowest dose possible for the shortest time needed.*

even before confirming the diagnosis with a temporal artery biopsy. As with polymyalgia rheumatica, the symptoms of giant cell arteritis quickly disappear with treatment; however, high doses of corticosteroids are typically maintained for 1 month. Once symptoms disappear and the sed rate is normal, there is much less risk of blindness. At that point, the doctor can begin to gradually reduce the corticosteroid dose.

In both polymyalgia rheumatica and giant cell arteritis, an increase in symptoms may develop when the corticosteroid dose is reduced to lower levels. The doctor may need to hold the lower dose for a longer period of time or even modestly increase it again, temporarily, to control the symptoms. Once the symptoms are in remission and the corticosteroid has been discontinued for several months, recurrence is less common. Whether taken on a long-term basis for polymyalgia rheumatica or for a shorter period for giant cell arteritis, corticosteroids carry a risk of side effects. Although long-term use and/or higher doses carry the greatest risk, people taking the drug at any dose or for any length of time should be aware of the potential side effects, which include:

- fluid retention and weight gain
- rounding of the face
- delayed wound healing
- bruising easily
- diabetes
- myopathy (muscle wasting)
- glaucoma
- increased blood pressure
- decreased calcium absorption in the bones, which can lead to osteoporosis
- irritation of the stomach
- increase in infections

People taking corticosteroids may have some side effects or none at all. Anyone who experiences side effects should report them to his or her doctor. When the medication is stopped, the side effects disappear. Because corticosteroid drugs reduce the body's natural production of corticosteroid hormones, which are necessary for the body to function properly, it is important not to stop taking the medication unless instructed by a doctor to do so. The patient and doctor must work together to gradually reduce the medication.

What Is the Outlook?

Most people with polymyalgia rheumatica and giant cell arteritis lead productive, active lives. The duration of drug treatment differs by patient. Once treatment is discontinued, polymyalgia may recur; but once again, symptoms respond rapidly to prednisone. When properly treated, giant cell arteritis rarely recurs.

Chapter 11

Back and Spinal Pain

Chapter Contents

Section 11.1

What You Should Know about Back Pain

This section includes text excerpted from "Back Pain,"
National Institute of Arthritis and Musculoskeletal and
Skin Diseases (NIAMS), August 2016.

Back pain is an all-too-familiar problem that can range from a dull, constant ache to a sudden, sharp pain that leaves you incapacitated. It can come on suddenly—from an accident, a fall, or lifting something heavy—or it can develop slowly, perhaps as the result of age-related changes to the spine. Regardless of how back pain happens or how it feels, you know it when you have it. And chances are, if you don't have back pain now, you will eventually.

How Common Is Back Pain?

In a 3-month period, more than one-fourth of U.S. adults experience at least 1 day of back pain. It is one of our society's most common medical problems.

What Are the Risk Factors for Back Pain?

Although anyone can have back pain, a number of factors increase your risk. They include:

Age. The first attack of low back pain typically occurs between the ages of 30 and 40. Back pain becomes more common with age.

Fitness level. Back pain is more common among people who are not physically fit. Weak back and abdominal muscles may not properly support the spine.

People who go out and exercise a lot after being inactive all week are more likely to suffer painful back injuries than people who make moderate physical activity a daily habit. Studies show that low-impact aerobic exercise is good for the disks that cushion the vertebrae, the individual bones that make up the spine.

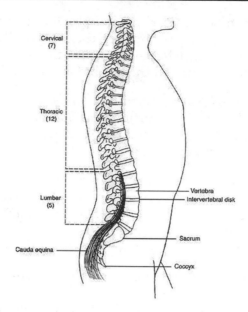

Figure 11.1. *Side View of Spine*

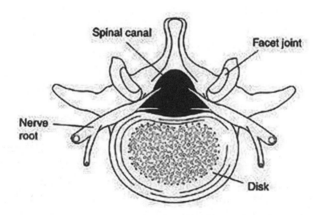

Figure 11.2. *Normal Vertebra (Cross Section)*

Diet. A diet high in calories and fat, combined with an inactive lifestyle, can lead to obesity, which can put stress on the back.

Heredity. Some causes of back pain, such as ankylosing spondylitis, a form of arthritis that affects the spine, have a genetic component.

Race. Race can be a factor in back problems. African American women, for example, are two to three times more likely than white women to develop spondylolisthesis, a condition in which a vertebra of the lower spine—also called the lumbar spine—slips out of place.

The presence of other diseases. Many diseases can cause or contribute to back pain. These include various forms of arthritis, such as osteoarthritis and rheumatoid arthritis, and cancers elsewhere in the body that may spread to the spine.

Occupational risk factors. Having a job that requires heavy lifting, pushing, or pulling, particularly when this involves twisting or vibrating the spine, can lead to injury and back pain. An inactive job or a desk job may also lead to or contribute to pain, especially if you have poor posture or sit all day in an uncomfortable chair.

Cigarette smoking. Although smoking may not directly cause back pain, it increases your risk of developing low back pain and low back pain with sciatica. (Sciatica is back pain that radiates to the hip and/or leg due to pressure on a nerve.) Furthermore, smoking can slow healing, prolonging pain for people who have had back injuries, back surgery, or broken bones.

What Are the Causes of Back Pain?

It is important to understand that back pain is a symptom of a medical condition, not a diagnosis itself. Medical problems that can cause back pain include the following:

- **Mechanical problems.** A mechanical problem is a problem with the way your spine moves or the way you feel when you move your spine in certain ways. Perhaps the most common mechanical cause of back pain is a condition called intervertebral disk degeneration, which simply means that the disks located between the vertebrae of the spine are breaking down with age. As they deteriorate, they lose their cushioning ability. This problem can lead to pain if the back is stressed. Other mechanical causes of back pain include spasms, muscle tension, and ruptured disks, which are also called herniated disks.

- **Injuries.** Spine injuries such as sprains and fractures can cause either short-lived or chronic pain. Sprains are tears in the ligaments that support the spine, and they can occur from twisting or lifting improperly. Fractured vertebrae are often the result of osteoporosis. Less commonly, back pain may be caused by more severe injuries that result from accidents or falls.

- **Acquired conditions and diseases.** Many medical problems can cause or contribute to back pain. They include scoliosis, a curvature of the spine that does not usually cause pain until middle age; spondylolisthesis; various forms of arthritis, including osteoarthritis, rheumatoid arthritis, and ankylosing spondylitis; and spinal stenosis, a narrowing of the spinal column that puts pressure on the spinal cord and nerves. Although osteoporosis itself is not painful, it can lead to painful fractures of the vertebrae. Other causes of back pain include pregnancy; kidney stones or infections; endometriosis, which is the buildup of uterine tissue in places outside the uterus; and fibromyalgia, a condition of widespread muscle pain and fatigue.

- **Infections and tumors.** Although they are not common causes of back pain, infections can cause pain when they involve the vertebrae, a condition called osteomyelitis, or when they involve the disks that cushion the vertebrae, which is called diskitis. Tumors also are relatively rare causes of back pain. Occasionally, tumors begin in the back, but more often they appear in the back as a result of cancer that has spread from elsewhere in the body.

Although the causes of back pain are usually physical, emotional stress can play a role in how severe pain is and how long it lasts. Stress can affect the body in many ways, including causing back muscles to become tense and painful.

Can Back Pain Be Prevented?

One of the best things you can do to prevent many types of back pain is to exercise regularly and keep your back muscles strong. Exercises that increase balance and strength can decrease your risk of falling and injuring your back or breaking bones. Exercises such as tai chi and yoga—or any weight-bearing exercise that challenges your balance—are good ones to try.

Eating a healthy diet also is important. For one thing, eating to maintain a healthy weight—or to lose weight, if you are overweight—helps you avoid putting unnecessary and injury-causing stress and strain on your back. To keep your spine strong, as with all bones, you need to get enough calcium and vitamin D every day. These nutrients help prevent osteoporosis, which is responsible for a lot of the bone fractures that lead to back pain. Calcium is found in dairy products; green, leafy vegetables; and fortified products, like orange juice. Your skin makes vitamin D when you are in the sun. If you are not outside much, you can obtain vitamin D from your diet: nearly all milk and some other foods are fortified with this nutrient. Most adults don't get enough calcium and vitamin D, so talk to your doctor about how much you need per day, and consider taking a nutritional supplement or a multivitamin.

Practicing good posture, supporting your back properly, and avoiding heavy lifting when you can may all help you prevent injury. If you do lift something heavy, keep your back straight. Don't bend over the item; instead, lift it by putting the stress on your legs and hips.

When Should I See a Doctor for Pain?

In most cases, it is not necessary to see a doctor for back pain because pain usually goes away with or without treatment. However, a trip to the doctor is probably a good idea if you have numbness or tingling, if your pain is severe and doesn't improve with medication and rest, or if you have pain after a fall or an injury. It is also important to see your doctor if you have pain along with any of the following problems: trouble urinating; weakness, pain, or numbness in your legs; fever; or unintentional weight loss. Such symptoms could signal a serious problem that requires treatment soon.

Which Type of Doctor Should I See?

Many different types of doctors treat back pain, from family physicians to doctors who specialize in disorders of the nerves and musculoskeletal system. In most cases, it is best to see your primary care doctor first. In many cases, he or she can treat the problem. In other cases, your doctor may refer you to an appropriate specialist.

How Is Back Pain Diagnosed?

Diagnosing the cause of back pain requires a medical history and a physical exam. If necessary, your doctor may also order medical tests, which may include X-rays. During the medical history, your doctor will ask questions about the nature of your pain and about any health problems you and close family members have or have had. Often a doctor can find the cause of your pain with a physical and medical history alone. However, depending on what the history and exam show, your doctor may order medical tests to help find the cause.

Following are some tests your doctor may order:

- X-rays
- Magnetic resonance imaging (MRI)
- Computed tomography (CT) scan
- Blood tests

Only with a medical history and exam—and sometimes medical tests—can a doctor diagnose the cause of back pain. Many times, the precise cause of back pain is never known. In these cases, it may be comforting to know that most back pain gets better whether or not you find out what is causing it.

What Is the Difference between Acute and Chronic Pain?

Pain that hits you suddenly—after falling from a ladder, being tackled on the football field, or lifting a load that is too heavy, for example—is acute pain. Acute pain comes on quickly and often leaves just as quickly. To be classified as acute, pain should last no longer than 6 weeks. Acute pain is the most common type of back pain.

Chronic pain, on the other hand, may come on either quickly or slowly, and it lingers a long time. In general, pain that lasts longer than 3 months is considered chronic. Chronic pain is much less common than acute pain.

How Is Back Pain Treated?

Treatment for back pain generally depends on what kind of pain you experience: acute or chronic.

Acute Back Pain

Acute back pain usually gets better on its own and without treatment, although you may want to try acetaminophen, aspirin, or ibuprofen to help ease the pain. Perhaps the best advice is to go about your usual activities as much as you can with the assurance that the problem will clear up. Getting up and moving around can help ease stiffness, relieve pain, and have you back doing your regular activities sooner. Exercises or surgery are not usually advisable for acute back pain.

Chronic Back Pain

Treatment for chronic back pain falls into two basic categories: the kind that requires an operation and the kind that does not. In the vast majority of cases, back pain does not require surgery. Doctors will nearly always try nonsurgical treatments before recommending surgery. In a very small percentage of cases—when back pain is caused by a tumor, an infection, or a nerve root problem called cauda equina syndrome, for example—prompt surgery is necessary to ease the pain and prevent further problems.

Following are some of the more commonly used treatments for chronic back pain:

Nonsurgical Treatments

- Hot or cold
- Exercise
  - Flexion
  - Extension
  - Stretching
  - Aerobic
- Medications
  - Analgesics
  - NSAIDs
  - Other medications such as muscle relaxants and certain antidepressants
- Traction
- Behavioral modification
- Complementary and alternative treatments

Surgical Treatments

Depending on the diagnosis, surgery may either be the first treatment of choice—although this is rare—or it is reserved for chronic back pain for which other treatments have failed. If you are in constant pain or if pain reoccurs frequently and interferes with your ability to sleep, to function at your job, or to perform daily activities, you may be a candidate for surgery.

Some of the diagnoses that may need surgery include:

- Herniated disks

- Spinal stenosis

- Spondylolisthesis

- Vertebral fractures

- Discogenic low back pain (degenerative disk disease)

Following are some of the most commonly performed back surgeries:

For Herniated Disks

- Laminectomy/discectomy

- Microdiscectomy

- Laser surgery

For Spinal Stenosis

- Laminectomy

For Spondylolisthesis

- Spinal fusion

For Vertebral Osteoporotic Fractures

- Vertebroplasty

- Kyphoplasty

For Diskogenic Low Back Pain (Degenerative Disk Disease)

- Intradiskal electrothermal therapy (IDET)

- Spinal fusion

- Disk replacement

Section 11.2

Spinal Stenosis

This section includes text excerpted from "Questions and
Answers about Spinal Stenosis," National Institute of Arthritis and
Musculoskeletal and Skin Diseases (NIAMS), August 2016.

Spinal stenosis is a narrowing of spaces in the spine (backbone)
that results in pressure on the spinal cord and/or nerve roots. This
disorder usually involves the narrowing of one or more of three areas
of the spine:

1. the canal in the center of the column of bones (vertebral or spinal column) through which the spinal cord and nerve roots run,

2. the canals at the base or roots of nerves branching out from the spinal cord, or

3. the openings between vertebrae (bones of the spine) through which nerves leave the spine and go to other parts of the body.

Who Gets Spinal Stenosis?

This disorder is most common in men and women over 50 years
of age. However, it may occur in younger people who are born with
a narrowing of the spinal canal or who suffer an injury to the spine.

What Structures of the Spine Are Involved?

The vertebrae link to each other and are cushioned by shock-absorbing disks that lie between them. Other structures of the spine include:

Facet joints. Joints located on the back of the main part of the
vertebra. They are formed by a portion of one vertebra and the vertebra above it. They connect the vertebrae to each other and permit
backward motion.

Ligaments. Elastic bands of tissue that support the spine by preventing the vertebrae from slipping out of line as the spine moves.

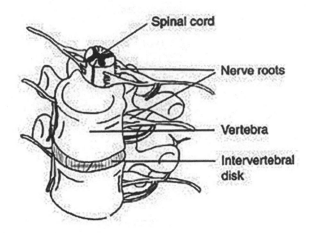

Figure 11.3. *Section of the Spine*

The spine is a column of 26 bones that extend in a line from the base of the skull to the pelvis (see figure. 11.3). Twenty-four of the bones are called vertebrae. The bones of the spine include 7 cervical vertebrae in the neck; 12 thoracic vertebrae at the back wall of the chest; 5 lumbar vertebrae at the inward curve (small) of the lower back; the sacrum, composed of 5 fused vertebrae between the hip bones; and the coccyx, composed of 3 to 5 fused bones at the lower tip of the vertebral column.

Spinal cord/nerve roots. A major part of the central nervous system that extends from the base of the brain down to the lower back and that is encased by the vertebral column. It consists of nerve cells and bundles of nerves. The cord connects the brain to all parts of the body via 31 pairs of nerves that branch out from the cord and leave the spine between vertebrae.

Cauda equina. A sack of nerve roots that continues from the lumbar region, where the spinal cord ends, and continues down to provide neurologic function to the lower part of the body. It resembles a "horse's tail."

What Causes Spinal Stenosis?

Degenerative Conditions

Spinal stenosis most often results from a gradual, degenerative aging process. Either structural changes or inflammation can begin the process. As people age, the ligaments of the spine may thicken and

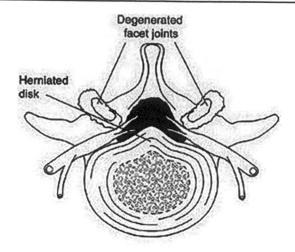

Figure 11.4. *Herniated Disk*

calcify (harden from deposits of calcium salts). Bones and joints may also enlarge: when surfaces of the bone begin to project out from the body, these projections are called osteophytes (bone spurs).

When the health of one part of the spine fails, it usually places increased stress on other parts of the spine. For example, a herniated (bulging) disk may place pressure on the spinal cord or nerve root. When a segment of the spine becomes too mobile, the capsules (enclosing membranes) of the facet joints thicken in an effort to stabilize the segment, and bone spurs may occur. This decreases the space available for nerve roots leaving the spinal cord.

Spondylolisthesis, a condition in which one vertebra slips forward on another, may result from a degenerative condition or an accident, or, very rarely, may be acquired at birth. Poor alignment of the spinal column when a vertebra slips forward onto the one below it can place pressure on the spinal cord or nerve roots at that place.

Aging with secondary changes is the most common cause of spinal stenosis. Two forms of arthritis that may affect the spine are osteoarthritis and rheumatoid arthritis.

- **Osteoarthritis**. Osteoarthritis is the most common form of arthritis and is more likely to occur in middle-aged and older people. It is a chronic, degenerative process that may involve multiple joints of the body. It wears away the surface cartilage layer of joints, and is often accompanied by overgrowth of bone, formation of bone spurs, and impaired function. If the degenerative process of osteoarthritis affects the facet joint(s) and the disk, the condition is sometimes referred to as spondylosis. This condition may be accompanied by disk degeneration, and an enlargement or overgrowth of bone that narrows the central and nerve root canals.

- **Rheumatoid Arthritis**. Rheumatoid arthritis usually affects people at an earlier age than osteoarthritis does and is associated with inflammation and enlargement of the soft tissues (the synovium) of the joints. Although not a common cause of spinal stenosis, damage to ligaments, bones, and joints that begins as synovitis (inflammation of the synovial membrane that lines the inside of the joint) has a severe and disrupting effect on joint function. The portions of the vertebral column with the greatest mobility (for example, the neck area) are often the ones most affected in people with rheumatoid arthritis.

Other Acquired Conditions

The following conditions that are not related to degenerative disease are causes of acquired spinal stenosis:

- Tumors of the spine are abnormal growths of soft tissue that may affect the spinal canal directly by inflammation or by growth of tissue into the canal. Tissue growth may lead to bone resorption (bone loss due to overactivity of certain bone cells) or displacement of bone.

- Trauma (accidents) may either dislocate the spine and the spinal canal or cause burst fractures that produce fragments of bone that penetrate the canal.

- Paget disease of bone is a chronic (long-term) disorder that typically results in enlarged and abnormal bones. Excessive bone breakdown and formation cause thick and fragile bone. As a result, bone pain, arthritis, noticeable bone structure changes, and fractures can occur. The disease can affect any bone of the body, but is often found in the spine. The blood supply that feeds healthy nerve tissue may be diverted to the area of involved bone. Also, structural problems of the involved vertebrae can cause narrowing of the spinal canal, producing a variety of neurological symptoms. Other developmental conditions may also result in spinal stenosis.

- Ossification of the posterior longitudinal ligament occurs when calcium deposits form on the ligament that runs up and down behind the spine and inside the spinal canal. These deposits turn the fibrous tissue of the ligament into bone. (Ossification means "forming bone.") These deposits may press on the nerves in the spinal canal.

What Are the Symptoms of Spinal Stenosis?

The space within the spinal canal may narrow without producing any symptoms. However, if narrowing places pressure on the spinal cord, cauda equina, or nerve roots, there may be a slow onset and progression of symptoms. The neck or back may or may not hurt. More often, people experience numbness, weakness, cramping, or general pain in the arms or legs. If the narrowed space within the spine is pushing on a nerve root, people may feel pain radiating down the leg (sciatica). Sitting or flexing the lower back should relieve symptoms. (The flexed position "opens up" the spinal column, enlarging the spaces between vertebrae at the back of the spine.) Flexing exercises are often advised, along with stretching and strengthening exercises.

People with more severe stenosis may have problems with bowel and bladder function and foot disorders. For example, cauda equina syndrome is a severe, and very rare, form of spinal stenosis. It occurs because of compression of the cauda equina, and symptoms may include loss of control of the bowel, bladder, or sexual function and/ or pain, weakness, or loss of feeling in one or both legs. Cauda equina syndrome is a serious condition requiring urgent medical attention.

How Is Spinal Stenosis Diagnosed?

The doctor may use a variety of approaches to diagnose spinal stenosis and rule out other conditions.

- Medical history
- Physical examination
- X-ray
- MRI (magnetic resonance imaging)
- Computerized axial tomography (CAT)
- Myelogram

Who Treats Spinal Stenosis?

Nonsurgical treatment of spinal stenosis may be provided by internists or general practitioners. The disorder is also treated by specialists such as rheumatologists and neurologists. Orthopaedic surgeons and neurosurgeons also provide nonsurgical treatment and perform spinal surgery if it is required. Allied health professionals such as physical therapists may also help treat patients.

What Are Some Nonsurgical Treatments for Spinal Stenosis?

In the absence of severe or progressive nerve involvement, a doctor may prescribe one or more of the following conservative treatments:

- Nonsteroidal anti–inflammatory drugs (NSAIDs), such as aspirin, naproxen, ibuprofen, or indomethacin, to reduce inflammation and relieve pain.

- Analgesics, such as acetaminophen, to relieve pain.

- Corticosteroid injections into the outermost of the membranes covering the spinal cord and nerve roots to reduce inflammation and treat acute pain that radiates to the hips or down a leg.

- Anesthetic injections, known as nerve blocks, near the affected nerve to temporarily relieve pain.

- Restricted activity (varies depending on extent of nerve involvement).

- Prescribed exercises and/or physical therapy to maintain motion of the spine, strengthen abdominal and back muscles, and build endurance, all of which help stabilize the spine. Some patients may be encouraged to try slowly progressive aerobic activity such as swimming or using exercise bicycles.

- A lumbar brace or corset to provide some support and help the patient regain mobility. This approach is sometimes used for patients with weak abdominal muscles or older patients with degeneration at several levels of the spine.

When Should Surgery Be Considered and What Is Involved?

In many cases, the conditions causing spinal stenosis cannot be permanently altered by nonsurgical treatment, even though these measures may relieve pain for a period of time. To determine how much nonsurgical treatment will help, a doctor may recommend such

143

treatment first. However, surgery might be considered immediately if a patient has numbness or weakness that interferes with walking, impaired bowel or bladder function, or other neurological involvement. The effectiveness of nonsurgical treatments, the extent of the patient's pain, and the patient's preferences may all factor into whether or not to have surgery.

The purpose of surgery is to relieve pressure on the spinal cord or nerves and restore and maintain alignment and strength of the spine. This can be done by removing, trimming, or adjusting diseased parts that are causing the pressure or loss of alignment. The most common surgery is called decompressive laminectomy: removal of the lamina (roof) of one or more vertebrae to create more space for the nerves. A surgeon may perform a laminectomy with or without fusing vertebrae or removing part of a disk. Various devices may be used to enhance fusion and strengthen unstable segments of the spine following decompression surgery.

Patients with spinal stenosis caused by spinal trauma or achondroplasia may need surgery at a young age. When surgery is required in patients with achondroplasia, laminectomy (removal of the roof) without fusion is usually sufficient.

What Are the Major Risks of Surgery?

All surgery, particularly that involving general anesthesia and older patients, carries risks. The most common complications of surgery for spinal stenosis are a tear in the membrane covering the spinal cord at the site of the operation, infection, or a blood clot that forms in the veins. These conditions can be treated but may prolong recovery. The presence of other diseases and the physical condition of the patient are also significant factors to consider when making decisions about surgery.

What Are Some Alternative Therapies for Spinal Stenosis?

Alternative (or complementary) therapies are diverse medical and healthcare systems, practices, and products that are not presently considered to be part of conventional medicine. Some examples of these therapies used to treat spinal stenosis follow:

- Chiropractic treatment
- Acupuncture

More research is needed before the effectiveness of these or other possible alternative therapies can be definitively stated. Healthcare providers may suggest these therapies in addition to more conventional treatments.

Chapter 12

Bone Pain

Chapter Contents

Section 12.1

Bone Cancer

This section contains text excerpted from the following
sources: Text in this section begins with excerpts from "Cancer
Pain (PDQ®)—Health Professional Version," National Cancer
Institute (NCI), May 17, 2017; Text under the heading
"Osteosarcoma" is excerpted from "Bone Cancer—Patient
Version," National Cancer Institute (NCI), May 15, 2017.

Bone pain due to metastatic disease is one of the most common causes of pain in cancer patients. Bone is highly innervated tissue with receptors sensitive to mechanical damage. The entrapment of nerve fibers in the collapsing bony matrix caused by increased osteoclastic activity and the release of inflammatory cytokines by cancer cells and immune cells are also central to the pathophysiology of bone pain. Patients typically describe the pain as continuous, deep, and throbbing, with brief episodes of more-severe pain often precipitated by movement (i.e., a type of incident pain).

Most patients will require morphine or an equivalent opioid for adequate pain relief, although incident pain is less responsive. Adjunctive agents such as nonsteroidal anti-inflammatory drugs and corticosteroids are often prescribed and appear moderately effective and safe. In addition to providing analgesia, the clinician introduces treatments designed to prevent further weakening of skeletal integrity, which may lead to loss of functional status or further pain. Bone-targeting agents such as the bisphosphonates (zoledronic acid or pamidronate) or denosumab have been demonstrated to reduce future skeletal-related events and to reduce the likelihood of increased pain or increased use of opioids in patients with advanced cancer.

Palliative radiation therapy produces complete or partial pain relief in up to 80 percent of treated patients; the median duration of relief exceeds 6 months.

Finally, orthopedic consultation is frequently necessary to determine whether operative intervention is required to prevent and/or treat pathological fractures.

Osteosarcoma

Osteosarcoma usually starts in osteoblasts, which are a type of bone cell that becomes new bone tissue. Osteosarcoma is most common in adolescents. It commonly forms in the ends of the long bones of the body, which include bones of the arms and legs. In children and adolescents, it often forms in the bones near the knee. Rarely, osteosarcoma may be found in soft tissue or organs in the chest or abdomen. Osteosarcoma is the most common type of bone cancer. Malignant fibrous histiocytoma (MFH) of bone is a rare tumor of the bone. It is treated like osteosarcoma.

Anything that increases your risk of getting a disease is called a risk factor. Having a risk factor does not mean that you will get cancer; not having risk factors doesn't mean that you will not get cancer. Talk with your child's doctor if you think your child may be at risk. Risk factors for osteosarcoma include the following:

- Past treatment with radiation therapy.

- Past treatment with anticancer drugs called alkylating agents.

- Having a certain change in the retinoblastoma gene.

- Having certain conditions, such as the following:

  - Bloom syndrome.

  - Diamond-Blackfan anemia.

  - Li-Fraumeni syndrome.

  - Paget disease.

  - Hereditary retinoblastoma.

  - Rothmund-Thomson syndrome.

  - Werner syndrome.

Signs and Symptoms of Osteosarcoma

Signs and symptoms of osteosarcoma and MFH include swelling over a bone or a bony part of the body and joint pain.

These and other signs and symptoms may be caused by osteosarcoma or MFH or by other conditions. Check with a doctor if your child has any of the following:

- Swelling over a bone or bony part of the body.

149

- Pain in a bone or joint.

- A bone that breaks for no known reason.

Diagnosis of Osteosarcoma

Imaging tests are done before the biopsy. The following tests and procedures may be used:

- Physical exam and history

- X-ray

- CT scan (CAT scan)

- MRI (magnetic resonance imaging)

A biopsy is done to diagnose osteosarcoma.

Cells and tissues are removed during a biopsy so they can be viewed under a microscope by a pathologist to check for signs of cancer. It is important that the biopsy be done by a surgeon who is an expert in treating cancer of the bone. It is best if that surgeon is also the one who removes the tumor. The biopsy and the surgery to remove the tumor are planned together. The way the biopsy is done affects which type of surgery can be done later.

The type of biopsy that is done will be based on the size of the tumor and where it is in the body. There are two types of biopsy that may be used:

- Core biopsy

- Incisional biopsy

The following test may be done on the tissue that is removed:

- Light and electron microscopy

The prognosis (chance of recovery) is affected by certain factors before and after treatment. The prognosis of untreated osteosarcoma and MFH depends on the following:

- Where the tumor is in the body and whether tumors formed in more than one bone.

- The size of the tumor.

- Whether the cancer has spread to other parts of the body and where it has spread.

- The type of tumor (based on how the cancer cells look under a microscope).
- The patient's age and weight at diagnosis.
- Whether the tumor has caused a break in the bone.
- Whether the patient has certain genetic diseases.

After osteosarcoma or MFH is treated, prognosis also depends on the following:

- How much of the cancer was killed by chemotherapy.
- How much of the tumor was taken out by surgery.
- Whether chemotherapy is delayed for more than 3 weeks after surgery takes place.
- Whether the cancer has recurred (come back) within 2 years of diagnosis.

Treatment options for osteosarcoma and MFH depend on the following:

- Where the tumor is in the body.
- The size of the tumor.
- The stage of the cancer.
- Whether the bones are still growing.
- The patient's age and general health.
- The desire of the patient and family for the patient to be able to participate in activities such as sports or have a certain appearance.
- Whether the cancer is newly diagnosed or has recurred after treatment.

Stages of Osteosarcoma

After osteosarcoma or malignant fibrous histiocytoma (MFH) has been diagnosed, tests are done to find out if cancer cells have spread to other parts of the body.

The process used to find out if cancer has spread to other parts of the body is called staging. For osteosarcoma and malignant fibrous histiocytoma (MFH), most patients are grouped according to whether cancer is found in only one part of the body or has spread.

151

The following tests and procedures may be used:

- X-ray
- CT scan (CAT scan)
- PET-CT scan
- MRI (magnetic resonance imaging)
- Bone scan

There are three ways that cancer spreads in the body.

Cancer can spread through tissue, the lymph system, and the blood.
Cancer may spread from where it began to other parts of the body.

When cancer spreads to another part of the body, it is called metastasis. Cancer cells break away from where they began (the primary tumor) and travel through the lymph system or blood.

The metastatic tumor is the same type of cancer as the primary tumor. For example, if osteosarcoma spreads to the lung, the cancer cells in the lung are actually osteosarcoma cells. The disease is metastatic osteosarcoma, not lung cancer. Many cancer deaths are caused when cancer moves from the original tumor and spreads to other tissues and organs. This is called metastatic cancer. This animation shows how cancer cells travel from the place in the body where they first formed to other parts of the body.

Osteosarcoma and MFH are described as either localized or metastatic.

Localized osteosarcoma or MFH has not spread out of the bone where the cancer started. There may be one or more areas of cancer in the bone that can be removed during surgery. Metastatic osteosarcoma or MFH has spread from the bone in which the cancer began to other parts of the body. The cancer most often spreads to the lungs. It may also spread to other bones.

Recurrent Osteosarcoma and Malignant Fibrous Histiocytoma of Bone

Recurrent osteosarcoma and malignant fibrous histiocytoma (MFH) of bone are cancers that have recurred (come back) after being treated. The cancer may come back in the bone or in other parts of the body. Osteosarcoma and MFH most often recur in the lung, bone, or both. When osteosarcoma recurs, it is usually within 18 months after treatment is completed.

Treatment of Osteosarcoma

Different types of treatment are available for children with osteosarcoma or malignant fibrous histiocytoma (MFH) of bone. Some treatments are standard (the currently used treatment), and some are being tested in clinical trials. A treatment clinical trial is a research study meant to help improve current treatments or obtain information on new treatments for patients with cancer. When clinical trials show that a new treatment is better than the standard treatment, the new treatment may become the standard treatment. Because cancer in children is rare, taking part in a clinical trial should be considered. Some clinical trials are open only to patients who have not started treatment.

Children with osteosarcoma or MFH should have their treatment planned by a team of healthcare providers who are experts in treating cancer in children.

Treatment will be overseen by a pediatric oncologist, a doctor who specializes in treating children with cancer. The pediatric oncologist works with other pediatric healthcare providers who are experts in treating osteosarcoma and MFH and who specialize in certain areas of medicine. These may include the following specialists:

- Pediatrician.

- Orthopedic surgeon.

- Radiation oncologist.

- Rehabilitation specialist.

- Pediatric nurse specialist.

- Social worker.

- Psychologist.

Treatment for osteosarcoma or malignant fibrous histiocytoma may cause side effects.

Side effects from cancer treatment that begin after treatment and continue for months or years are called late effects. Late effects of cancer treatment may include the following:

- Physical problems.

- Changes in mood, feelings, thinking, learning, or memory.

- Second cancers (new types of cancer).

153

Some late effects may be treated or controlled. It is important to talk with your child's doctors about the effects cancer treatment can have on your child.

Four types of standard treatment are used:

1. Surgery

   - Wide local excision

   - Limb-sparing surgery

   - Amputation

   - Rotationplasty

2. Chemotherapy

3. Radiation therapy

   - External radiation therapy

   - Internal radiation therapy

4. Samarium

New types of treatment are being tested in clinical trials.

Targeted therapy

Targeted therapy is a treatment that uses drugs or other substances to find and attack specific cancer cells without harming normal cells. Kinase inhibitor therapy and monoclonal antibody therapy are types of targeted therapy being studied in clinical trials for osteosarcoma. Kinase inhibitor therapy blocks a protein needed for cancer cells to divide. Sorafenib is a type of kinase inhibitor therapy being studied for the treatment of recurrent osteosarcoma.

Monoclonal antibody therapy is a cancer treatment that uses antibodies made in the laboratory, from a single type of immune system cell. These antibodies can identify substances on cancer cells or normal substances that may help cancer cells grow. The antibodies attach to the substances and kill the cancer cells, block their growth, or keep them from spreading. Monoclonal antibodies are given by infusion. They may be used alone or to carry drugs, toxins, or radioactive material directly to cancer cells. Denosumab, dinutuximab, and glembatumumab are monoclonal antibodies being studied for the treatment of recurrent osteosarcoma.

Section 12.2

Paget Disease of Bone

This section contains text excerpted from the following
sources: Text in this section begins with excerpts from
"Paget Disease of Bone," Genetics Home Reference (GHR),
National Institutes of Health (NIH), September 2015;
Text under the heading "Types of Pain" is excerpted from
"Paget's Disease of Bone," National Institute of Arthritis and
Musculoskeletal and Skin Diseases (NIAMS), May 2015.

Paget disease of bone is a disorder that causes bones to grow larger
and weaker than normal. Affected bones may be misshapen and easily
broken (fractured).

The classic form of Paget disease of bone typically appears in middle
age or later. It usually occurs in one or a few bones and does not spread
from one bone to another. Any bones can be affected, although the
disease most commonly affects bones in the spine, pelvis, skull, or legs.

Many people with classic Paget disease of bone do not experience
any symptoms associated with their bone abnormalities. The disease
is often diagnosed unexpectedly by X-rays or laboratory tests done for
other reasons. People who develop symptoms are most likely to experience pain. The affected bones may themselves be painful, or pain
may be caused by arthritis in nearby joints. Arthritis results when
the distortion of bones, particularly weight-bearing bones in the legs,
causes extra wear and tear on the joints. Arthritis most frequently
affects the knees and hips in people with this disease.

Other complications of Paget disease of bone depend on which bones
are affected. If the disease occurs in bones of the skull, it can cause an
enlarged head, hearing loss, headaches, and dizziness. If the disease
affects bones in the spine, it can lead to numbness and tingling (due
to pinched nerves) and abnormal spinal curvature. In the leg bones,
the disease can cause bowed legs and difficulty walking.

A rare type of bone cancer called osteosarcoma has been associated
with Paget disease of bone. This type of cancer probably occurs in less
than 1 in 1,000 people with this disease.

Early-onset Paget disease of bone is a less common form of the
disease that appears in a person's teens or twenties. Its features are

similar to those of the classic form of the disease, although it is more likely to affect the skull, spine, and ribs (the axial skeleton) and the small bones of the hands. The early-onset form of the disorder is also associated with hearing loss early in life.

Types of Pain

Paget disease can cause several different kinds of pain, as described below:

- **Bone pain.** Small breaks called microfractures can occur in pagetic bone. These breaks can cause pain, especially in weight-bearing bone such as the spine, pelvis, or leg.

- **Joint pain.** Cartilage (a hard but slippery tissue that cushions the joints) can be damaged when Paget disease reaches the end of a long bone or changes the shape of bones located near joints. This can result in osteoarthritis and joint pain.

- **Muscle pain.** When bone is changed by Paget disease, the muscles that support the bone may have to work harder and at different angles, causing muscle pain.

- **Nervous system pain.** Bones enlarged by Paget disease can put pressure on the brain, spinal cord, or nerves. This can cause headache; pain in the neck, back, and legs; and sciatica, a "shooting" pain that travels down the sciatic nerve from the lower back to the leg.

Available Treatments

It is important for most people with Paget disease to receive medical treatment as soon as possible. Today's treatments can help reduce pain and possibly prevent the development of further complications. Several types of medicines are used to address the pain caused by Paget disease. A doctor may recommend drugs designed to control the Paget disease or to relieve pain. The doctor also may recommend drugs to address painful complications of Paget disease, such as arthritis.

When severe pain cannot be controlled with medicine, surgery on the affected bone or joint may be needed. An appropriate program of regular exercise also can help people with Paget disease reduce or eliminate pain. Medicines used to treat Paget disease help slow the rate at which affected bone is changed, thereby reducing pain. The U.S. Food and Drug Administration (FDA) has approved several bisphosphonates and calcitonin for the treatment of Paget disease.

Several over-the-counter (nonprescription) drugs can be used to reduce the pain associated with Paget disease. Each of these medicines is taken orally (by mouth), usually in tablet form. Although there are many brand names for these drugs, they can be purchased on the basis of their key ingredient, which is:

- ibuprofen

- naproxen

- aspirin

- acetaminophen

In some cases physicians will recommend the use of pain-relieving medicine that requires a prescription.

Surgery to Manage Pain

Although surgery is rarely required for Paget disease, it should be considered in certain circumstances. Hip or knee replacement surgery may help people with severe pain from Paget disease-related arthritis. Surgery can also realign affected leg bones to reduce the stress and pain at knee and ankle joints or help broken bones heal in a better position.

The Value of Exercise

Physical exercise is an important tool for persons with Paget disease. Regular exercise can help patients:

- maintain bone strength

- avoid weight gain (and the pressure added weight puts on weakened bone)

- keep weight-bearing joints mobile and free of pain

To make sure that pagetic bone is not harmed, patients should discuss their plans with a doctor before beginning any exercise program.

There Is No Need to Be in Pain

Although there is no cure for Paget disease, people with the disorder do not have to live with constant pain. As this section describes, available therapies—especially when started early—can greatly reduce or, in some cases, eliminate the pain associated with the disease.

Section 12.3

Osteonecrosis

This section includes text excerpted from "Questions and Answers about Osteonecrosis (Avascular Necrosis)," National Institute of Arthritis and Musculoskeletal and Skin Diseases (NIAMS), October 2015.

Osteonecrosis is a disease resulting from the temporary or permanent loss of blood supply to the bones. Without blood, the bone tissue dies, and ultimately the bone may collapse. If the process involves the bones near a joint, it often leads to collapse of the joint surface. Osteonecrosis is also known as avascular necrosis, aseptic necrosis, and ischemic necrosis.

Although it can happen in any bone, osteonecrosis most commonly affects the ends (epiphysis) of the femur, the bone extending from the knee joint to the hip joint. Other sites include the upper arm bone, knees, shoulders, and ankles. The disease may affect just one bone, more than one bone at the same time, or more than one bone at different times. Osteonecrosis of the jaw (ONJ) is a rare condition that has been linked to the use of bisphosphonate medications. ONJ has different causes and treatments than osteonecrosis found in other parts of the skeleton.

The amount of disability that results from osteonecrosis depends on what part of the bone is affected, how large an area is involved, and how effectively the bone rebuilds itself. Normally, bone continuously breaks down and rebuilds—old bone is replaced with new bone. This process, which takes place after an injury as well as during normal growth, keeps the skeleton strong and helps it to maintain a balance of minerals. In the course of osteonecrosis, however, the healing process is usually ineffective and the bone tissues break down faster than the body can repair them. If left untreated, the disease progresses, the bone collapses, and the joint surface breaks down, leading to pain and arthritis.

What Causes Osteonecrosis?

Osteonecrosis is caused by impaired blood supply to the bone, but it is not always clear what causes that impairment. Osteonecrosis often occurs in people with certain medical conditions or risk factors (such as high-dose corticosteroid use or excessive alcohol intake). However, it also affects people with no health problems and for no known reason. Following are some potential causes of osteonecrosis and other health conditions associated with its development.

Steroid Medications

Aside from injury, one of the most common causes of osteonecrosis is the use of corticosteroid medications such as prednisone. Corticosteroids are commonly used to treat inflammatory diseases such as systemic lupus erythematosus (SLE), rheumatoid arthritis, inflammatory bowel disease, severe asthma, and vasculitis. Studies suggest that long-term use of oral or intravenous corticosteroids is associated with nontraumatic osteonecrosis. Patients should discuss concerns about steroid use with their doctor.

Doctors are not sure exactly why the use of corticosteroids sometimes leads to osteonecrosis. They speculate that the drugs may interfere with the body's ability to break down fatty substances called lipids. These substances then build up in and clog the blood vessels, causing them to narrow and to reduce the amount of blood that gets to the bone. Some studies suggest that corticosteroid-related osteonecrosis is more severe and more likely to affect both hips (when occurring in the hip) than osteonecrosis resulting from other causes.

Alcohol Use

Excessive alcohol use is another common cause of osteonecrosis. People who drink alcohol in excess can develop fatty substances that may block blood vessels, causing a decreased blood supply to the bones.

Injury

When a fracture, a dislocation, or some other joint injury occurs, the blood vessels may be damaged. This can interfere with the blood circulation to the bone and lead to trauma-related osteonecrosis. In fact, studies suggest that hip dislocation and hip fractures are major risk factors for osteonecrosis.

Increased pressure within the bone may be another cause of osteonecrosis. When there is too much pressure within the bone, the blood vessels narrow, making it hard for them to deliver enough blood to the bone cells. The cause of increased pressure is not fully understood.

Other Risk Factors

Other risk factors for osteonecrosis include radiation therapy, chemotherapy, and organ transplantation (particularly kidney transplantation). Osteonecrosis is also associated with a number of medical conditions, including cancer, SLE, blood disorders such as sickle cell disease, HIV infection, Gaucher disease, and Caisson disease.

Who Is Likely to Develop Osteonecrosis?

Although osteonecrosis affects both men and women, it mainly affects men. However, in cases related to SLE, the disease mostly affects women. It can occur in people of any age, from children to the elderly. However, it is more common in people in their thirties, forties, and fifties.

What Are the Symptoms?

In the early stages of osteonecrosis, people may not have any symptoms. As the disease progresses, however, most experience joint pain. At first, the pain occurs only when putting weight on the affected joint. Later, it occurs even when resting. Pain usually develops gradually, and may be mild or severe. If osteonecrosis progresses and the bone and surrounding joint surface collapse, pain may develop or increase dramatically. Pain may be severe enough to limit range of motion in the affected joint. In some cases, particularly those involving the hip, disabling osteoarthritis may develop. The period between the first symptoms and loss of joint function is different for each person, but it typically ranges from several months to more than a year.

How Is Osteonecrosis Diagnosed?

After performing a complete physical examination and asking about the patient's medical history, the doctor may use one or more bone imaging techniques to diagnose osteonecrosis. As with many other diseases, early diagnosis increases the chances of treatment success. The tests described below may be used to determine the amount of bone affected and how far the disease has progressed.

- X-Ray
- Magnetic Resonance Imaging (MRI)
- Computed/Computerized Tomography (CT scan)
- Bone Scan
- Biopsy
- Functional Evaluation of Bone

What Treatments Are Available?

Appropriate treatment for osteonecrosis is necessary to keep joints from breaking down. Without treatment, most people with the disease will experience severe pain and limitation in movement. To determine the most appropriate treatment, the doctor considers the following:

- the age of the patient
- the stage of the disease (early or late)
- the location and whether bone is affected over a small or large area
- the underlying cause of osteonecrosis; with an ongoing cause such as corticosteroid or alcohol use, treatment may not work unless use of the substance is stopped

The goal in treating osteonecrosis is to improve the patient's use of the affected joint, stop further damage to the bone, and ensure bone and joint survival. To reach these goals, the doctor may use one or more of the following surgical or nonsurgical treatments.

Nonsurgical Treatments

- Medications
- Reduced weight bearing
- Range-of-motion exercises
- Electrical stimulation

Surgical Treatment

A number of different surgical procedures are used to treat osteonecrosis. Most people with osteonecrosis will eventually need surgery.

- Core decompression

- Osteotomy

- Bone graft

- Arthroplasty/total joint replacement

For most people with osteonecrosis, treatment is an ongoing process. Depending upon the stage of the disease, doctors may first recommend the least complex or nonoperative treatment plans, such as medication or reduced weight bearing. If these modalities are unsuccessful, surgical treatments may be needed. It is important that patients carefully follow instructions about activity limitations and work closely with their doctors to ensure that appropriate treatments are used.

Chapter 13

Fibromyalgia

Fibromyalgia syndrome is a common and chronic disorder characterized by widespread pain, diffuse tenderness, and a number of other symptoms. The word "fibromyalgia" comes from the Latin term for fibrous tissue (fibro) and the Greek ones for muscle (myo) and pain (algia).

Although fibromyalgia is often considered an arthritis-related condition, it is not truly a form of arthritis (a disease of the joints) because it does not cause inflammation or damage to the joints, muscles, or other tissues. Like arthritis, however, fibromyalgia can cause significant pain and fatigue, and it can interfere with a person's ability to carry on daily activities. Also like arthritis, fibromyalgia is considered a rheumatic condition, a medical condition that impairs the joints and/ or soft tissues and causes chronic pain.

In addition to pain and fatigue, people who have fibromyalgia may experience a variety of other symptoms including:

- cognitive and memory problems (sometimes referred to as "fibro fog")

- sleep disturbances

- morning stiffness

- headaches

This chapter includes text excerpted from "Questions and Answers about Fibromyalgia," National Institute of Arthritis and Musculoskeletal and Skin Diseases (NIAMS), July 2014.

- irritable bowel syndrome
- painful menstrual periods
- numbness or tingling of the extremities
- restless legs syndrome
- temperature sensitivity
- sensitivity to loud noises or bright lights.

A person may have two or more coexisting chronic pain conditions. Such conditions can include chronic fatigue syndrome, endometriosis, fibromyalgia, inflammatory bowel disease, interstitial cystitis, temporomandibular joint dysfunction, and vulvodynia. It is not known whether these disorders share a common cause.

Who Gets Fibromyalgia?

Scientists estimate that fibromyalgia affects 5 million Americans age 18 or older. For unknown reasons, between 80 and 90 percent of those diagnosed with fibromyalgia are women; however, men and children also can be affected. Most people are diagnosed during middle age, although the symptoms often become present earlier in life.

People with certain rheumatic diseases, such as rheumatoid arthritis, systemic lupus erythematosus (commonly called lupus), or ankylosing spondylitis (spinal arthritis) may be more likely to have fibromyalgia, too.

Several studies indicate that women who have a family member with fibromyalgia are more likely to have fibromyalgia themselves, but the exact reason for this—whether it is heredity, shared environmental factors, or both—is unknown. Researchers are trying to determine whether variations in certain genes cause some people to be more sensitive to stimuli, which lead to pain syndromes.

What Causes Fibromyalgia?

The causes of fibromyalgia are unknown, but there are probably a number of factors involved. Many people associate the development of fibromyalgia with a physically or emotionally stressful or traumatic event, such as an automobile accident. Some connect it to repetitive injuries. Others link it to an illness. For others, fibromyalgia seems to occur spontaneously.

Many researchers are examining other causes, including problems with how the central nervous system (the brain and spinal cord) processes pain.

Some scientists speculate that a person's genes may regulate the way his or her body processes painful stimuli. According to this theory, people with fibromyalgia may have a gene or genes that cause them to react strongly to stimuli that most people would not perceive as painful. There have already been several genes identified that occur more commonly in fibromyalgia patients, and National Institute of Arthritis and Musculoskeletal and Skin Diseases (NIAMS)-supported researchers are currently looking at other possibilities.

How Is Fibromyalgia Diagnosed?

Research shows that people with fibromyalgia typically see many doctors before receiving the diagnosis. One reason for this may be that pain and fatigue, the main symptoms of fibromyalgia, overlap with those of many other conditions. Therefore, doctors often have to rule out other potential causes of these symptoms before making a diagnosis of fibromyalgia. Another reason is that there are currently no diagnostic laboratory tests for fibromyalgia; standard laboratory tests fail to reveal a physiologic reason for pain. Because there is no generally accepted, objective test for fibromyalgia, some doctors unfortunately may conclude a patient's pain is not real, or they may tell the patient there is little they can do.

A doctor familiar with fibromyalgia, however, can make a diagnosis based on criteria established by the American College of Rheumatology (ACR): a history of widespread pain lasting more than 3 months, and other general physical symptoms including fatigue, waking unrefreshed, and cognitive (memory or thought) problems. In making the diagnosis, doctors consider the number of areas throughout the body in which the patient has had pain in the past week.

How Is Fibromyalgia Treated?

Fibromyalgia can be difficult to treat. Not all doctors are familiar with fibromyalgia and its treatment, so it is important to find a doctor who is. Many family physicians, general internists, or rheumatologists (doctors who specialize in arthritis and other conditions that affect the joints or soft tissues) can treat fibromyalgia.

Fibromyalgia treatment often requires a team approach, with your doctor, a physical therapist, possibly other health professionals, and most importantly, yourself, all playing an active role. It can be hard to assemble this team, and you may struggle to find the right professionals to treat you. When you do, however, the combined expertise of these various professionals can help you improve your quality of life.

You may find several members of the treatment team you need at a clinic. There are pain clinics that specialize in pain and rheumatology clinics that specialize in arthritis and other rheumatic diseases, including fibromyalgia.

Only three medications, duloxetine, milnacipran, and pregabalin are approved by the U.S. Food and Drug Administration (FDA) for the treatment of fibromyalgia.[1] Duloxetine was originally developed for and is still used to treat depression. Milnacipran is similar to a drug used to treat depression but is FDA approved only for fibromyalgia. Pregaballin is a medication developed to treat neuropathic pain (chronic pain caused by damage to the nervous system).

Doctors also treat fibromyalgia with a variety of other medications developed and approved for other purposes.

Analgesics

Analgesics are painkillers. They range from over-the-counter products to prescription medicines. For a subset of people with fibromyalgia, narcotic medications are prescribed for severe muscle pain. However, there is no solid evidence showing that for most people narcotics actually work to treat the chronic pain of fibromyalgia, and most doctors hesitate to prescribe them for long-term use because of the potential that the person taking them will become physically or psychologically dependent on them.

Nonsteroidal Anti-Inflammatory Drugs (NSAIDs)

As their name implies, nonsteroidal anti-inflammatory drugs, including aspirin, ibuprofen, and naproxen sodium, are used to treat inflammation.[2] Although inflammation is not a symptom of fibromyalgia, NSAIDs also relieve pain. The drugs work by inhibiting substances in the body called prostaglandins, which play a role in pain and inflammation. These medications, some of which are available without a prescription, may help ease the muscle aches of fibromyalgia. They may also relieve menstrual cramps and the headaches often associated with fibromyalgia.

Complementary and Alternative Therapies

Many people with fibromyalgia also report varying degrees of success with complementary and alternative therapies, including massage, movement therapies (such as Pilates and the Feldenkrais method), chiropractic treatments, acupuncture, and various herbs and dietary supplements for different fibromyalgia symptoms.

Although some of these supplements are being studied for fibromyalgia, there is little, if any, scientific proof yet that they help. FDA does not regulate the sale of dietary supplements, so information about side effects, proper dosage, and the amount of a preparation's active ingredients may not be well known. If you are using or would like to try a complementary or alternative therapy, you should first speak with your doctor, who may know more about the therapy's effectiveness, as well as whether it is safe to try in combination with your medications.

[1] *All medicines can have side effects. Some medicines and side effects are mentioned in this publication. Some side effects may be more severe than others. You should review the package insert that comes with your medicine and ask your healthcare provider or pharmacist if you have any questions about the possible side effects.*

[2] *Warning: Side effects of NSAIDs include stomach problems; skin rashes; high blood pressure; fluid retention; and liver, kidney, and heart problems. The longer a person uses NSAIDs, the more likely he or she is to have side effects, ranging from mild to serious. Many other drugs cannot be taken when a patient is being treated with NSAIDs, because NSAIDs alter the way the body uses or eliminates these other drugs. Check with your healthcare provider or pharmacist before you take NSAIDs. NSAIDs should only be used at the lowest dose possible for the shortest time needed.*

Will Fibromyalgia Get Better with Time?

Fibromyalgia is a chronic condition, meaning it lasts a long time — possibly a lifetime. However, it may be comforting to know that fibromyalgia is not a progressive disease. It is never fatal, and it will not cause damage to the joints, muscles, or internal organs. In many people, the condition does improve over time.

What Can I Do to Try to Feel Better?

Besides taking medicine prescribed by your doctor, there are many things you can do to minimize the impact of fibromyalgia on your life. These include:

- Getting enough sleep
- Exercising
- Making changes at work
- Eating well

  Tips for good sleep:
- Keep regular sleep habits
- Avoid caffeine and alcohol in the late afternoon and evening
- Time your exercise
- Avoid daytime naps
- Reserve your bed for sleeping
- Keep your bedroom dark, quiet, and cool
- Avoid liquids and spicy meals before bed
- Wind down before bed

Chapter 14

Knees and Their Problems

Chapter Contents

Section 14.1

Knee Basics

This section includes text excerpted from "Questions and Answers about Knee Problems," National Institute of Arthritis and Musculoskeletal and Skin Diseases (NIAMS), March 2016.

What Do the Knees Do? How Do They Work?

The knee is the joint where the bones of the upper leg meet the bones of the lower leg, allowing hinge-like movement while providing stability and strength to support the weight of the body. Flexibility, strength, and stability are needed for standing and for motions like walking, running, crouching, jumping, and turning.

Several kinds of supporting and moving parts, including bones, cartilage, muscles, ligaments, and tendons, help the knees do their job. Each of these structures is subject to disease and injury. When a knee problem affects your ability to do things, it can have a big impact on your life. Knee problems can interfere with many things, from participation in sports to simply getting up from a chair and walking.

Joint Basics

The point at which two or more bones are connected is called a joint. In all joints, the bones are kept from grinding against each other by a lining called cartilage. Bones are joined to bones by strong, elastic bands of tissue called ligaments. Muscles are connected to bones by tough cords of tissue called tendons. Muscles pull on tendons to move joints. Although muscles are not technically part of a joint, they're important because strong muscles help support and protect joints.

What Are the Parts of the Knee?

Like any joint, the knee is composed of bones and cartilage, ligaments, tendons, and muscles. Take a closer look at the different parts of the knee in the illustration below.

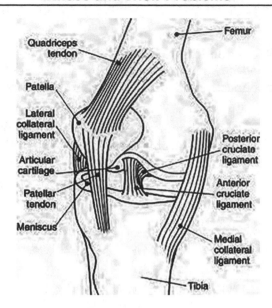

Figure 14.1. *Lateral View of the Knee*

Bones and Cartilage

The knee joint is the junction of three bones: the femur (thigh bone or upper leg bone), the tibia (shin bone or larger bone of the lower leg), and the patella (kneecap). The patella is 2 to 3 inches wide and 3 to 4 inches long. It sits over the other bones at the front of the knee joint and slides when the knee moves. It protects the knee and gives leverage to muscles.

The ends of the three bones in the knee joint are covered with articular cartilage, a tough, elastic material that helps absorb shock and allows the knee joint to move smoothly. Separating the bones of the knee are pads of connective tissue called menisci. The menisci are two crescent-shaped discs, each called a meniscus, positioned between the tibia and femur on the outer and inner sides of each knee. The two menisci in each knee act as shock absorbers, cushioning the lower part of the leg from the weight of the rest of the body as well as enhancing stability.

Muscles

There are two groups of muscles at the knee. The four quadriceps muscles on the front of the thigh work to straighten the knee from a bent position. The hamstring muscles, which run along the back of the thigh from the hip to just below the knee, help to bend the knee.

171

Tendons and Ligaments

The quadriceps tendon connects the quadriceps muscle to the patella and provides the power to straighten the knee. The following four ligaments connect the femur and tibia and give the joint strength and stability:

- The medial collateral ligament, which runs along the inside of the knee joint, provides stability to the inner (medial) part of the knee.

- The lateral collateral ligament, which runs along the outside of the knee joint, provides stability to the outer (lateral) part of the knee.

- The anterior cruciate ligament, in the center of the knee, limits rotation and the forward movement of the tibia.

- The posterior cruciate ligament, also in the center of the knee, limits backward movement of the tibia.

The knee capsule is a protective, fiber-like structure that wraps around the knee joint. Inside the capsule, the joint is lined with a thin, soft tissue called synovium.

What Causes Knee Problems?

Knee problems can be the result of disease or injury.

Disease

A number of diseases can affect the knee. The most common is arthritis. Although arthritis technically means "joint inflammation," the term is used loosely to describe many different diseases that can affect the joints. Some of the most common forms of arthritis and their effects on the knees are described a bit later in this section.

Injury

Knee injuries can occur as the result of a direct blow or sudden movements that strain the knee beyond its normal range of motion. Sometimes knees are injured slowly over time. Problems with the hips or feet, for example, can cause you to walk awkwardly, which throw off the alignment of the knees and leads to damage. Knee problems can also be the result of a lifetime of normal wear and tear. Much like the treads on a tire, the joint simply wears out over time. This section discusses some of the most common knee injuries, but first describes the structure of the knee joint.

How Are Knee Problems Diagnosed?

Doctors diagnose knee problems based on the findings of a medical history, physical exam, and diagnostic tests.

- Medical History
- Physical Examination
- Diagnostic Tests
  - X-ray (radiography)
  - Computerized axial tomography (CT) scan
  - Ultrasound
  - Magnetic resonance imaging (MRI)
  - Arthroscopy
  - Joint aspiration
  - Biopsy

What Kinds of Doctors Evaluate and Treat Knee Problems?

After an examination by your primary care doctor, he or she may refer you to a rheumatologist, an orthopaedic surgeon, or both.

You may also be referred to a physiatrist. Minor injuries or arthritis may be treated by an internist or your primary care doctor.

About Total Knee Replacement

Joint replacement is becoming more common, and hips and knees are the most commonly replaced joints. The new joint, called a prosthesis, can be made of plastic, metal, or ceramic materials. It may be cemented into place or uncemented. An uncemented prosthesis is designed so that bones will grow into it.

First made available in the late 1950s, early total knee replacements did a poor job of mimicking the natural motion of the knee. For that reason, these procedures resulted in high failure and complication rates. Advances in total knee replacement technology in the past several years have enhanced the design and fit of knee implants.

Total knee replacement may be indicated when X-rays and other tests show joint damage; when moderate-to-severe, persistent pain does not improve adequately with nonsurgical treatment; and when the limited range of motion in their knee joint diminishes their quality of life.

Most patients appear to experience rapid and substantial reduction in pain, feel better in general, and enjoy improved joint function. Although most total knee replacement surgeries are successful, failure does occur and revision is sometimes necessary.

How Can People Prevent Knee Problems?

Some knee problems, such as those resulting from an accident, cannot be foreseen or prevented. However, people can prevent many knee problems by following these suggestions:

- Before exercising or participating in sports, warm up by walking or riding a stationary bicycle, then do stretches. Stretching the muscles in the front of the thigh (quadriceps) and back of the thigh (hamstrings) reduces tension on the tendons and relieves pressure on the knee during activity.

- Strengthen the leg muscles by doing specific exercises (for example, by walking up stairs or hills or by riding a stationary bicycle). A supervised workout with weights is another way to strengthen the leg muscles that support the knee.

- Avoid sudden changes in the intensity of exercise. Increase the force or duration of activity gradually.

- Wear shoes that fit properly and are in good condition. This will help maintain balance and leg alignment when walking or running. Flat feet or overpronated feet (feet that roll inward) can cause knee problems. People can often reduce some of these problems by wearing special shoe inserts (orthotics).

- Maintain a healthy weight to reduce stress on the knee. Obesity increases the risk of osteoarthritis of the knee.

What Types of Exercise Are Best for People with Knee Problems?

Ideally, everyone should get three types of exercise regularly:

- **Range-of-motion exercises** to help maintain normal joint movement and relieve stiffness.

- **Strengthening exercises** to help keep or increase muscle strength. Keeping muscles strong with exercises, such as walking up stairs, doing leg lifts or dips, or riding a stationary bicycle, helps support and protect the knee.

- **Aerobic or endurance exercises** to improve function of the heart and circulation and to help control weight. Weight control can be important to people who have arthritis because extra weight puts pressure on many joints. Some studies show that aerobic exercise can reduce inflammation in some joints.

If you already have knee problems, your doctor or physical therapist can help with a plan of exercise that will help the knee(s) without increasing the risk of injury or further damage. As a general rule, you should choose gentle exercises such as swimming, aquatic exercise, or walking rather than jarring exercises such as jogging or high-impact aerobics.

Section 14.2

Common Knee Problems

This section includes text excerpted from "Questions and Answers about Knee Problems," National Institute of Arthritis and Musculoskeletal and Skin Diseases (NIAMS), March 2016.

There are many diseases and types of injuries that can affect the knee. These are some of the most common, along with their diagnoses and treatment.

Arthritis

There are some 100 different forms of arthritis, rheumatic diseases, and related conditions. Virtually all of them have the potential to affect the knees in some way; however, the following are the most common.

- Osteoarthritis
- Rheumatoid arthritis

- Other rheumatic diseases
  - Gout
  - Systemic lupus erythematosus (lupus)
  - Ankylosing spondylitis
  - Psoriatic arthritis
  - Reactive arthritis

Symptoms

The symptoms are different for the different forms of arthritis. For example, people with rheumatoid arthritis, gout, or other inflammatory conditions may find the knee swollen, red, and even hot to the touch. Any form of arthritis can cause the knee to be painful and stiff.

Diagnosis

The doctor may confirm the diagnosis by conducting a careful history and physical examination. Blood tests may be helpful for diagnosing rheumatoid arthritis, but other tests may also be needed. Analyzing fluid from the knee joint, for example, may be helpful in diagnosing gout. X-rays may be taken to determine loss or damage to cartilage or bone.

Treatment

Like the symptoms, treatment varies depending on the form of arthritis affecting the knee. For osteoarthritis, treatment is targeted at relieving symptoms and may include pain-reducing medicines such as aspirin or acetaminophen; nonsteroidal anti-inflammatory drugs (NSAIDs) such as ibuprofen; or, in some cases, injections of corticosteroid medications directly into the knee joint.

People with diseases such as rheumatoid arthritis, ankylosing spondylitis, or psoriatic arthritis often require disease-modifying antirheumatic drugs (DMARDs) or biologic response modifiers (biologics) to control the underlying disease that is the source of their knee problems. These drugs are typically prescribed after less potent treatments, such as NSAIDs or intra-articular injections, are deemed ineffective. People with any type of arthritis may benefit from exercises to strengthen the muscles that support the knee and from weight loss, if needed, to relieve excess stress on the joints. If arthritis causes serious damage to a knee or there is incapacitating pain or loss of use of the knee from arthritis, joint surgery may be considered. Traditionally, this has been done with what is known as a total knee replacement. However, newer surgical procedures are continuously being developed that include resurfacing or replacing only the damaged cartilage surfaces while leaving the rest of the joint intact.

Chondromalacia

Chondromalacia, also called chondromalacia patellae, refers to softening and breakdown of the articular cartilage of the kneecap. This disorder occurs most often in young adults and can be caused by injury, overuse, misalignment of the patella, or muscle weakness. Instead of gliding smoothly across the lower end of the thigh bone, the kneecap rubs against it, thereby roughening the cartilage underneath the kneecap. The damage may range from a slightly abnormal surface of the cartilage to a surface that has been worn away to the bone. Chondromalacia related to injury occurs when a blow to the kneecap tears off either a small piece of cartilage or a large fragment containing a piece of bone (osteochondral fracture).

Symptoms

The most frequent symptom of chondromalacia is a dull pain around or under the kneecap that worsens when walking down stairs or hills. A person may also feel pain when climbing stairs or when the knee bears weight as it straightens. The disorder is common in runners and is also seen in skiers, cyclists, and soccer players.

Diagnosis

Your description of symptoms and an X-ray or MRI usually help the doctor make a diagnosis. Although arthroscopy can confirm the diagnosis, it's not performed unless conservative treatment has failed.

Treatment

Many doctors recommend that people with chondromalacia perform low-impact exercises that strengthen muscles, particularly muscles of the inner part of the quadriceps, without injuring joints. Swimming, riding a stationary bicycle, and using a cross-country ski machine are examples of good exercises for this condition. If these treatments don't improve the condition, surgery may be indicated.

Meniscal Injuries (Injuries to the Menisci)

The menisci can be easily injured by the force of rotating the knee while bearing weight. A partial or total tear may occur when a person quickly twists or rotates the upper leg while the foot stays still (for example, when dribbling a basketball around an opponent or turning to hit a tennis ball). If the tear is tiny, the meniscus stays connected to the front and back of the knee; if the tear is large, the meniscus may be left hanging by a thread of cartilage. The seriousness of a tear depends on its location and extent.

Symptoms

Generally, when people injure a meniscus, they feel some pain, particularly when the knee is straightened. If the pain is mild, the person may continue moving. Severe pain may occur if a fragment of the meniscus catches between the femur and the tibia. Swelling may occur soon after injury if there is damage to blood vessels. Swelling may also occur several hours later if there is inflammation of the joint lining (synovium). Sometimes, an injury that occurred in the past but was not treated becomes painful months or years later, particularly if the knee is injured a second time. After any injury, the knee may click, lock, feel weak, or give way. Although symptoms of meniscal injury may disappear on their own, they frequently persist or return and require treatment.

Diagnosis

In addition to listening to your description of the onset of pain and swelling, the doctor may perform a physical examination and request X-rays or an ultrasound of the knee. An MRI may be recommended to confirm the diagnosis. Occasionally, the doctor may use arthroscopy to help diagnose a meniscal tear.

Treatment

If the tear is minor and the pain and other symptoms go away, the doctor may recommend a muscle-strengthening program. The following exercises are designed to build up the quadriceps and hamstring muscles and increase flexibility and strength after injury to the meniscus:

- Warming up the joint by riding a stationary bicycle, then straightening and raising the leg (but not straightening it too much).

- Extending the leg while sitting (a weight may be worn on the ankle for this exercise).

- Raising the leg while lying on the stomach.

- Exercising in a pool (walking as fast as possible in chest-deep water, performing small flutter kicks while holding onto the side of the pool, and raising each leg to 90 degrees in chest-deep water while pressing the back against the side of the pool).

Before beginning any type of exercise program, consult your doctor or physical therapist to learn which exercises are appropriate for you and how to do them correctly, because doing the wrong exercise or exercising improperly can cause problems. A healthcare professional can also advise you on how to warm up safely and when to avoid exercising a joint affected by arthritis. If your lifestyle is limited by the symptoms or the problem, surgery may be indicated.

Cruciate Ligament Injuries

Cruciate ligament injuries are sometimes referred to as sprains. They don't necessarily cause pain, but they are disabling. The anterior cruciate ligament is most often stretched or torn (or both) by a sudden twisting motion (for example, when the feet are planted one way and the knees are turned another). The posterior cruciate ligament is most often injured by a direct impact, such as in an automobile accident or football tackle.

Symptoms

You may hear a popping sound, and the leg may buckle when you try to stand on it.

Diagnosis

The doctor may perform several tests to see whether the parts of the knee stay in proper position when pressure is applied in different directions. A thorough examination is essential. An MRI is accurate in detecting a complete tear, but arthroscopy may be the only reliable means of detecting a partial one.

Treatment

For an incomplete tear, the doctor may recommend an exercise program to strengthen surrounding muscles. He or she may also prescribe a brace to protect the knee during activity. For a completely torn anterior cruciate ligament in an active athlete and motivated person, the doctor is likely to recommend surgery.

Medial and Lateral Collateral Ligament Injuries

The medial collateral ligament is more easily injured than the lateral collateral ligament. The cause of collateral ligament injuries is most often a blow to the outer side of the knee that stretches and tears the ligament on the inner side of the knee. Such blows frequently occur in contact sports such as football or hockey.

Symptoms

When injury to the medial collateral ligament occurs, you may feel a pop and the knee may buckle sideways. Pain and swelling are common.

Diagnosis

A thorough examination is needed to determine the type and extent of the injury. In diagnosing a collateral ligament injury, the doctor exerts pressure on the side of the knee to determine the degree of pain and the looseness of the joint. An MRI is helpful in diagnosing injuries to these ligaments.

Treatment

Most sprains of the collateral ligaments will heal if you follow a prescribed exercise program. In addition to exercise, the doctor may recommend ice packs to reduce pain and swelling, and a small sleeve-type brace to protect and stabilize the knee. A sprain may take 2 to 4 weeks to heal. A severely sprained or torn collateral ligament may be accompanied by a torn anterior cruciate ligament, which usually requires surgical repair.

Tendon Injuries

Knee tendon injuries range from tendinitis (inflammation of a tendon) to a ruptured (torn) tendon. If a person overuses a tendon during certain activities such as dancing, cycling, or running, the tendon stretches and becomes inflamed. Tendinitis of the patellar tendon is sometimes called "jumper's knee" because in sports that require jumping, such as basketball, the muscle contraction and force of hitting the ground after a jump strain the tendon. After repeated stress, the tendon may become inflamed or tear.

Symptoms

People with tendinitis often have tenderness at the point where the patellar tendon meets the bone. In addition, they may feel pain during running, hurried walking, or jumping. A complete rupture of the quadriceps or patellar tendon is not only painful, but also makes it difficult for a person to bend, extend, or lift the leg against gravity.

Diagnosis

If there is not much swelling, the doctor will be able to feel a defect in the tendon near the tear during a physical examination. An X-ray will show that the patella is lower than normal in a quadriceps tendon tear and higher than normal in a patellar tendon tear. The doctor may use an ultrasound or MRI to confirm a partial or total tear.

Treatment

Initially, the treatment for tendinitis involves rest, elevating the knee, applying ice, and taking NSAID medications such as aspirin or ibuprofen to relieve pain and decrease inflammation and swelling. A series of rehabilitation exercises is also useful. If the quadriceps or patellar tendon is completely ruptured, a surgeon will reattach the ends.

Rehabilitating a partial or complete tear of a tendon requires an exercise program that is similar to but less vigorous than that prescribed for ligament injuries. The goals of exercise are to restore the ability to bend and straighten the knee and to strengthen the leg to prevent repeat injury.

Osgood-Schlatter Disease

Osgood-Schlatter disease is a condition caused by repetitive stress or tension on part of the growth area of the upper tibia (the apophysis). It is characterized by inflammation of the patellar tendon and surrounding soft tissues at the point where the tendon attaches to the tibia. The disease may also be associated with an injury in which the tendon is stretched so much that it tears away from the tibia and takes a fragment of bone with it. The disease most commonly affects active young people, particularly boys between the ages of 10 and 15, who play games or sports that include frequent running and jumping.

Symptoms

People with this disease experience pain just below the knee joint that usually worsens with activity and is relieved by rest. A bony bump that is particularly painful when pressed may appear on the upper edge of the tibia (below the kneecap). Usually, the motion of the knee is not affected. Pain may last a few months and may recur until the child's growth is completed.

Diagnosis

Osgood-Schlatter disease is most often diagnosed by the symptoms. An X-ray may be normal, or show an injury, or, more typically, show that the growth area is in fragments.

Treatment

Osgood-Schlatter disease is temporary and the pain usually goes away without treatment. Applying ice to the knee when pain begins helps relieve inflammation and is sometimes used along with stretching and strengthening exercises. The doctor may advise you to limit participation in vigorous sports. Children who wish to continue moderate or less stressful sports activities may need to wear knee pads for protection and apply ice to the knee after activity. If there is a great deal of pain, sports activities may be limited until the discomfort becomes tolerable.

Iliotibial Band Syndrome

Iliotibial band syndrome is an inflammatory condition caused when a band of tissue rubs over the outer bone (lateral condyle) of the knee. Although iliotibial band syndrome may be caused by direct injury to the knee, it is most often caused by the stress of long-term overuse, such as sometimes occurs in sports training and, particularly, in running.

Symptoms

A person with this syndrome feels an ache or burning sensation at the side of the knee during activity. Pain may be localized at the side of the knee or radiate up the side of the thigh. A person may also feel a snap when the knee is bent and then straightened. Swelling is usually absent, and knee motion is normal.

Diagnosis

The diagnosis of this disorder is typically based on the symptoms, such as pain at the outer bone, and exclusion of other conditions with similar symptoms.

Treatment

Usually, iliotibial band syndrome disappears if the person reduces activity and performs stretching exercises followed by muscle-strengthening exercises. In rare cases when the syndrome doesn't disappear, surgery may be necessary to split the tendon so it isn't stretched too tightly over the bone.

Osteochondritis Dissecans

Osteochondritis dissecans results from a loss of the blood supply to an area of bone underneath a joint surface. It usually involves the knee. The affected bone and its covering of cartilage gradually loosen and cause pain. This problem usually arises spontaneously in an active adolescent or young adult. It may be caused by a slight blockage of a small artery or to an unrecognized injury or tiny fracture that damages the overlying cartilage. A person with this condition may eventually develop osteoarthritis. Lack of a blood supply can cause bone to break down (osteonecrosis). The involvement of several joints or the appearance of osteochondritis dissecans in several family members may indicate that the disorder is inherited.

Symptoms

If normal healing doesn't occur, cartilage separates from the diseased bone and a fragment breaks loose into the knee joint, causing weakness, sharp pain, and locking of the joint.

Diagnosis

An X-ray, MRI, or arthroscopy can determine the condition of the cartilage and can be used to diagnose osteochondritis dissecans.

Treatment

In most cases, healing occurs after a period of rest and limited activity. Physical therapy can be beneficial. When conservative measures do not help or cartilage fragments are loose, surgery may be indicated.

Plica Syndrome

Plica syndrome occurs when plicae (bands of synovial tissue) are irritated by overuse or injury. Synovial plicae are the remains of tissue pouches found in the early stages of fetal development. As the fetus develops, these pouches normally combine to form one large synovial cavity. If this process is incomplete, plicae remain as four folds or bands of synovial tissue within the knee. Injury, chronic overuse, or inflammatory conditions are associated with this syndrome.

Symptoms

Symptoms of plica syndrome include pain and swelling, a clicking sensation, and locking and weakness of the knee.

Diagnosis

Because the symptoms are similar to those of some other knee problems, plica syndrome is often misdiagnosed. Diagnosis usually depends on excluding other conditions that cause similar symptoms.

Treatment

The goal of treatment for plica syndrome is to reduce inflammation of the synovium and thickening of the plicae. The doctor usually prescribes medicine to reduce inflammation. People are also advised to reduce activity, apply ice and an elastic bandage to the knee, and do strengthening exercises. If treatment fails to relieve symptoms, the doctor may recommend arthroscopic or open surgery to remove the plicae.

Chapter 15

Muscle Pain

Chapter Contents

Section 15.1

Chronic Myofascial Pain

Chronic myofascial pain (CMP), also known as myofascial pain syndrome (MPS), is a chronic, painful condition that affects the muscles, in particular the covering layer of the muscle, known as the fascia. When repetitive or excessive stress is placed on a muscle, it can create sensitive areas called myofascial trigger points (MTrPs) that can cause pain throughout the muscle. These trigger points can also cause pain in unrelated parts of the body, a phenomena called "referred pain."

Myofacial pain is dull, aching, and deep. Along with pain, individuals may experience sleep problems as well as decreased muscle flexibility and strength. The trigger point may be active (consistently painful) or latent (pain and tenderness only when touched).

Possible Causes of Trigger Points

Although what causes trigger points is not completely understood, potential contributing factors include:

- Poorly conditioned muscles
- Chronic overload of muscles associated with repetitive movements
- Poor ergonomics and postural stress such as sitting for prolonged duration of time
- A difference in length between the patient's legs
- Lifting or moving objects without using proper techniques
- Increased muscle tension due to anxiety or depression
- Fatigue, trauma, and cold weather

Diagnosing CMP

Healthcare providers diagnose CMP by completing a physical examination of the painful areas and collecting a detailed history from the patient. During the examination, the doctors may apply gentle pressure in a certain way to the trigger points to check for a referred pattern of pain or a muscle twitch. They will also feel for the texture of the muscle fibers and do tests to determine the strength and flexibility of the muscles.

CMP is common in people between the ages of 30 and 60, affecting both men and women equally. Recent research has identified myofascial trigger points as a contributing factor in chronic headaches, tension type headaches, neck pain, and shoulder disorders.

Managing Myofascial Pain Syndrome

Treatment consists of 3 main components:

1. Reducing the chronic overload of the muscles. Identify the factors and correct it.

2. Eliminate the trigger point. There are several methods used to do this.

3. Strengthen the affected group of muscles.

Treatment Options for Chronic Myofascial Pain

Medications

- Pain relievers—Over-the-counter pain relievers, including ibuprofen (Advil, Motrin IB, others) and naproxen sodium (Aleve), may relieve pain.

- Antidepressants—Can reduce pain and improve sleep.

- Sedatives—Can help to relax muscles; however, they should be used under a doctor's supervision since they can be addictive

Physical Therapy

A physical therapist may treat chronic myofascial pain using one or more of the following methods:

- Stretching exercises—loosens tight muscles and releases trigger points

- Strengthening exercises—builds up muscle strength and prevents early muscle fatigue

- Massage therapy—helps muscles relax and prevents spasms or cramps.

- Hot packs or hot shower

- Ultrasound—Uses high frequency sound waves to promote healing in the muscle tissue and helps release triggers.

Needle Procedures

There are 2 types of needle procedures:

- Wet needling. Therapeutic practice in which a numbing agent or steroid is injected by needle into the trigger point to relieve the pain.

- Dry needling. Involves inserting an acupuncture needle into the trigger point. This results in a reduction of substances that interact with nearby nociceptors (the parts of nerves that sense pain) and ultimately provides pain relief.

Self-Care Measures

Along with the treatment, patients can employ a variety of measures that can prevent recurrence and aid in better treatment outcomes:

- Exercise: Regular exercise and an active lifestyle can help patients cope with pain

- Relaxation: Various relaxation methods can help reduce tension and stress. Deep breathing exercises, listening to soothing music, mediation, and talking with friends can help.

- Taking time for yourself: Taking care of yourself by eating healthy and getting enough sleep will help relieve pain and the associated stress

- Support group: Talking to a counselor or joining a support group can help patients cope with pain

References

1. "Chronic Myofascial Pain (CMP)," Cleveland Clinic, March 1, 2013.

2. "Dry needling," Physiopedia, n.d.

3. "Myofascial pain syndrome," MayoClinic, December 9, 2014.

Section 15.2

Delayed Onset Muscle Soreness

This section contains text excerpted from the following sources:
Text in this section begins with excerpts from "Physical Activity and
Your Heart," National, Heart, Lung and Blood Institute (NHLBI),
June 22, 2016; Text under the heading "What Is Delayed Onset
Muscle Soreness (DOMS)?" is excerpted from "The Effects of High
Dose Fish Oil Supplementation on Delayed Onset Muscle Soreness
and Inflammatory Markers," Clinicaltrials.gov, National Institutes of
Health (NIH), December 9, 2008. Reviewed June 2017; Text under the
heading "DOMS: Symptoms and Treatment" is excerpted from "Fitness
Work and Capacity," National Wildfire Coordinating Group (NWCG),
December 2009. Reviewed June 2017; Text under the heading "Prevent
Muscle Soreness" is excerpted from "Why Warm Up, Cool Down and
Stretch?" U.S. Department of Veterans Affairs (VA), March 16, 2014.

According to the U.S. Department of Health and Human Services'
Physical Activity Guidelines for Americans physical activity generally
refers to movement that enhances health. Exercise is a type of physical
activity that's planned and structured. Lifting weights, taking an aerobics class, and playing on a sports team are examples of exercise. The
four main types of physical activity are aerobic, muscle-strengthening,
bone-strengthening, and stretching.

Aerobic Activity

Aerobic activity moves your large muscles, such as those in your
arms and legs. Running, swimming, walking, bicycling, dancing, and
doing jumping jacks are examples of aerobic activity. Aerobic activity
is also called endurance activity. Aerobic activity makes your heart
beat faster than usual. You also breathe harder during this type of
activity. Over time, regular aerobic activity makes your heart and
lungs stronger and able to work better.

Other Types of Physical Activity

The other types of physical activity—muscle-strengthening, bone
strengthening, and stretching—benefit your body in other ways.

Muscle-strengthening activities improve the strength, power, and endurance of your muscles. Doing pushups and situps, lifting weights, climbing stairs, and digging in the garden are examples of muscle-strengthening activities.

With bone-strengthening activities, your feet, legs, or arms support your body's weight, and your muscles push against your bones. This helps make your bones strong. Running, walking, jumping rope, and lifting weights are examples of bone-strengthening activities.

Muscle-strengthening and bone-strengthening activities also can be aerobic, depending on whether they make your heart and lungs work harder than usual. For example, running is both an aerobic activity and a bone-strengthening activity.

Stretching helps improve your flexibility and your ability to fully move your joints. Touching your toes, doing side stretches, and doing yoga exercises are examples of stretching.

What Is Delayed Onset Muscle Soreness (DOMS)?

DOMS is associated with the eccentric phase of exercise, where the muscle is actively creating force while lengthening. The onset of muscle soreness is part of an inflammatory response due to the muscular damage caused by the exercise. Research has shown that fish oils have anti-inflammatory properties. Direct intake of various polyunsaturated fatty acids (PUFA) alters the cell membrane fatty acid composition, which, in turn modulates cell/tissue response to infection, injury and inflammatory events. These properties may be beneficial to relieve muscle soreness.

DOMS: Symptoms and Treatment

The delayed onset muscle soreness that begins about 24 hours after your first exposure to vigorous effort may be due to microscopic tears in the muscle membrane or tissue. The soreness peaks several days after the first day of activity, then diminishes slowly. It can reduce strength and influence performance for 1 or 2 weeks. It is accompanied by swelling and leakage of enzymes from the muscle, but not by the accumulation of lactic acid, which is gone within an hour of exercise. Soreness can be minimized with a gradual transition to weightlifting, starting with light weights. Static stretching of the affected muscles and the use of an anti-inflammatory drug can help relieve soreness. Soreness only occurs when you begin a new activity, but it may reoccur if you lay off for many weeks or do lifts with new muscle groups.

Prevent Muscle Soreness

You can help prevent injury and reduce muscle soreness if you warm up before and cool down after physical activity. Warming-up prepares your muscles and heart for activity. Cooling-down slows your heart rate gradually and helps prepare your muscles for the next time you're active.

Warm-ups take 5 to 15 minutes.

1. Do your planned activity, such as walking, but at a lower intensity (slower pace) for a brief time. This may mean walking slowly for a few minutes before speeding up.

2. Do a few minutes of gentle stretching if you plan to do something more vigorous than walking.

Cool-downs take 5 to 15 minutes.

1. To cool down, continue your activity, but slow down the pace for a brief time to slow your heart rate.

2. Stretch all major muscle groups used during the activity. Stretching the muscles while they are warm will help increase flexibility.

Stretch: Stretching is important for a good warm-up and cool-down and is one of the best ways to prevent and avoid muscle soreness, cramps, and injury.

Here are some helpful tips for proper stretching:

- Do a short warm-up before stretching, such as walking or marching in place. Stretching is more beneficial when your muscles are warm.

- Stretch in both directions (i.e., if you stretch to the left, don't forget to stretch to the right).

- Avoid fast, jerky movements. Stretch slowly and smoothly.

- Stretches should not be painful. Gentle stretching is best. When you repeat the stretch, you should be able to stretch a little further without pain.

- Hold each stretch for 15-60 seconds. Do not bounce.

- Repeat each stretch 4 or more times.

- Breathe slowly in and out. Do not hold your breath.

- Relax, enjoy, and feel good about yourself.
- Stretch often, if possible every day

Section 15.3

Muscle Cramps

"Muscle Cramps," © 2017 Omnigraphics.
Reviewed June 2017.

Overview

Our body muscles regularly contract and relax to produce movement. However, when a muscle suddenly contracts involuntarily and does not relax, what you are experiencing is a spasm. Spasm is an inbuilt protective mechanism that happens normally when an injury occurs. But when a spasm happens suddenly for no reason, it is considered a muscle cramp. The muscle will tighten and remain contracted for a few seconds to minutes before relaxing again. While painful and debilitating when they occur, muscle cramps are harmless.

Muscle cramps are extremely common. Researchers estimate that at least 95 percent of individuals have experienced cramps at some point in their lives. Research has also indicated that episodes of cramping increases with aging.

Muscle cramps commonly occur in the following groups of muscles:

- Muscles at the back of your lower leg or calf (gastrocnemius). Commonly called a "charley horse."

- Muscles at the back of thigh (hamstrings)

- Muscles at the front of thigh (quadriceps)

Some people also experience cramps in feet, arms, abdomen, and ribs occasionally.

Types and Causes of Muscle Cramps

Muscle cramps are classified into 3 types based on their cause:

1. True cramps

True cramp is the common skeletal muscle cramp, and can involve a part or all of a single muscle or group of muscles. Studies have shown that true cramps happen when associated nerves become overstimulated and result in involuntary muscle contractions. True cramps can occur under the following circumstances:

- Injury—When the muscle contracts as an involuntary protective mechanism resulting from injury. This is a normal physiological reaction: the spasm minimizes movement and protects the injured body part.

- High intensity activity—True cramps may result when muscles are fatigued due to a vigorous or strenuous activity such as participating in sports or taking part in an unaccustomed activity.

- Rest cramps—Called a nocturnal cramp, this type of muscle cramp is commonly seen in older adults and usually happens in the night, disrupting an individual's sleep. Though the actual cause of a rest cramp is unknown, it has been noted that when a movement shortening the length of a muscle is initiated (like in pointing the toe down, which shortens the calf muscle), a rest cramp is stimulated.

- Dehydration—Endurance athletes who do not replace fluids lost through perspiration, especially those in warm climates, can suffer from muscle cramps. Depletion of body fluids from diuretics and poor fluid intake can also lead to dehydration-induced cramps in older adults. Loss of sodium in body fluids is also associated with cramps.

- Low blood calcium or magnesium—In some pregnant women, low levels of calcium and magnesium can result in muscle cramps.

2. Tetany

Tetany, or tetanic cramping, occurs when the all nerve cells in the body are stimulated and all muscles contract. Tetany is normally associated with chronic depletion of blood calcium and magnesium. Sometimes the muscle contraction is accompanied by numbness and a tingling sensation around the mouth and other areas.

3. Dystonic cramps

A less common type of muscle cramp, dystonia is a type of movement disorder in which an individual's muscles contract uncontrollably.

Muscles not required for a particular movement or activity start contracting involuntarily, disrupting the desired movement. Dystonia is commonly seen in smaller muscles of the body like eyelids, fingers, toes, jaw, neck, and larynx. Individuals who engage in repetitive activities, such as typing or playing a musical instrument, are more likely to suffer from this sort of muscle cramp.

Diagnosis

The doctor will collect a detailed history and perform a physical examination of the muscle or muscle groups that are involved. He or she may prescribe a routine blood test to rule out any other problems.

Treatment

Most muscle cramps, particularly true cramps, go away without any intervention and, if needed, can be treated with home care measures and remedies. Stop any physical activity when you get a cramp. Do gentle stretches and massage the affected muscle. For example, in the case of a calf cramp, stand facing a wall few feet away and lean in to the wall, keeping the knees and back straight with the heels in full contact with the floor. Also, in a lying position, you can put a towel around your feet and pull the towel towards you, keeping the knee straight. Hot packs can also be applied to relax the muscles.

Also, make sure you are well hydrated, especially when you are doing sports or vigorous activity and replenish electrolytes if needed. For severe, repetitive cramps that disrupt sleep, doctors may prescribe medications such as muscle relaxants.

References

1. Shiel Jr., William C., MD, FACP, FACR. "Muscle Cramps," eMedicineHealth, July 26, 2016.

2. Stöppler, Melissa Conrad, MD. "Muscle Cramps," MedicineNet, June 6, 2017.

3. Wilkerson, Rick, DO. "Muscle Cramps," American Academy of Orthopaedic Surgeons, May 2010.

Chapter 16

Neck Pain

Chapter Contents

Section 16.1

What Causes a Pain in the Neck?

This section contains text excerpted from the following sources:
Text in this section begins with excerpts from "Neck Injuries and
Disorders," U.S. National Library of Medicine (NLM), National
Institutes of Health (NIH), January 3, 2017; Text under the heading
"Causes of Neck Pain" is excerpted from "ACR Appropriateness
Criteria® Chronic Neck Pain," Agency for Healthcare Research and
Quality (AHRQ), U.S. Department of Health and Human Services
(HHS), August 9, 2013. Reviewed June 2017; Text beginning with
the heading "Diagnosis of Neck Pain" is excerpted from "Cervical
Musculoligamentous Injury (Sprain/Strain)," Rhode Island Judiciary,
June 21, 2007. Reviewed June 2017; Text under the heading "CAM
Practices for Neck Pain" is excerpted from "Review of CAM Practices
for Back and Neck Pain Shows Modest Results," National Center for
Complementary and Integrative Health (NCCIH), January 31, 2012.
Reviewed June 2017.

Any part of your neck—muscles, bones, joints, tendons, ligaments,
or nerves—can cause neck problems. Neck pain is very common. Pain
may also come from your shoulder, jaw, head, or upper arms. Muscle
strain or tension often causes neck pain. The problem is usually overuse, such as from sitting at a computer for too long. Sometimes you
can strain your neck muscles from sleeping in an awkward position or
overdoing it during exercise. Falls or accidents, including car accidents,
are another common cause of neck pain. Whiplash, a soft tissue injury
to the neck, is also called neck sprain or strain. Treatment depends on
the cause, but may include applying ice, taking pain relievers, getting
physical therapy or wearing a cervical collar. You rarely need surgery

Causes of Neck Pain

The patient with chronic neck pain presents both diagnostic and
therapeutic dilemmas for the clinician because of considerable contro-
versy in the literature over its etiology, as well as the role of imaging
in its evaluation. The literature focuses on two general categories:
post-traumatic and mechanical/degenerative, but in most cases, multiple etiological factors are present. Post-traumatic etiologies include

the so-called "whiplash" syndrome, defined as any injury to the cervical vertebrae and adjacent soft tissues as a result of sudden jerking. This classically includes extension-flexion mechanisms sustained in rear-end motor vehicle collisions (MVC) as well as abrupt lateral flexion mechanisms. Mechanical/degenerative conditions include spondylosis, disc degeneration, acute disc herniation and facet joint osteoarthritis. These conditions may also result from prior acute injury. Chronic neck pain and/or neurologic symptoms may also be seen in patients with prior cervical spine surgery as well as in the setting of ossification of the posterior longitudinal ligament (OPLL). Finally, there are anecdotal reports in the literature about other etiologies of chronic neck pain that include carotid or vertebral artery dissection, arteriovenous malformations, and tumors.

Diagnosis of Neck Pain

Pertinent Historical and Physical Findings

The onset of neck pain and paraspinal muscle spasm begins either suddenly after the injury occurs or develops gradually over the next 24 hours. This pain is usually aggravated by motion of the neck and/or shoulder and frequently relieved by rest. The pain usually does not radiate below the shoulder. It can be accompanied by paresthesia or a sense of weakness in the upper extremities related to the muscle spasm in the neck. Physical findings include tenderness to palpation, spasm of the paravertebral muscles and aggravation of the pain with motion. Neurological examination and nerve root stretch tests are usually negative.

Appropriate Diagnostic Tests and Examinations

In general, anteroposterior, lateral, oblique, flexion and extension x-rays of the cervical spine and open mouth view to visualize the odontoid process are appropriate. Other x-rays may be added to the roentgenographic series as indicated. Straightening of the cervical spine is frequently observed on the lateral X-ray.

Treatment of Neck Pain

Non-Operative Treatment

Almost all patients with cervical musculoligamentous (sprain/strain) can be treated satisfactorily. No indications exist for the use of surgery in the treatment of cervical musculoligamentous injury.

Treatment Options

- Pain medication, non-narcotic

- Muscle relaxants

- Anti-inflammatory drugs, non-steroidal

- Physical therapy and/or rehabilitive services

- Occasional trigger point injections may be helpful

- Spinal manipulative therapy

Rehabilitation Procedures

Therapy may be initiated as early as the day of injury; indications for and focus of (early) intervention include:

- acute management of pain/spasms;

- limited use of passive modalities, except unlimited ice;

- instruction in ROM/stretching exercises for neck/shoulder muscles;

- assessment of return to work readiness and identifying necessary work modifications;

- patient education in healing process and body mechanics.

If the patient has not responded to the above-outlined treatments in four weeks time, the patient must be referred to a Neurologist, Neurosurgeon, Orthopedic Surgeon, or Physiatrist. The specialist referred to above may order further diagnostic procedures, since the failure to respond to conservative treatment brings with it the distinct possibility of a different diagnosis such as a cervical disc.

CAM Practices for Neck Pain

According to a review published by the Agency for Healthcare Research and Quality (AHRQ), the benefits of complementary and alternative therapies for back and neck pain—such as acupuncture, massage, and spinal manipulation—are modest in size but provide more benefit than usual medical care. While these effects are most evident following the end of treatment, the authors of the report noted that very few studies looked at long-term outcomes.

Researchers at the University of Ottawa Evidence-Based Practice Center reviewed the scientific literature on the efficacy, safety, and cost-effectiveness of acupuncture, spinal manipulation, mobilization, and massage techniques for the management of back, neck, and thoracic pain. General findings from the analysis include the following:

- CAM therapies tended to reduce pain and/or disability more than usual medical care (such as anti-inflammatory medications and exercise), physical therapy, or no treatment.

- Acupuncture was associated with a significant reduction in chronic low-back pain intensity compared with placebo, but only immediately after treatment.

- For chronic neck pain, acupuncture did not result in any different benefits compared with placebo (simulated acupuncture), pain medication, mobilization or traction, or laser therapy for reducing pain or disability after treatment.

- Spinal manipulation was significantly more effective than placebo, or equivalent to pain medication, for reducing the intensity of low-back pain.

- Mobilization was better than placebo for reducing acute or subacute neck pain, but not for chronic neck pain. Mobilization did not result in any different benefits compared with placebo in reducing low-back pain or flexibility after treatment.

- Massage significantly reduced the intensity of acute or subacute low-back pain, but not chronic pain, compared with placebo.

Section 16.2

Whiplash and Whiplash-Associated Disorders (WADs)

This section includes text excerpted from documents published by three public domain sources. Text under heading marked 1 is excerpted from "Whiplash Information Page," National Institute of Neurological Disorders and Stroke (NINDS), February 13, 2017; Text under heading marked 2 is excerpted from "Preventing Chronic Whiplash Pain," Clinicaltrials.gov, National Institutes of Health (NIH), August 9, 2013. Reviewed June 2017; Text under heading marked 3 is excerpted from "A Study of Whiplash Injury Occurrence Mechanisms Using Human Finite Element Model," U.S. Department of Transportation (DOT), February 6, 2014.

What Is Whiplash Injury?[1]

Whiplash-a soft tissue injury to the neck-is also called neck sprain or neck strain. It is characterized by a collection of symptoms that occur following damage to the neck, usually because of sudden extension and flexion. The disorder commonly occurs as the result of an automobile accident and may include injury to intervertebral joints, discs, and ligaments, cervical muscles, and nerve roots. Symptoms such as neck pain may be present directly after the injury or may be delayed for several days. In addition to neck pain, other symptoms may include neck stiffness, injuries to the muscles and ligaments (myofascial injuries), headache, dizziness, abnormal sensations such as burning or prickling (paresthesias), or shoulder or back pain. In addition, some people experience cognitive, somatic, or psychological conditions such as memory loss, concentration impairment, nervousness/irritability, sleep disturbances, fatigue, or depression. Generally, prognosis for individuals with whiplash is good. The neck and head pain clears within a few days or weeks. Most patients recover within 3 months after the injury, however, some may continue to have residual neck pain and headaches and effective pain management needs to be a top priority for researchers and for the healthcare system.

Symptoms and Prognosis of WAD[2]

More than 1.8 million people in the United States suffer from chronic pain and disability following motor vehicle accidents (MVAs) each year. The majority of these cases start with a relatively minor neck injury. Multiple studies have described the clinical features of WAD, which include neck, shoulder, arm, low back, and head pain; tinnitus; visual symptoms; dizziness; temporomandibular joint pain; and paraesthesias. Onset of these symptoms after the injury is usually delayed for several hours and worsens within 24 to 48 hours. Neck pain is the most frequent symptom, and between 14% and 42% of patients with WAD develop chronic neck pain symptoms. Studies suggest that the neck pain will either resolve in the first few months or persist indefinitely. One variable that may predict outcome after an MVA is the acute emotional response immediately after the MVA. A severe emotional reaction accompanied by neck pain and stiffness after an MVA could lead an injured person to avoid subsequent physical activity through such mechanisms as fear avoidance and fear of reinjury. Research investigating the evolution of chronic pain due to musculoskeletal injury suggests that initial emotional reactivity, particularly fear of reinjury and subsequent activity avoidance, contributes significantly to unremitting pain and persistent disability. Research based on this model has shown that early interventions targeting normalization of excessive emotionality and restriction of activities associated with fear following injury effectively prevent chronic pain due to back injury.

Mechanisms for the Occurrence of Whiplash Injury[3]

1. One hypothesis is that whiplash injuries are caused by severe hyperextension such that the head's extension angle exceeds 90°. This was the initial theory. Later, the introduction of the headrest failed to prevent whiplash injuries perfectly, so other hypotheses were proposed.

2. In another one, pain is caused by the spinal nerves or the dorsal roots as the result of increased pressure in the spinal canal and the cervical region during extension in whiplash.

3. Hypothesis based on facet joint surface impingement between upper and lower vertebrae.

During a rear-end collision, shear forces and axial compressive forces are exerted on the cervical vertebrae. According to this hypothesis, the center of rotation by extension during whiplash moves upward, so facet joint injury occurs as the result of the facet joint impingement when the lower articular process of the upper cervical vertebra contacts the upper articular process of the lower cervical vertebra. Also, cervical-region pain occurs as the result of the inflammation that occurs after the synovial folds with the articular capsule of the joint are stimulated by the facet joint impingement.

iv. Hypothesis based on the shear deformation of the capsules that covers the facet joint.

In this hypothesis, the compressive loading of the cervical vertebrae as the result of the straightening of the thoracic spinal column by the contact to seat during a rear-end collision causes the cervical vertebrae to slide relative to each other, thereby stretching the joint capsule which results in inflammation and pain.

Treatment[1]

Treatment for individuals with whiplash may include pain medications, nonsteroidal anti-inflammatory drugs, antidepressants, muscle relaxants, and a cervical collar (usually worn for 2 to 3 weeks). Range of motion exercises, physical therapy, and cervical traction may also be prescribed. Supplemental heat application may relieve muscle tension.

Section 16.3

Massage Therapy for Managing Neck Pain

This section includes text excerpted from "Multiple 60-Minute Massages per Week Offer Relief for Chronic Neck Pain," National Center for Complementary and Integrative Health (NCCIH), June 2, 2014.

Results of an National Center for Complementary and Alternative Medicine (NCCAM)-funded study found that multiple 60-minute massages per week were more effective than fewer or shorter sessions for people with chronic neck pain, suggesting that several hour-long massages per week may be the best "dose" for people with this condition.

Researchers enrolled 228 people with chronic neck pain into five randomly assigned groups receiving various "doses" of massage: a 4-week course of 30-minute sessions two or three times each week, or 60-minute sessions one, two, or three times each week. Other participants were assigned to a 4-week wait list, which served as the control group. Therapists used a wide range of massage techniques and were not allowed to make any self-care recommendations.

The researchers found that 30-minute massages two or three times per week did not provide significant benefits compared with the wait-list control group. However, beneficial effects of 60-minute massages increased with dose and were particularly evident for participants receiving massages two or three times per week. Compared with the control group, participants were three times more likely to have clinically meaningful improvement in neck function if they received 60-minute massages twice per week and five times more likely if they received 60-minute massages three times per week. However, the researchers noted that longer and more frequent massages might be challenging for many patients due to financial and time constraints. They also noted that future studies of massage for neck pain should include multiple 60-minute massages per week for the first 4 weeks of treatment, self-care recommendations, and longer-term follow-up.

Chapter 17

Repetitive Motion Disorders

Chapter Contents

Section 17.1

Bursitis and Tendinitis

This section includes text excerpted from "Questions and Answers about Bursitis and Tendinitis," National Institute of Arthritis and Musculoskeletal and Skin Diseases (NIAMS), February 2017.

Bursitis and tendinitis are both common conditions that involve inflammation of the soft tissue around muscles and bones, most often in the shoulder, elbow, wrist, hip, knee, or ankle. A bursa is a small, fluid-filled sac that acts as a cushion between a bone and other moving parts: muscles, tendons, or skin. Bursae are found throughout the body. Bursitis occurs when a bursa becomes inflamed (redness and increased fluid in the bursa).

A tendon is a flexible band of fibrous tissue that connects muscles to bones. Tendinitis is inflammation of a tendon. Tendons transmit the pull of the muscle to the bone to cause movement. They are found throughout the body, including the hands, wrists, elbows, shoulders, hips, knees, ankles, and feet. Tendons can be small, like those found in the hand, or large, like the Achilles tendon in the heel.

What Causes These Conditions?

Bursitis is commonly caused by overuse or direct trauma to a joint. Bursitis may occur at the knee or elbow, from kneeling or leaning on the elbows longer than usual on a hard surface, for example. Tendinitis is most often the result of a repetitive injury or motion in the affected area. These conditions occur more often with age. Tendons become less flexible with age, and therefore, more prone to injury.

People such as carpenters, gardeners, musicians, and athletes who perform activities that require repetitive motions or place stress on joints are at higher risk for tendinitis and bursitis.

An infection, arthritis, gout, thyroid disease, and diabetes can also bring about inflammation of a bursa or tendon.

What Parts of the Body Are Affected?

Tendinitis causes pain and tenderness just outside a joint. Some common names for tendinitis identify with the sport or movement that typically increases risk for tendon inflammation. They include tennis elbow, golfer's elbow, pitcher's shoulder, swimmer's shoulder, and jumper's knee. Some common examples are given below.

Tennis Elbow and Golfer's Elbow

Tennis elbow refers to an injury to the outer elbow tendon. Golfer's elbow is an injury to the inner tendon of the elbow. These conditions can also occur with any activity that involves repetitive wrist turning or hand gripping, such as tool use, hand shaking, or twisting movements. Carpenters, gardeners, painters, musicians, manicurists, and dentists are at higher risk for these forms of tendinitis. Pain occurs near the elbow, sometimes radiating into the upper arm or down to the forearm. Another name for tennis elbow is lateral epicondylitis. Golfer's elbow is also called medial epicondylitis.

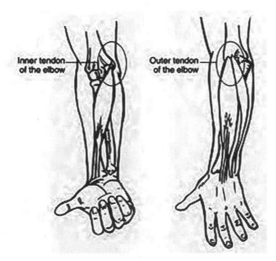

Inner tendon of the elbow

Outer tendon of the elbow

Figure 17.1. *Structure of the Elbow*

Shoulder Tendinitis, Bursitis, and Impingement Syndrome

Two types of tendinitis can affect the shoulder. Biceps tendinitis causes pain in the front or side of the shoulder and may travel down to the elbow and forearm. Pain may also occur when the arm is raised overhead. The biceps muscle, in the front of the upper arm, helps stabilize the upper arm bone (humerus) in the shoulder socket. It also helps accelerate and decelerate the arm during overhead movement in activities like tennis or pitching.

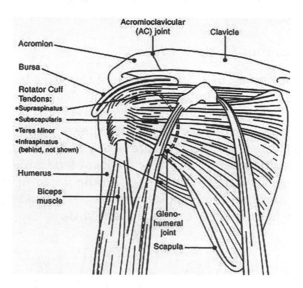

Figure 17.2. *Structure of the Shoulder*

Rotator cuff tendinitis causes shoulder pain at the tip of the shoulder and the upper, outer arm. The pain can be aggravated by reaching, pushing, pulling, lifting, raising the arm above shoulder level, or lying on the affected side. The rotator cuff is primarily a group of four muscles that attach the arm to the shoulder joint and allow the arm to rotate and elevate. If the rotator cuff and bursa are irritated, inflamed, and swollen, they may become compressed between the head of the humerus and the acromion, the outer edge of the shoulder blade. Repeated motion involving the arms, or the aging process involving shoulder motion over many years, may also irritate and wear down the tendons, muscles, and surrounding structures. Squeezing of the rotator cuff is called shoulder impingement syndrome.

Inflammation caused by rheumatoid arthritis may cause rotator cuff tendinitis and bursitis. Sports involving overuse of the shoulder and occupations requiring frequent overhead reaching are other potential causes of irritation to the rotator cuff or bursa, and may lead to inflammation and impingement.

Knee Tendinitis or Jumper's Knee

If a person overuses a tendon during activities such as dancing, cycling, or running, it may elongate or undergo microscopic tears and become inflamed. Trying to break a fall may also cause the quadriceps muscles to contract and tear the quadriceps tendon above the knee cap (patella) or the patellar tendon below it. This type of injury is most likely to happen in older people whose tendons tend to be weaker and less flexible. Tendinitis of the patellar tendon is sometimes called jumper's knee because in sports that require jumping, such as basketball, the muscle contraction and force of hitting the ground after a jump strain the tendon. After repeated stress, the tendon may become inflamed or tear.

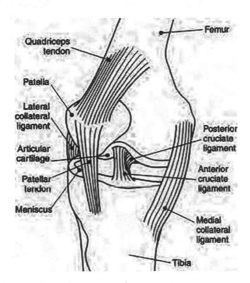

Figure 17.3. *View of the Knee*

People with tendinitis of the knee may feel pain during running, hurried walking, or jumping. Knee tendinitis can increase risk for ruptures or large tears to the tendon. A complete rupture of the quadriceps or patellar tendon is not only painful, but also makes it difficult for a person to bend, extend, or lift the leg, or to bear weight on the involved leg.

Achilles Tendinitis

Achilles tendon injuries involve an irritation, stretch, or tear to the tendon connecting the calf muscle to the back of the heel. Achilles tendinitis is a common overuse injury, but can also be caused by tight or weak calf muscles or any condition that causes the tendon to become less flexible and more rigid, such as reactive arthritis or normal aging.

Achilles tendon injuries can happen to anyone who regularly participates in an activity that causes the calf muscle to contract, like climbing stairs or using a stair-stepper, but are most common in middle-aged "weekend warriors" who may not exercise regularly. Among professional athletes, most Achilles injuries seem to occur in quick-acceleration or jumping sports like football, tennis, and basketball, and almost always end the season's competition for the athlete.

Achilles tendinitis can be a chronic condition. It can also cause what appears to be a sudden injury. Tendinitis is the most common factor contributing to Achilles tendon tears. When a tendon is weakened by age or overuse, trauma can cause it to rupture. These injuries can be so sudden and agonizing that they have been known to bring down charging professional football players in shocking fashion.

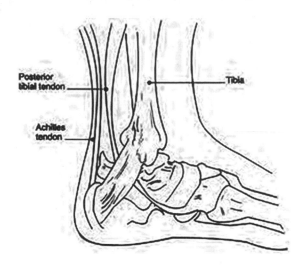

Figure 17.4. *Lateral View of the Ankle*

How Are These Conditions Diagnosed?

- Medical history and physical examination

- Selective tissue tension tests

- X-rays

- Magnetic resonance imaging (MRI)

To rule out infection, the doctor may remove and test fluid from the inflamed area.

What Kind of Healthcare Professional Treats These Conditions?

A primary care physician or a physical therapist can treat the common causes of tendinitis and bursitis. Complicated cases or those resistant to conservative therapies may require referral to a specialist, such as an orthopaedist or rheumatologist.

How Are Bursitis and Tendinitis Treated?

Treatment focuses on healing the injured bursa or tendon. The first step in treating both of these conditions is to reduce pain and inflammation with rest, compression, elevation, and anti-inflammatory medicines such as aspirin, naproxen, or ibuprofen. Ice may also be used in acute injuries, but most cases of bursitis or tendinitis are considered chronic, and ice is not helpful. When ice is needed, an ice pack can be applied to the affected area for 15 to 20 minutes every 4 to 6 hours for 3 to 5 days. Longer use of ice and a stretching program may be recommended by a healthcare provider.

Activity involving the affected joint is also restricted to encourage healing and prevent further injury. In some cases (e.g., in tennis elbow), elbow bands may be used to compress the forearm muscle to provide some pain relief, limiting the pull of the tendon on the bone. Other protective devices, such as foot orthoses for the ankle and foot or splints for the knee or hand, may temporarily reduce stress to the affected tendon or bursa and facilitate quicker healing times, while allowing general activity levels to continue as usual.

Gentle stretching and strengthening exercises are added gradually. Massage of the soft tissue may be helpful. These may be preceded or followed by use of an ice pack. The type of exercises recommended may vary depending on the location of the affected bursa or tendon. If there is no improvement, the doctor may inject a corticosteroid medicine into the area surrounding the inflamed bursa or tendon. Although corticosteroid injections are a common treatment, they must be used with caution because they may lead to weakening or rupture of the tendon (especially weight-bearing tendons such as the Achilles [ankle], posterior tibial [arch of the foot], and patellar [knee] tendons). If there is still no improvement after 6 to 12 months, the doctor may perform either arthroscopic or open surgery to repair damage and relieve pressure on the tendons and bursae.

If the bursitis is caused by an infection, the doctor will prescribe antibiotics. If a tendon is completely torn, surgery may be needed to repair the damage. After surgery on a quadriceps or patellar tendon, for example, the patient will wear a cast or brace or immobilizing device for 3 to 6 weeks and use crutches. For a partial tear, the doctor might apply a cast without performing surgery. Rehabilitating a partial or complete tear of a tendon requires an exercise program to restore the ability to bend and straighten the knee and to strengthen the leg to prevent repeat injury. A rehabilitation program may last up to 6 months, although the patient can return to many activities before then.

Can Bursitis and Tendinitis Be Prevented?

To help prevent inflammation or reduce the severity of its recurrence:

- Begin new activities or exercise regimens slowly.

- Gradually increase physical demands following several well-tolerated exercise sessions.

- Exercise regularly.

- Strengthen muscles around the joint.

- Take breaks from repetitive tasks often.

- Stop activities that cause pain.

- Cushion the affected joint. Use foam for kneeling or elbow pads. Increase the gripping surface of tools with gloves or padding. Apply grip tape or an oversized grip to golf clubs.

- Use two hands to hold heavy tools; use a two-handed backhand in tennis.

- Don't sit still for long periods.

- Practice good posture and position the body properly when going about daily activities.

- If a history of tendinitis is present, consider seeking guidance from your doctor or therapist before engaging in new exercises and activities.

Section 17.2

Carpal Tunnel Syndrome

This section includes text excerpted from "Carpal
Tunnel Syndrome Fact Sheet," National Institute of
Neurological Disorders and Stroke (NINDS), January 2017.

What Is Carpal Tunnel Syndrome (CTS)?

Carpal tunnel syndrome (CTS) occurs when the median nerve, which runs from the forearm into the palm of the hand, becomes pressed or squeezed at the wrist. The carpal tunnel—a narrow, rigid passageway of ligament and bones at the base of the hand—houses the median nerve and the tendons that bend the fingers. The median nerve provides feeling to the palm side of the thumb and to the index, middle, and part of the ring fingers (although not the little finger). It also controls some small muscles at the base of the thumb.

Sometimes, thickening from the lining of irritated tendons or other swelling narrows the tunnel and causes the median nerve to be compressed. The result may be numbness, weakness, or sometimes pain in the hand and wrist, or occasionally in the forearm and arm. CTS is the most common and widely known of the entrapment neuropathies, in which one of the body's peripheral nerves is pressed upon.

What Are the Symptoms of CTS?

Symptoms usually start gradually, with frequent burning, tingling, or itching numbness in the palm of the hand and the fingers, especially the thumb and the index and middle fingers. Some carpal tunnel sufferers say their fingers feel useless and swollen, even though little or no swelling is apparent. The symptoms often first appear in one or both hands during the night, since many people sleep with flexed wrists. A person with carpal tunnel syndrome may wake up feeling the need to "shake out" the hand or wrist. As symptoms worsen, people might feel tingling during the day. Decreased grip strength may make it difficult to form a fist, grasp small objects, or perform other manual tasks. In chronic and/or untreated cases, the muscles at the base of the thumb may waste away. Some people are unable to tell between hot and cold by touch.

What Are the Causes of CTS?

Carpal tunnel syndrome is often the result of a combination of factors that reduce the available space for the median nerve within the carpal tunnel, rather than a problem with the nerve itself. Contributing factors include trauma or injury to the wrist that cause swelling, such as sprain or fracture; an overactive pituitary gland; an underactive thyroid gland; and rheumatoid arthritis. Mechanical problems in the wrist joint, work stress, repeated use of vibrating hand tools, fluid retention during pregnancy or menopause, or the development of a cyst or tumor in the canal also may contribute to the compression. Often, no single cause can be identified.

Who Is at Risk of Developing CTS?

Women are three times more likely than men to develop carpal tunnel syndrome, perhaps because the carpal tunnel itself may be smaller in women than in men. The dominant hand is usually affected first and produces the most severe pain. Persons with diabetes or other metabolic disorders that directly affect the body's nerves and make them more susceptible to compression are also at high risk. Carpal tunnel syndrome usually occurs only in adults.

The risk of developing carpal tunnel syndrome is not confined to people in a single industry or job, but is especially common in those performing assembly line work—manufacturing, sewing, finishing, cleaning, and meat, poultry, or fish packing. In fact, carpal tunnel syndrome is three times more common among assemblers than among data-entry personnel.

How Is CTS Diagnosed?

Early diagnosis and treatment are important to avoid permanent damage to the median nerve.

- Medical history and physical examination
- Routine laboratory tests and X-rays
- Specific tests
  - Tinel test
  - Phalen's maneuver (wrist-flexion test)

- Electrodiagnostic tests
- Ultrasound imaging
- Magnetic resonance imaging (MRI)

How Is CTS Treated?

Treatments for carpal tunnel syndrome should begin as early as possible, under a doctor's direction. Underlying causes such as diabetes or arthritis should be treated first.

Non-Surgical Treatments

- Splinting
- Avoiding daytime activities that may provoke symptoms
- Over-the-counter drugs
- Prescription medicines
- Alternative therapies

Surgery

Carpal tunnel release is one of the most common surgical procedures in the United States. Generally, surgery involves severing a ligament around the wrist to reduce pressure on the median nerve. Surgery is usually done under local or regional anesthesia (involving some sedation) and does not require an overnight hospital stay. Many people require surgery on both hands. While all carpal tunnel surgery involves cutting the ligament to relieve the pressure on the nerve, there are two different methods used by surgeons to accomplish this.

- Open release surgery
- Endoscopic surgery

Following surgery, the ligaments usually grow back together and allow more space than before. Although symptoms may be relieved immediately after surgery, full recovery from carpal tunnel surgery can take months. Almost always there is a decrease in grip strength, which improves over time. Some individuals may develop infections, nerve damage, stiffness, and pain at the scar. Most people need to modify work activity for several weeks following surgery, and some people may need to adjust job duties or even change jobs after recovery from surgery.

Although recurrence of carpal tunnel syndrome following treatment is rare, fewer than half of individuals report their hand(s) feeling completely normal following surgery. Some residual numbness or weakness is common.

How Can CTS Be Prevented?

At the workplace, workers can do on-the-job conditioning, perform stretching exercises, take frequent rest breaks, and ensure correct posture and wrist position. Wearing fingerless gloves can help keep hands warm and flexible. Workstations, tools and tool handles, and tasks can be redesigned to enable the worker's wrist to maintain a natural position during work. Jobs can be rotated among workers. Employers can develop programs in ergonomics, the process of adapting workplace conditions and job demands to the capabilities of workers. However, research has not conclusively shown that these workplace changes prevent the occurrence of carpal tunnel syndrome.

Chapter 18

Shoulder Problems

What Are the Most Common Shoulder Problems?

The most movable joint in the body, the shoulder is also one of the most potentially unstable joints. As a result, it is the site of many common problems. They include sprains, strains, dislocations, separations, tendinitis, bursitis, torn rotator cuffs, frozen shoulder, fractures, and arthritis. Specific shoulder problems will be discussed later in this chapter.

How Common Are Shoulder Problems?

According to the Centers for Disease Control (CDC) and Prevention, nearly 1.2 million people in the United States visited an emergency room in 2010 for shoulder problems.

What Are the Structures of the Shoulder and How Does It Function?

To better understand shoulder problems and how they occur, it helps to begin with an explanation of the shoulder's structure and how it functions.

This chapter includes text excerpted from "Questions and Answers about Shoulder Problems," National Institute of Arthritis and Musculoskeletal and Skin Diseases (NIAMS), April 2014.

The shoulder joint is composed of three bones: the clavicle (collarbone), the scapula (shoulder blade), and the humerus (upper arm bone). Two joints facilitate shoulder movement. The acromioclavicular joint is located between the acromion (the part of the scapula that forms the highest point of the shoulder) and the clavicle. The glenohumeral joint, commonly called the shoulder joint, is a ball-and-socket-type joint that helps move the shoulder forward and backward and allows the arm to rotate in a circular fashion or hinge out and up away from the body. (The "ball," or humerus, is the top, rounded portion of the upper arm bone; the "socket," or glenoid, is a dish-shaped part of the outer edge of the scapula into which the ball fits.) The capsule is a soft tissue envelope that encircles the glenohumeral joint. It is lined by a thin, smooth synovial membrane.

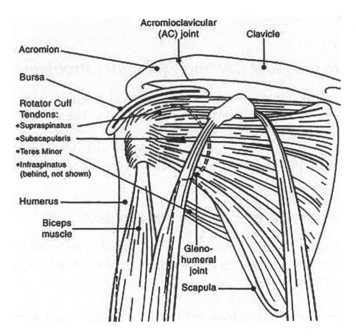

Figure 18.1. *Structure of the Shoulder*

In contrast to the hip joint, which more closely approximates a true ball-and-socket joint, the shoulder joint can be compared to a golf ball and tee, in which the ball can easily slip off the flat tee. Because the bones provide little inherent stability to the shoulder joint, it is highly dependent on surrounding soft tissues such as capsule ligaments and the muscles surrounding the rotator cuff to hold the ball in place. Whereas the hip joint is inherently quite stable because of the encircling bony anatomy, it also is relatively immobile. The shoulder, on the other hand, is relatively unstable but highly mobile, allowing an individual to place the hand in numerous positions. It is, in fact, one of the most mobile joints in the human body.

The bones of the shoulder are held in place by muscles, tendons, and ligaments. Tendons are tough cords of tissue that attach the shoulder muscles to bone and assist the muscles in moving the shoulder. Ligaments attach shoulder bones to each other, providing stability. For example, the front of the joint capsule is anchored by three glenohumeral ligaments. The rotator cuff is a structure composed of tendons that work along with associated muscles to hold the ball at the top of the humerus in the glenoid socket and provide mobility and strength to the shoulder joint. Two filmy sac-like structures called bursae permit smooth gliding between bones, muscles, and tendons. They cushion and protect the rotator cuff from the bony arch of the acromion.

What Are the Origins and Causes of Shoulder Problems?

The shoulder is easily injured because the ball of the upper arm is larger than the shoulder socket that holds it. To remain stable, the shoulder must be anchored by its muscles, tendons, and ligaments.

Although the shoulder is easily injured during sporting activities and manual labor, the primary source of shoulder problems appears to be the natural age-related degeneration of the surrounding soft tissues such as those found in the rotator cuff. The incidence of rotator cuff problems rises dramatically as a function of age and is generally seen among individuals who are more than 60 years old. Often, the dominant and nondominant arm will be affected to a similar degree. Overuse of the shoulder can lead to more rapid age-related deterioration.

Shoulder pain may be localized or may be felt in areas around the shoulder or down the arm. Disease within the body (such as gallbladder, liver, or heart disease, or disease of the cervical spine of the neck) also may generate pain that travels along nerves to the shoulder. However, these other causes of shoulder pain are beyond the scope of this chapter, which will focus on problems within the shoulder itself.

How Are Shoulder Problems Diagnosed?

As with any medical issue, a shoulder problem is generally diagnosed using a three-part process.

- Medical history
- Physical examination
- Tests
  - Standard X-ray
  - Arthrogram
  - Ultrasound
  - MRI (magnetic resonance imaging)

Other diagnostic tests, such as one that involves injecting an anesthetic into and around the shoulder joint, are discussed in detail in other parts of this chapter.

What Should I Know about Specific Shoulder Problems, Including Their Symptoms and Treatment?

The symptoms of shoulder problems, as well as their diagnosis and treatment, vary widely, depending on the specific problem. The following is important information to know about some of the most common shoulder problems.

Dislocation

The shoulder joint is the most frequently dislocated major joint of the body. In a typical case of a dislocated shoulder, either a strong force pulls the shoulder outward (abduction) or extreme rotation of the joint pops the ball of the humerus out of the shoulder socket. Dislocation commonly occurs when there is a backward pull on the arm that either catches the muscles unprepared to resist or overwhelms the muscles. When a shoulder dislocates frequently, the condition is referred to as shoulder instability. A partial dislocation in which the upper arm bone is partially in and partially out of the socket is called a subluxation.

- **Signs and symptoms.** The shoulder can dislocate either forward, backward, or downward. When the shoulder dislocates, the arm appears out of position. Other symptoms include pain, which may be worsened by muscle spasms, swelling, numbness, weakness, and bruising. Problems seen with a dislocated shoulder are tearing of the ligaments or tendons reinforcing the joint capsule and, less commonly, bone and/or nerve damage.

- **Diagnosis.** Doctors usually diagnose a dislocation by a physical examination; X-rays may be taken to confirm the diagnosis and to rule out a related fracture.

- **Treatment.** Doctors treat a dislocation by putting the ball of the humerus back into the joint socket, a procedure called a closed reduction. The arm is then stabilized for several weeks in a sling or a device called a shoulder immobilizer. Usually the doctor recommends resting the shoulder and applying ice three or four times a day. After pain and swelling have been controlled, the patient enters a rehabilitation program that includes exercises. The goal is to restore the range of motion of the shoulder, strengthen the muscles, and prevent future dislocations. These exercises may progress from simple motion to the use of weights.

After treatment and recovery, a previously dislocated shoulder may remain more susceptible to reinjury, especially in young, active individuals. Ligaments may have been stretched or torn, and the shoulder may tend to dislocate again. A shoulder that dislocates severely or often, injuring surrounding tissues or nerves, usually requires surgical repair to tighten stretched ligaments or reattach torn ones.

Sometimes the doctor performs surgery through a tiny incision into which a small scope (arthroscope) is inserted to observe the inside of the joint. After this procedure, called arthroscopic surgery, the shoulder is generally stabilized for about 6 weeks. Full recovery takes several months. In other cases, the doctor may repair the dislocation using a traditional open surgery approach.

Separation

A shoulder separation occurs where the collarbone (clavicle) meets the shoulder blade (scapula). When ligaments that hold the joint together are partially or completely torn, the outer end of the clavicle may slip out of place, preventing it from properly meeting the scapula. Most often, the injury is caused by a blow to the shoulder or by falling on an outstretched hand.

- **Signs and symptoms.** Shoulder pain or tenderness and, occasionally, a bump in the middle of the top of the shoulder (over the acromioclavicular or AC joint) are signs that a separation may have occurred.

- **Diagnosis.** Doctors may diagnose a separation by performing a physical examination. They may confirm the diagnosis and determine the severity of the separation by taking an X-ray. While the X-ray is being taken, the patient makes the separation more pronounced by holding a light weight that pulls on the muscles.

- **Treatment.** A shoulder separation is usually treated conservatively by rest and wearing a sling. Soon after injury, an ice bag may be applied to relieve pain and swelling. After a period of rest, a therapist helps the patient perform exercises that put the shoulder through its range of motion. Most shoulder separations heal within 2 or 3 months without further intervention. However, if ligaments are severely torn, surgical repair may be required to hold the clavicle in place. A doctor may wait to see if conservative treatment works before deciding whether surgery is required.

Rotator Cuff Disease: Tendinitis and Bursitis

These conditions are closely related and may occur alone or in combination.

Tendinitis is inflammation (redness, soreness, and swelling) of a tendon. In tendinitis of the shoulder, the rotator cuff and/or biceps tendon become inflamed, usually as a result of being pinched by surrounding structures. The injury may vary from mild inflammation to involvement of most of the rotator cuff. When the rotator cuff tendon becomes inflamed and thickened, it may get trapped under the acromion. Squeezing of the rotator cuff is called impingement syndrome.

Bursitis, or inflammation of the bursa sacs that protect the shoulder, may accompany tendinitis and impingement syndrome. Inflammation caused by a disease such as rheumatoid arthritis may cause rotator cuff tendinitis and bursitis. Sports involving overuse of the shoulder and occupations requiring frequent overhead reaching are other potential causes of irritation to the rotator cuff or bursa and may lead to inflammation and impingement.

If the rotator cuff and bursa are irritated, inflamed, and swollen, they may become squeezed between the head of the humerus and the acromion. Repeated motion involving the arms, or the effects of the aging process on shoulder movement over many years, may also irritate and wear down the tendons, muscles, and surrounding structures.

- **Signs and symptoms.** Signs of these conditions include the slow onset of discomfort and pain in the upper shoulder or upper third of the arm and/or difficulty sleeping on the shoulder.

Tendinitis and bursitis also cause pain when the arm is lifted away from the body or overhead. If tendinitis involves the biceps tendon (the tendon located in front of the shoulder that helps bend the elbow and turn the forearm), pain will occur in the front or side of the shoulder and may travel down to the elbow and forearm. Pain may also occur when the arm is forcefully pushed upward overhead.

- **Diagnosis.** Diagnosis of tendinitis and bursitis begins with a medical history and physical examination. X-rays do not show tendons or the bursae, but may be helpful in ruling out bony abnormalities or arthritis. The doctor may remove and test fluid from the inflamed area to rule out infection. Impingement syndrome may be confirmed when injection of a small amount of anesthetic (lidocaine hydrochloride) into the space under the acromion relieves pain.

- **Treatment.** The first step in treating these conditions is to reduce pain and inflammation with rest, ice, and anti-inflammatory medicines such as aspirin and ibuprofen (Advil, Motrin). In some cases, the doctor or therapist will use ultrasound (gentle sound-wave vibrations) to warm deep tissues and improve blood flow. Gentle stretching and strengthening exercises are added gradually. These may be preceded or followed by use of an ice pack. If there is no improvement, the doctor may inject a corticosteroid medicine into the space under the acromion. Although steroid injections are a common treatment, they must be used with caution because they may lead to tendon rupture. If there is still no improvement after 6 to 12 months, the doctor may recommend either arthroscopic or open surgery to repair damage and relieve pressure on the tendons and bursae.

Torn Rotator Cuff

Rotator cuff tendons often become inflamed from overuse, aging, or a fall on an outstretched hand or another traumatic cause. Sports or occupations requiring repetitive overhead motion or heavy lifting can also place a significant strain on rotator cuff muscles and tendons. Over time, as a function of aging, tendons become weaker and degenerate. Eventually, this degeneration can lead to complete tears of both muscles and tendons. These tears are surprisingly common. In fact, a tear of the rotator cuff is not necessarily an abnormal situation in older individuals if there is no significant pain or disability.

Fortunately, these tears do not lead to any pain or disability in most people. However, some individuals can develop very significant pain as a result of these tears and they may require treatment.

- **Signs and symptoms.** Typically, a person with a rotator cuff injury feels pain over the deltoid muscle at the top and outer side of the shoulder, especially when the arm is raised or extended out from the side of the body. Motions like those involved in getting dressed can be painful. The shoulder may feel weak, especially when trying to lift the arm into a horizontal position. A person may also feel or hear a click or pop when the shoulder is moved. Pain or weakness on outward or inward rotation of the arm may indicate a tear in a rotator cuff tendon. The patient also feels pain when lowering the arm to the side after the shoulder is moved backward and the arm is raised.

- **Diagnosis.** A doctor may detect weakness but may not be able to determine from a physical examination where the tear is located. X-rays, if taken, may appear normal. An MRI or ultrasound can help detect a full tendon tear or a partial tendon tear.

- **Treatment.** Doctors usually recommend that patients with a rotator cuff injury rest the shoulder, apply heat or cold to the sore area, and take medicine to relieve pain and inflammation. Other treatments might be added, such as electrical stimulation of muscles and nerves, ultrasound, or a cortisone injection near the inflamed area of the rotator cuff. If surgery is not an immediate consideration, exercises are added to the treatment program to build flexibility and strength and restore the shoulder's function. If there is no improvement with these conservative treatments and functional impairment persists, the doctor may perform arthroscopic or open surgical repair of the torn rotator cuff.

Treatment for a torn rotator cuff usually depends on the severity of the injury, the age and health status of the patient, and the length of time a given patient may have had the condition. Patients with rotator cuff tendinitis or bursitis that does not include a complete tear of the tendon can usually be treated without surgery. Nonsurgical treatments include the use of anti-inflammatory medication and occasional steroid injections into the area of the inflamed rotator cuff, followed by rehabilitative rotator cuff-strengthening exercises. These treatments are best undertaken with the guidance of a healthcare professional such as a physical therapist, who works in conjunction with the treating physician.

Surgical repair of rotator cuff tears is best for the following individuals:

- Younger patients, especially those with small tears. Surgery leads to a high degree of successful healing and reduces concerns about the tear getting worse over time.

- Individuals whose rotator cuff tears are caused by an acute, severe injury. These people should seek immediate treatment that includes surgical repair of the tendon.

Generally speaking, individuals who are older and have had shoulder pain for a longer period of time can be treated with nonoperative measures even in the presence of a complete rotator cuff tear. These people are often treated similarly to those who have pain but do not have a rotator cuff tear. Again, anti-inflammatory medication, use of steroid injections, and rehabilitative exercises can be very effective. When treated surgically, rotator cuff tears can be repaired by either arthroscopic or traditional open surgical techniques.

Frozen Shoulder (Adhesive Capsulitis)

As the name implies, movement of the shoulder is severely restricted in people with a "frozen shoulder." This condition, which doctors call adhesive capsulitis, is frequently caused by injury that leads to lack of use due to pain. Rheumatic disease progression and recent shoulder surgery can also cause frozen shoulder. Intermittent periods of use may cause inflammation. Adhesions (abnormal bands of tissue) grow between the joint surfaces, restricting motion. There is also a lack of synovial fluid, which normally lubricates the gap between the arm bone and socket to help the shoulder joint move. It is this restricted space between the capsule and ball of the humerus that distinguishes adhesive capsulitis from a less complicated painful, stiff shoulder. People with diabetes, stroke, lung disease, rheumatoid arthritis, and heart disease, or those who have been in an accident, are at a higher risk for frozen shoulder. People between the ages of 40 and 70 are most likely to experience it.

- **Signs and symptoms.** With a frozen shoulder, the joint becomes so tight and stiff that it is nearly impossible to carry out simple movements, such as raising the arm. Stiffness and discomfort may worsen at night.

- **Diagnosis.** A doctor may suspect a frozen shoulder if a physical examination reveals limited shoulder movement. X-rays usually appear normal.

- **Treatment.** Treatment of this disorder focuses on restoring joint movement and reducing shoulder pain. Usually, treatment begins with nonsteroidal anti-inflammatory drugs and the application of heat, followed by gentle stretching exercises. These stretching exercises, which may be performed in the home with the help of a physical therapist, are the treatment of choice. In some cases, transcutaneous electrical nerve stimulation (TENS) with a small battery-operated unit may be used to reduce pain by blocking nerve impulses. If these measures are unsuccessful, an intra-articular injection of steroids into the glenoid-humeral joint can result in marked improvement of the frozen shoulder in a large percentage of cases. In those rare people who do not improve from nonoperative measures, manipulation of the shoulder under general anesthesia and an arthroscopic procedure to cut the remaining adhesions can be highly effective in most cases.

Fracture

A fracture involves a partial or total crack through a bone. The break in a bone usually occurs as a result of an impact injury, such as a fall or blow to the shoulder. A fracture usually involves the clavicle or the neck (area below the ball) of the humerus.

- **Signs and symptoms.** A shoulder fracture that occurs after a major injury is usually accompanied by severe pain. Within a short time, there may be redness and bruising around the area. Sometimes a fracture is obvious because the bones appear out of position.

- **Diagnosis.** X-rays can confirm the diagnosis of a shoulder fracture and the degree of its severity.

- **Treatment.** When a fracture occurs, the doctor tries to bring the bones into a position that will promote healing and restore arm movement. If someone's clavicle is fractured, he or she must initially wear a strap and sling around the chest to keep the clavicle in place. After removing the strap and sling, the doctor will prescribe exercises to strengthen the shoulder and restore movement. Surgery is occasionally needed for certain clavicle fractures.

Fracture of the neck of the humerus is usually treated with a sling or shoulder stabilizer. If the bones are out of position, surgery may be necessary to reset them. Exercises are also part of restoring shoulder strength and motion.

Arthritis of the Shoulder

Arthritis is a degenerative disease caused by either wear and tear of the cartilage (osteoarthritis) or an inflammation (rheumatoid arthritis) of one or more joints. Arthritis not only affects joints, but may also affect supporting structures such as muscles, tendons, and ligaments.

- **Signs and symptoms.** The usual signs of arthritis of the shoulder are pain, particularly over the acromioclavicular joint, and a decrease in shoulder motion.

- **Diagnosis.** A doctor may suspect the patient has arthritis when there is both pain and swelling in the joint. The diagnosis may be confirmed by a physical examination and X-rays. Blood tests may be helpful for diagnosing rheumatoid arthritis, but other tests may be needed as well. Analysis of synovial fluid from the shoulder joint may be helpful in diagnosing some kinds of arthritis. Although arthroscopy permits direct visualization of damage to cartilage, tendons, and ligaments, and may confirm a diagnosis, it is usually done only if a repair procedure is to be performed.

- **Treatment.** Treatment of shoulder arthritis depends in part on the type of arthritis. Osteoarthritis of the shoulder is usually treated with nonsteroidal anti-inflammatory drugs, such as aspirin and ibuprofen. Rheumatoid arthritis may require physical therapy and additional medications such as corticosteroids.

When nonoperative treatment of arthritis of the shoulder fails to relieve pain or improve function, or when there is severe wear and tear of the joint causing parts to loosen and move out of place, shoulder joint replacement (arthroplasty) may provide better results. In this operation, a surgeon replaces the shoulder joint with an artificial ball for the top of the humerus and a cap (glenoid) for the scapula. Passive shoulder exercises (where someone else moves the arm to rotate the shoulder joint) are started soon after surgery. Patients begin exercising on their own about 3 to 6 weeks after surgery. Eventually, stretching and strengthening exercises become a major part of the rehabilitation program. The success of the operation often depends on the condition of rotator cuff muscles before surgery and the degree to which the patient follows the exercise program.

Treat Shoulder Injuries with RICE (Rest, Ice, Compression, and Elevation)

If you injure a shoulder, try the following:

- **Rest.** Reduce or stop using the injured area for 48 hours.

- **Ice.** Put an ice pack on the injured area for 20 minutes at a time, 4 to 8 times per day. Use a cold pack, ice bag, or a plastic bag filled with crushed ice that has been wrapped in a towel.

- **Compression.** Compress the area with bandages, such as an elastic wrap, to help stabilize the shoulder. This may help reduce the swelling.

- **Elevation.** Keep the injured area elevated above the level of the heart. Use a pillow to help elevate the injury.

If pain and stiffness persist, see a doctor.

Chapter 19

Sprains and Strains

What Is the Difference between a Sprain and a Strain?

A sprain is a stretch and/or tear of a ligament (a band of fibrous tissue that connects two or more bones at a joint). One or more ligaments can be injured at the same time. The severity of the injury will depend on the extent of injury (whether a tear is partial or complete) and the number of ligaments involved.

A strain is an injury to either a muscle or a tendon (fibrous cords of tissue that connect muscle to bone). Depending on the severity of the injury, a strain may be a simple overstretch of the muscle or tendon, or it can result from a partial or complete tear.

What Causes a Sprain?

A sprain can result from a fall, a sudden twist, or a blow to the body that forces a joint out of its normal position and stretches or tears the ligament supporting that joint. Typically, sprains occur when people fall and land on an outstretched arm, slide into a baseball base, land on the side of their foot, or twist a knee with the foot planted firmly on the ground.

This chapter includes text excerpted from "Questions and Answers about Sprains and Strains," National Institute of Arthritis and Musculoskeletal and Skin Diseases (NIAMS), January 2015.

Where Do Sprains Usually Occur?

Although sprains can occur in both the upper and lower parts of the body, the most common site is the ankle. It is estimated that more than 628,000 ankle sprains occur in the United States each year.

The ankle joint is supported by several lateral (outside) ligaments and medial (inside) ligaments (see figure. 19.1). Most ankle sprains happen when the foot turns inward as a person runs, turns, falls, or lands on the ankle after a jump. This type of sprain is called an inversion injury. The knee is another common site for a sprain. A blow to the knee or a fall is often the cause; sudden twisting can also result in a sprain (see figure. 19.2).

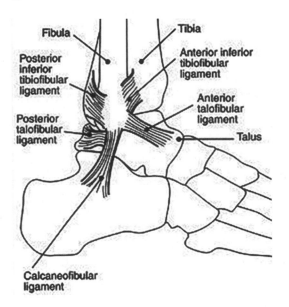

Figure 19.1. *Lateral View of the Ankle*

Sprains frequently occur at the wrist, typically when people fall and land on an outstretched hand. A sprain to the thumb is common in skiing and other sports. This injury often occurs when a ligament near the base of the thumb (the ulnar collateral ligament of the metacarpophalangeal joint) is torn (see figure. 19.3).

What Are the Signs and Symptoms of a Sprain?

The usual signs and symptoms include pain, swelling, bruising, instability, and loss of the ability to move and use the joint (called functional ability). However, these signs and symptoms can vary in

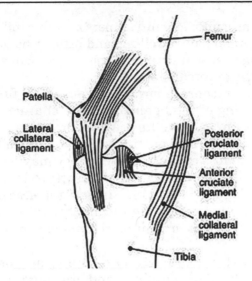

Figure 19.2. *Lateral View of the Knee*

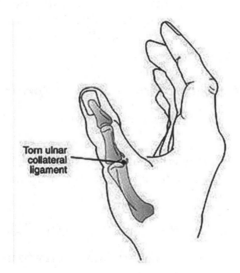

Figure 19.3. *Lateral View of the Thumb*

intensity, depending on the severity of the sprain. Sometimes people feel a pop or tear when the injury happens.

Doctors closely observe an injured site and ask questions to obtain information to diagnose the severity of a sprain. In general, a grade I or mild sprain is caused by overstretching or slight tearing of the

231

ligaments with no joint instability. A person with a mild sprain usually experiences minimal pain, swelling, and little or no loss of functional ability. Bruising is absent or slight, and the person is usually able to put weight on the affected joint.

A grade II or moderate sprain is caused by further, but still incomplete, tearing of the ligament and is characterized by bruising, moderate pain, and swelling. A person with a moderate sprain usually has more difficulty putting weight on the affected joint and experiences some loss of function. An X-ray may be needed to help the healthcare provider determine if a fracture is causing the pain and swelling. Magnetic resonance imaging is occasionally used to help differentiate between a significant partial injury and a complete tear in a ligament, or can be recommended to rule out other injuries.

People who sustain a grade III or severe sprain completely tear or rupture a ligament. Pain, swelling, and bruising are usually severe, and the patient is unable to put weight on the joint. An X-ray is usually taken to rule out a broken bone. When diagnosing any sprain, the healthcare provider will ask the patient to explain how the injury happened. He or she will examine the affected area and check its stability and its ability to move and bear weight.

When to See a Healthcare Provider for a Sprain

- You have severe pain and cannot put any weight on the injured joint.

- The injured area looks crooked or has lumps and bumps (other than swelling) that you do not see on the uninjured joint.

- You cannot move the injured joint.

- You cannot walk more than four steps without significant pain.

- Your limb buckles or gives way when you try to use the joint.

- You have numbness in any part of the injured area.

- You see redness or red streaks spreading out from the injury.

- You injure an area that has been injured several times before.

- You have pain, swelling, or redness over a bony part of your foot.

- You are in doubt about the seriousness of the injury or how to care for it.

What Causes a Strain?

A strain is caused by twisting or pulling a muscle or tendon. Strains can be acute or chronic. An acute strain is associated with a recent trauma or injury; it also can occur after improperly lifting heavy objects or overstressing the muscles. Chronic strains are usually the result of overuse: prolonged, repetitive movement of the muscles and tendons.

Where Do Strains Usually Occur?

Two common sites for a strain are the back and the hamstring muscle (located in the back of the thigh). Contact sports such as soccer, football, hockey, boxing, and wrestling put people at risk for strains. Gymnastics, tennis, rowing, golf, and other sports that require extensive gripping can increase the risk of hand and forearm strains. Elbow strains sometimes occur in people who participate in racquet sports, throwing, and contact sports.

What Are the Signs and Symptoms of a Strain?

Typically, people with a strain experience pain, limited motion, muscle spasms, and possibly muscle weakness. They also can have localized swelling, cramping, or inflammation and, with a minor or moderate strain, usually some loss of muscle function. Patients typically have pain in the injured area and general weakness of the muscle when they attempt to move it. Severe strains that partially or completely tear the muscle or tendon are often very painful and disabling.

How Are Sprains and Strains Treated?

Reduce Swelling and Pain

Treatments for sprains and strains are similar and can be thought of as having two stages. The goal during the first stage is to reduce swelling and pain. At this stage, healthcare providers usually advise patients to follow a formula of rest, ice, compression, and elevation (RICE) for the first 24 to 48 hours after the injury. The healthcare provider also may recommend an over-the-counter or prescription medication to help decrease pain and inflammation.[1]

For people with a moderate or severe sprain, particularly of the ankle, a hard cast may be applied. This often occurs after the initial swelling has subsided. Severe sprains and strains may require surgery to repair the torn ligaments, muscle, or tendons. Surgery is usually performed by an orthopaedic surgeon.

It is important that moderate and severe sprains and strains be evaluated by a healthcare provider to allow prompt, appropriate treatment to begin. This box lists some signs that should alert people to consult their healthcare provider. However, a person who has any concerns about the seriousness of a sprain or strain should always contact a healthcare provider for advice.

[1] *All medicines can have side effects. Some medicines and side effects are mentioned in this chapter. Some side effects may be more severe than others. You should review the package insert that comes with your medicine and ask your healthcare provider or pharmacist if you have any questions about the possible side effects.*

RICE Therapy

- **Rest.** Reduce regular exercise or activities of daily living as needed. Your healthcare provider may advise you to put no weight on an injured area for 48 hours. If you cannot put weight on an ankle or knee, crutches may help. If you use a cane or one crutch for an ankle injury, use it on the uninjured side to help you lean away and relieve weight on the injured ankle.

- **Ice.** Apply an ice pack to the injured area for 20 minutes at a time, four to eight times a day. A cold pack, ice bag, or plastic bag filled with crushed ice and wrapped in a towel can be used. To avoid cold injury and frostbite, do not apply the ice for more than 20 minutes.

- **Compression.** Compression of an injured ankle, knee, or wrist may help reduce swelling. Examples of compression bandages are elastic wraps, special boots, air casts, and splints. Ask your healthcare provider for advice on which one to use and how tight to apply the bandage safely.

- **Elevation.** If possible, keep the injured ankle, knee, elbow, or wrist elevated on a pillow, above the level of the heart, to help decrease swelling.

Begin Rehabilitation

The second stage of treating a sprain or strain is rehabilitation, with the overall goal of improving the condition of the injured area and restoring its function. The healthcare provider will prescribe an exercise program designed to prevent stiffness, improve range of motion, and restore the joint's normal flexibility and strength. Some patients may need physical therapy during this stage. When the acute pain and swelling have diminished, the healthcare provider will instruct the patient to do a series of exercises several times a day. These are very important because they help reduce swelling, prevent stiffness, and restore normal, pain-free range of motion. The healthcare provider can recommend many different types of exercises, depending on the injury. A patient with an injured knee or foot will work on weight-bearing and balancing exercises. The duration of the program depends on the extent of the injury, but the regimen commonly lasts for several weeks.

Another goal of rehabilitation is to increase strength and regain flexibility. Depending on the patient's rate of recovery, this process begins about the second week after the injury. The healthcare provider will instruct the patient to do a series of exercises designed to meet these goals. During this phase of rehabilitation, patients progress to more demanding exercises as pain decreases and function improves.

The final goal is the return to full daily activities, including sports when appropriate. Patients must work closely with their healthcare provider or physical therapist to determine their readiness to return to full activity. Sometimes people are tempted to resume full activity or play sports despite pain or muscle soreness. Returning to full activity before regaining normal range of motion, flexibility, and strength increases the chance of reinjury and may lead to a chronic problem.

The amount of rehabilitation and the time needed for full recovery after a sprain or strain depend on the severity of the injury and individual rates of healing. For example, a mild ankle sprain may require 3 to 6 weeks of rehabilitation; a moderate sprain could require 2 to 3 months. With a severe sprain, it can take 8 to 12 months to return to full activities. Extra care should be taken to avoid re-injury.

Can Sprains and Strains Be Prevented?

People can do many things to help lower their risk of sprains and strains:

- Avoid exercising or playing sports when tired or in pain.
- Maintain a healthy, well-balanced diet to keep muscles strong.
- Maintain a healthy weight.

- Practice safety measures to help prevent falls. For example, keep stairways, walkways, yards, and driveways free of clutter; anchor scatter rugs; and salt or sand icy sidewalks and driveways in the winter.

- Wear shoes that fit properly.

- Replace athletic shoes as soon as the tread wears out or the heel wears down on one side.

- Do stretching exercises daily.

- Be in proper physical condition to play a sport.

- Warm up and stretch before participating in any sport or exercise.

- Wear protective equipment when playing.

- Run on even surfaces.

Chapter 20

Sports Injuries

Chapter Contents

Section 20.1

Sports Injuries: An Overview

This section includes text excerpted from "Handout on Health: Sports
Injuries," National Institute of Arthritis and Musculoskeletal and
Skin Diseases (NIAMS), February 2016.

In recent years, increasing numbers of people of all ages have been
heeding their health professional's advice to get active for all of the
health benefits exercise has to offer. But for some people—particularly
those who overdo or who don't properly train or warm up—these benefits can come at a price: sports injuries.

Fortunately, most musculoskeletal sports injuries can be treated
effectively, and most people who suffer injuries can return to a sat-
isfying level of physical activity after an injury. Even better, many
sports injuries can be prevented if people take the proper precautions.

What Are Sports Injuries?

The term "sports injury," in the broadest sense, refers to the kinds
of injuries that most commonly occur during sports or exercise. Some
sports injuries result from accidents; others are due to poor training
practices, improper equipment, lack of conditioning, or insufficient
warm-up and stretching.

Following are some of the most common sports injuries.

- Muscle sprains and strains

- Tears of the ligaments that hold joints together

- Tears of the tendons that support joints and allow them to move

- Dislocated joints

- Fractured bones, including vertebrae

Sprains and Strains

A sprain is a stretch or tear of a ligament, the band of connective tissues that joins the end of one bone with another. Sprains are

caused by trauma such as a fall or blow to the body that knocks a joint out of position and, in the worst case, ruptures the supporting ligaments. Sprains can range from first degree (minimally stretched ligament) to third degree (a complete tear). Areas of the body most vulnerable to sprains are ankles, knees, and wrists. Signs of a sprain include varying degrees of tenderness or pain; bruising; inflammation; swelling; inability to move a limb or joint; or joint looseness, laxity, or instability.

A strain is a twist, pull, or tear of a muscle or tendon, a cord of tissue connecting muscle to bone. It is an acute, noncontact injury that results from overstretching or over-contraction. Symptoms of a strain include pain, muscle spasm, and loss of strength. Although it's hard to tell the difference between mild and moderate strains, severe strains not treated professionally can cause damage and loss of function.

Knee Injuries

Because of its complex structure and weight-bearing capacity, the knee is a commonly injured joint.

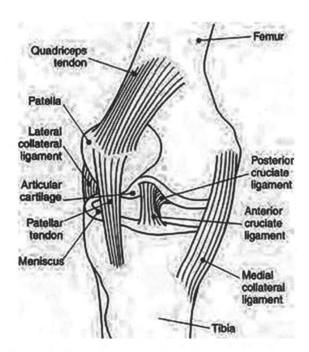

Figure 20.1. *Lateral View of the Knee*

Knee injuries can range from mild to severe. Some of the less severe, yet still painful and functionally limiting, knee problems are runner's knee (pain or tenderness close to or under the kneecap at the front or side of the knee), iliotibial band syndrome (pain on the outer side of the knee), and tendinitis, also called tendinosis (marked by degeneration within a tendon, usually where it joins the bone).

More severe injuries include bone bruises or damage to the cartilage or ligaments. There are two types of cartilage in the knee. One is the meniscus, a crescent-shaped disc that absorbs shock between the thigh (femur) and lower leg bones (tibia and fibula). The other is a surface-coating (or articular) cartilage. It covers the ends of the bones where they meet, allowing them to glide against one another. The four major ligaments that support the knee are the anterior cruciate ligament (ACL), the posterior cruciate ligament (PCL), the medial collateral ligament (MCL), and the lateral collateral ligament (LCL).

Knee injuries can result from a blow to or twist of the knee; from improper landing after a jump; or from running too hard, too much, or without proper warm-up.

Compartment Syndrome

In many parts of the body, muscles (along with the nerves and blood vessels that run alongside and through them) are enclosed in a "compartment" formed of a tough membrane called fascia. When muscles become swollen, they can fill the compartment to capacity, causing interference with nerves and blood vessels as well as damage to the muscles themselves. The resulting painful condition is referred to as compartment syndrome.

Compartment syndrome may be caused by a one-time traumatic injury (acute compartment syndrome), such as a fractured bone or a hard blow to the thigh, by repeated hard blows (depending upon the sport), or by ongoing overuse (chronic exertional compartment syndrome), which may occur, for example, in long-distance running.

Shin Splints

Although the term "shin splints" has been widely used to describe any sort of leg pain associated with exercise, the term actually refers to pain along the tibia or shin bone, the large bone in the front of the lower leg. This pain can occur at the front outside part of the lower leg, including the foot and ankle (anterior shin splints) or at the inner edge of the bone where it meets the calf muscles (medial shin splints).

Shin splints are primarily seen in runners, particularly those just starting a running program. Risk factors for shin splints include overuse or incorrect use of the lower leg; improper stretching, warm-up, or exercise technique; overtraining; running or jumping on hard surfaces; and running in shoes that don't have enough support. These injuries are often associated with flat (overpronated) feet.

Achilles Tendon Injuries

An Achilles tendon injury results from a stretch, tear, or irritation to the tendon connecting the calf muscle to the back of the heel. These injuries can be so sudden and agonizing that they have been known to bring down charging professional football players in shocking fashion.

The most common cause of Achilles tendon tears is a problem called tendinitis, a degenerative condition caused by aging or overuse. When a tendon is weakened, trauma can cause it to rupture.

Achilles tendon injuries are common in middle-aged "weekend warriors" who may not exercise regularly or take time to stretch properly before an activity. Among professional athletes, most Achilles injuries seem to occur in quick-acceleration, jumping sports like football and basketball, and almost always end the season's competition for the athlete.

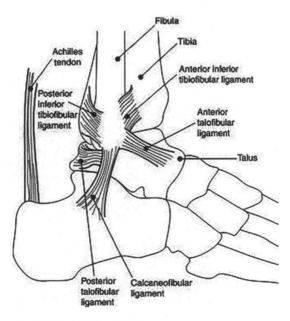

Figure 20.2. *Lateral View of the Ankle*

Fractures

A fracture is a break in the bone that can occur from either a quick, one-time injury to the bone (acute fracture) or from repeated stress to the bone over time (stress fracture).

Acute fractures. Acute fractures can be simple (a clean break with little damage to the surrounding tissue) or compound (a break in which the bone pierces the skin with little damage to the surrounding tissue). Most acute fractures are emergencies. One that breaks the skin is especially dangerous because there is a high risk of infection.

Stress fractures. Stress fractures occur largely in the feet and legs and are common in sports that require repetitive impact, primarily running/jumping sports such as gymnastics or track and field. Running creates forces two to three times a person's body weight on the lower limbs.

The most common symptom of a stress fracture is pain at the site that worsens with weight-bearing activity. Tenderness and swelling often accompany the pain.

Dislocations

When the two bones that come together to form a joint become separated, the joint is described as being dislocated. Contact sports such

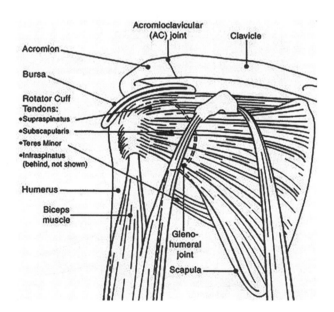

Figure 20.3. *The Shoulder Joint*

as football and basketball, as well as high-impact sports and sports that can result in excessive stretching or falling, cause the majority of dislocations. A dislocated joint is an emergency situation that requires medical treatment.

The joints most likely to be dislocated are some of the hand joints. Aside from these joints, the joint most frequently dislocated is the shoulder. Dislocations of the knees, hips, and elbows are uncommon.

What Is the Difference between Acute and Chronic Injuries?

Regardless of the specific structure affected, musculoskeletal sports injuries can generally be classified in one of two ways: acute or chronic.

Acute Injuries

Acute injuries, such as a sprained ankle, strained back, or fractured hand, occur suddenly during activity. Signs of an acute injury include the following:

- sudden, severe pain
- swelling
- inability to place weight on a lower limb
- extreme tenderness in an upper limb
- inability to move a joint through its full range of motion
- extreme limb weakness
- visible dislocation or break of a bone

Chronic Injuries

Chronic injuries usually result from overusing one area of the body while playing a sport or exercising over a long period. The following are signs of a chronic injury:

- pain when performing an activity
- a dull ache when at rest
- swelling

What Should I Do If I Suffer an Injury?

Whether an injury is acute or chronic, there is never a good reason to try to "work through" the pain of an injury. When you have pain from a particular movement or activity, STOP! Continuing the activity only causes further harm.

Some injuries require prompt medical attention, while others can be self-treated. Here's what you need to know about both types:

Seeking Medical Treatment

You should call a health professional if:

- The injury causes severe pain, swelling, or numbness.

- You can't tolerate any weight on the area.

- The pain or dull ache of an old injury is accompanied by increased swelling or joint abnormality or instability.

Treatment Steps to Follow at Home

If you don't have any of the above symptoms, it's probably safe to treat the injury at home—at least at first. If pain or other symptoms worsen, it's best to check with your healthcare provider. Use the RICE method to relieve pain and inflammation and speed healing. Follow these four steps immediately after injury and continue for at least 48 hours.

- **Rest**. Reduce regular exercise or activities of daily living as needed. If you cannot put weight on an ankle or knee, crutches may help. If you use a cane or one crutch for an ankle injury, use it on the uninjured side to help you lean away and relieve weight on the injured ankle.

- **Ice**. Apply an ice pack to the injured area for 20 minutes at a time, four to eight times a day. A cold pack, ice bag, or plastic bag filled with crushed ice and wrapped in a towel can be used. To avoid cold injury and frostbite, do not apply the ice for more than 20 minutes. (Note: Do not use heat immediately after an injury. This tends to increase internal bleeding or swelling. Heat can be used later on to relieve muscle tension and promote relaxation.)

- **Compression**. Compression of the injured area may help reduce swelling. Compression can be achieved with elastic wraps, special boots, air casts, and splints. Ask your healthcare provider for advice on which one to use.

- **Elevation**. If possible, keep the injured ankle, knee, elbow, or wrist elevated on a pillow, above the level of the heart, to help decrease swelling.

The Body's Healing Process

From the moment a bone breaks or a ligament tears, your body goes to work to repair the damage. Here's what happens at each stage of the healing process:

- **At the moment of injury.** Chemicals are released from damaged cells, triggering a process called inflammation. Blood vessels at the injury site become dilated; blood flow increases to carry nutrients to the site of tissue damage.

- **Within hours of injury.** White blood cells (leukocytes) travel down the bloodstream to the injury site where they begin to tear down and remove damaged tissue, allowing other specialized cells to start developing scar tissue.

- **Within days of injury.** Scar tissue is formed on the skin or inside the body. The amount of scarring may be proportional to the amount of swelling, inflammation, or bleeding within. In the next few weeks, the damaged area will regain a great deal of strength as scar tissue continues to form.

- **Within a month of injury.** Scar tissue may start to shrink, bringing damaged, torn, or separated tissues back together. However, it may be several months or more before the injury is completely healed.

Who Should I See for My Injury?

Although severe injuries will need to be seen immediately in an emergency room, particularly if they occur on the weekend or after office hours, most musculoskeletal sports injuries can be evaluated and, in many cases, treated by your primary healthcare provider.

Depending on your preference and the severity of your injury or the likelihood that your injury may cause ongoing, long-term problems, you may want to see, or have your primary healthcare professional refer you to, one of the following:

- An **orthopaedic surgeon** is a doctor specializing in the diagnosis and treatment of the musculoskeletal system, which includes bones, joints, ligaments, tendons, muscles, and nerves.

- A **physical therapist/physiotherapist** is a healthcare professional who can develop a rehabilitation program. Your primary care physician may refer you to a physical therapist after you begin to recover from your injury to help strengthen muscles and joints and prevent further injury.

How Are Sports Injuries Treated?

Although using the RICE technique described previously can be helpful for any sports injury, RICE is often just a starting point. Here are some other treatments your doctor or other healthcare provider may administer, recommend, or prescribe to help your injury heal.[1]

- Nonsteroidal Anti-Inflammatory Drugs (NSAIDs)
- Immobilization
  - Slings
  - Splints and casts
  - Leg immobilizers

Surgery

In some cases, surgery is needed to repair torn connective tissues or to realign bones with compound fractures. The vast majority of musculoskeletal sports injuries, however, do not require surgery.

Rehabilitation (Exercise)

A key part of rehabilitation from sports injuries is a graduated exercise program designed to return the injured body part to a normal level of function.

With most injuries, early mobilization—getting the part moving as soon as possible—will speed healing. Generally, early mobilization starts with gentle range-of-motion exercises and then moves on to stretching and strengthening exercises when you can without increasing pain. For example, if you have a sprained ankle, you may be able to work on range of motion for the first day or two after the sprain by gently tracing letters with your big toe. Once your range of motion is fairly good, you can start doing gentle stretching and strengthening exercises. When you are ready, weights may be added to your exercise routine to further strengthen the injured area. The key is to avoid movement that causes pain.

As damaged tissue heals, scar tissue forms, which shrinks and brings torn or separated tissues back together. As a result, the injury site becomes tight or stiff, and damaged tissues are at risk of reinjury. That's why stretching and strengthening exercises are so important. You should continue to stretch the muscles daily and as the first part of your warm-up before exercising.

When planning your rehabilitation program with a healthcare professional, remember that progression is the key principle. Start with just a few exercises, do them often, and then gradually increase how much you do. A complete rehabilitation program should include exercises for flexibility, endurance, and strength; instruction in balance and proper body mechanics related to the sport; and a planned return to full participation.

Throughout the rehabilitation process, avoid painful activities and concentrate on those exercises that will improve function in the injured part. Don't resume your sport until you are sure you can stretch the injured tissues without any pain, swelling, or restricted movement, and monitor any other symptoms. When you do return to your sport, start slowly and gradually build up to full participation. For more advice on how to prevent injuries as you return to active exercise.

Rest

Although it is important to get moving as soon as possible, you must also take time to rest following an injury. All injuries need time to heal; proper rest will help the process. Your healthcare professional can guide you regarding the proper balance between rest and rehabilitation.

Other Therapies

Other therapies used in rehabilitating sports injuries include:

- Cold/cryotherapy
- Heat/thermotherapy
- Ultrasound
- Massage

Most of these therapies are administered or supervised by a licensed healthcare professional.

Tips for Preventing Injury

Whether you've never had a sports injury and you're trying to keep it that way or you've had an injury and don't want another, the following tips can help.

- Avoid bending knees past 90 degrees when doing half knee bends.

- Avoid twisting knees by keeping feet as flat as possible during stretches.

- When jumping, land with your knees bent.

- Do warm-up exercises not just before vigorous activities like running, but also before less vigorous ones such as golf.

- Don't overdo.

- Do warm-up stretches before activity. Stretch the Achilles tendon, hamstring, and quadriceps areas and hold the positions. Don't bounce.

- Cool down following vigorous sports. For example, after a race, walk or walk/jog for 5 minutes so your pulse comes down gradually.

- Wear properly fitting shoes that provide shock absorption and stability.

- Use the softest exercise surface available, and avoid running on hard surfaces like asphalt and concrete. Run on flat surfaces. Running uphill may increase the stress on the Achilles tendon and the leg itself.

Section 20.2

Musculoskeletal Sports Injuries in Youth

This section includes text excerpted from "Preventing
Musculoskeletal Sports Injuries in Youth: A Guide for Parents,"
National Institute of Arthritis and Musculoskeletal and Skin
Diseases (NIAMS), September 2016.

Although sports participation provides numerous physical and social benefits, it also has a downside: the risk of sports-related injuries. According to the Centers for Disease Control and Prevention, more than 2.6 million children 0 to 19 years old are treated in the emergency department each year for sports and recreation-related injuries.

These injuries are by far the most common cause of musculoskeletal injuries in children treated in emergency departments. They are also the single most common cause of injury-related primary care office visits.

The Most Common Musculoskeletal Sports-Related Injuries in Kids

Although sports injuries can range from scrapes and bruises to serious brain and spinal cord injuries, most fall somewhere between the two extremes. Here are some of the more common types of injuries.

Sprains and Strains

A sprain is an injury to a ligament, one of the bands of tough, fibrous tissue that connects two or more bones at a joint and prevents excessive movement of the joint. An ankle sprain is the most common athletic injury.

A strain is an injury to either a muscle or a tendon. A muscle is a tissue composed of bundles of specialized cells that, when stimulated by nerve messages, contract and produce movement. A tendon is a tough, fibrous cord of tissue that connects muscle to bone. Muscles in any part of the body can be injured.

Growth Plate Injuries

In some sports accidents and injuries, the growth plate may be injured. The growth plate is the area of developing tissues at the end of the long bones in growing children and adolescents. When growth is complete, sometime during adolescence, the growth plate is replaced by solid bone. The long bones in the body include:

- the long bones of the hand and fingers (metacarpals and phalanges)

- both bones of the forearm (radius and ulna)

- the bone of the upper leg (femur)

- the lower leg bones (tibia and fibula)

- the foot bones (metatarsals and phalanges)

If any of these areas becomes injured, it's important to seek professional help from an orthopaedic surgeon, a doctor who specializes in bone injuries.

Repetitive Motion Injuries

Painful injuries such as stress fractures (a hairline fracture of the bone that has been subjected to repeated stress) and tendinitis (inflammation of a tendon) can occur from overuse of muscles and tendons. Some of these injuries don't always show up on X-rays, but they do cause pain and discomfort. The injured area usually responds to rest, ice, compression, and elevation (RICE). Other treatments can include crutches, cast immobilization, and physical therapy.

Preventing and Treating Musculoskeletal Injuries

Injuries can happen to any child who plays sports, but there are some things that can help prevent and treat injuries.

Prevention

- Enroll your child in organized sports through schools, community clubs, and recreation areas that are properly maintained. Any organized team activity should demonstrate a commitment to injury prevention. Coaches should be trained in first aid and cardiopulmonary resuscitation (CPR), and should have a plan for responding to emergencies. Coaches should be well versed in the proper use of equipment, and should enforce rules on equipment use.

- Organized sports programs may have adults on staff who are certified athletic trainers. These individuals are trained to prevent, recognize, and provide immediate care for athletic injuries.

- Make sure your child has—and consistently uses—proper gear for a particular sport. This may reduce the chances of being injured.

- Make warm-ups and cool-downs part of your child's routine before and after sports participation. Warm-up exercises make the body's tissues warmer and more flexible. Cool-down exercises loosen muscles that have tightened during exercise.

- Make sure your child has access to water or a sports drink while playing. Encourage him or her to drink frequently and stay properly hydrated. Remember to include sunscreen and a hat (when possible) to reduce the chance of sunburn, which is a type of injury to the skin. Sun protection may also decrease the chances of malignant melanoma—a potentially deadly skin cancer—or other skin cancers that can occur later in life.

- Learn and follow safety rules and suggestions for your child's particular sport. You'll find some more sport-specific safety suggestions below.

Treatment

- Treatment for sports-related injuries will vary by injury. But if your child suffers a soft tissue injury (such as a sprain or strain) or a bone injury, the best immediate treatment is easy to remember: RICE (rest, ice, compression, elevation) the injury. Get professional treatment if any injury is severe. A severe injury means having an obvious fracture or dislocation of a joint, prolonged swelling, or prolonged or severe pain.

Keep Kids Exercising

It's important that kids continue some type of regular exercise after the injury heals. Exercise may reduce their chances of obesity, which has become more common in children. It may also reduce the risk of diabetes, a disease that can be associated with a lack of exercise and poor eating habits. Exercise also helps build social skills and provides a general sense of well-being. Sports participation is an important part of learning how to build team skills.

As a parent, it is important for you to encourage your children to be physically active. It's also important to match your child to the sport, and not push him or her too hard into an activity that he or she may not like or be capable of doing. Teach your children to follow the rules and to play it safe when they get involved in sports, so they'll spend more time having fun in the game and be less likely to be sidelined with an injury. You should be mindful of the risks associated with different sports and take important measures to reduce the chance of injury.

Sport-Specific Safety Information

Here are some winning ways to help prevent an injury from occurring.

Basketball

- **Common injuries and locations.** Sprains, strains, bruises, fractures, scrapes, dislocations, cuts, injuries to teeth, ankles, and knees. (Injury rates are higher in girls, especially for the anterior cruciate ligament or ACL, the wide ligament that limits rotation and forward movement of the shin bone.)

- **Safest playing with.** Eye protection, elbow and knee pads, mouth guard, athletic supporters for males, proper shoes, water. If playing outdoors, wear sunscreen and, when possible, a hat.

- **Injury prevention.** Strength training (particularly knees and shoulders), aerobics (exercises that develop the strength and endurance of heart and lungs), warm-up exercises, proper coaching, use of safety equipment.

Track and Field

- **Common injuries.** Strains, sprains, scrapes from falls.

- **Safest playing with.** Proper shoes, athletic supporters for males, sunscreen, water.

- **Injury prevention.** Proper conditioning and coaching.

Football

- **Common injuries and locations.** Bruises, sprains, strains, pulled muscles, tears to soft tissues such as ligaments, broken bones, internal injuries (bruised or damaged organs), concussions, back injuries, sunburn. Knees and ankles are the most common injury sites.
- **Safest playing with.** Helmet, mouth guard, shoulder pads, athletic supporters for males, chest/rib pads, forearm, elbow, and thigh pads, shin guards, proper shoes, sunscreen, water.
- **Injury prevention.** Proper use of safety equipment, warm-up exercises, proper coaching techniques and conditioning.

Baseball and Softball

- **Common injuries.** Soft tissue strains, impact injuries that include fractures caused by sliding and being hit by a ball, sunburn.
- **Safest playing with.** Batting helmet; shin guards; elbow guards; athletic supporters for males; mouth guard; sunscreen; cleats; hat; detachable, "breakaway bases" rather than traditional, stationary ones.
- **Injury prevention.** Proper conditioning and warm-ups.

Soccer

- **Common injuries.** Bruises, cuts and scrapes, headaches, sunburn.
- **Safest playing with.** Shin guards, athletic supporters for males, cleats, sunscreen, water.
- **Injury prevention.** Aerobic conditioning and warm-ups, and—when age appropriate—proper training in "heading" (that is, using the head to strike or make a play with the ball).

Gymnastics

- **Common injuries.** Sprains and strains of soft tissues.
- **Safest playing with.** Athletic supporters for males, safety harness, joint supports (such as neoprene wraps), water.
- **Injury prevention.** Proper conditioning and warm-ups.

Treat Injuries with "RICE"

Rest. Reduce or stop using the injured area for at least 48 hours. If you have a leg injury, you may need to stay off of it completely.

Ice. Put an ice pack on the injured area for 20 minutes at a time, four to eight times per day. Use a cold pack, ice bag, or a plastic bag filled with crushed ice that has been wrapped in a towel.

Compression. Ask your child's doctor about elastics wraps, air casts, special boots, or splints that can be used to compress an injured ankle, knee, or wrist to reduce swelling.

Elevation. Keep the injured area elevated above the level of the heart to help decrease swelling. Use a pillow to help elevate an injured limb.

Play It Safe in the Heat

- Schedule regular fluid breaks during practice and games. Kids need to drink 8 ounces of fluid—preferably water—every 20 minutes, and more after playing.

- Have your child wear light-colored, "breathable" clothing.

- Make player substitutions more frequently in the heat.

- Use misting sprays on the body to keep cool.

- Know the signs of heat-related problems, including confusion; dilated pupils, dizziness, fainting; headache, heavy perspiration; nausea, pale and moist or hot, dry skin, weak pulse, and weakness. If your child experiences any combination of these symptoms or doesn't seem quite right, seek medical attention immediately.

Safety Tips for All Sports

- Be in proper physical condition to play the sport.

- Follow the rules of the sport.

- Wear appropriate protective gear (for example, shin guards for soccer, a hard-shell helmet when facing a baseball or softball pitcher, a helmet and body padding for ice hockey).

- Know how to use athletic equipment.

- Always warm up before playing.

- Avoid playing when very tired or in pain.

- Get a preseason physical examination.

- Make sure adequate water or other liquids are available to maintain proper hydration.

Section 20.3

Sports Injuries among Girls

This section includes text excerpted from "Avoiding Injuries," girlshealth.gov, Office on Women's Health (OWH), March 27, 2015.

Avoiding Knee Injuries

Knee injuries happen pretty often to young people. One of the most common knee injuries is a torn anterior cruciate ligament, called ACL for short. Teenage girls get these injuries a lot more than guys do. Why? Possibly because of the way girls' bodies are made or because of the way girls use them.

If you have a torn ACL, you might have one or all of the following symptoms:

- A "popping" sound at the time of the injury

- Pain

- Not being able to put weight on your knee

- Swelling

If you think you have any kind of injury to your knee, you should stop using it. Tell your parent or guardian right away (or, if you are at school, tell your coach or teacher). Treatment for a torn ACL may include surgery and physical therapy. Don't play again until your doctor says you can.

Your best bet is to try to prevent an ACL injury. Talk to your coach or gym teacher about what you can do. Special exercises can help build strength and flexibility, for example. You also can learn safer ways to do riskier movements, like making sure to bend your knees when you jump.

Protecting Your Bones

Your teenage years are the most important time for building strong bones. Physical activity, calcium, and vitamin D help build strong bones. Having strong bones can help prevent osteoporosis, which is a disease that can put you at risk for broken bones when you get older.

Sometimes, girls can develop osteoporosis when they're young. This doesn't happen very often. But it can happen if you get a lot of exercise from activities like competitive sports but you don't eat enough healthy food. Osteoporosis can ruin a female athlete's career because it may lead to frequent or serious injuries.

If you exercise a lot like in a competitive sport, make sure to eat a variety of healthy foods, including ones with calcium and vitamin D to protect your bones.

Not sure how much food you need? Every person is different, but generally teenage girls who are active for about an hour a day need between 2,000 and 2,400 calories every day. (For example, a 16-year-old girl who is a healthy weight and runs for an hour five days a week can eat around 2,200 calories each day.) Use the SuperTracker to get a personal plan with recommended calories and amounts of types of food to eat.

Do you do high-impact activities, like running or gymnastics? Vitamin D also may help lower your risk of getting tiny cracks in your bones, called stress fractures. You can do other things to help protect your bones from stress fractures, too. These include:

- Making sure to use the right equipment, like wearing running shoes for running

- Strengthening your muscles, so they can help protect your bones

- Taking a break from your high-impact activity at least one day each week

- Increasing how hard you work out only a little bit at a time

- Making sure to rest if you start to feel pain

Concussion and Girls

A concussion is a type of brain injury. It can happen when your head gets hit. But it also can happen when another part of your body gets hit in a way that the force goes all the way to your brain. Concussion is a possible risk for girls who play basketball, soccer, lacrosse, and other sports.

To lower the chances of getting a concussion, always make sure to follow any rules of your sport and to use the right equipment.

Symptoms of a concussion can happen right away or several hours later. They include:

- Headache

- Not being able to remember things well

- Feeling dazed, confused, or dizzy

- Nausea or vomiting

- Blurred vision

- Being sensitive to noise or light

- Having slurred speech or saying things that don't make sense

- Not being able to concentrate

- Feeling overly tired

- Passing out (but often a person with a concussion doesn't pass out)

Girls may have different concussion symptoms than boys. In a recent study, girls were more likely to feel drowsy and sensitive to noise. Those signs can be harder to notice than boys' symptoms, which most often were confusion and not remembering things.

If you get a concussion, you must rest your body and your mind. If you think you might have a concussion, you should stop playing right away. If you have a concussion, make sure to follow all your doctor's instructions for healing, even if you start to feel better. When can you play again? When a doctor or other licensed health professional trained in concussions says you can.

Safety and Team Sports

Team sports are fun and a great way to stay fit. One sport that has been growing in popularity—but also in riskiness—is cheerleading. Whatever your sport, remember to follow all the safety rules.

Things to Do If You've Had an Injury

It's very important to be careful about injuries. Make sure to:

- Stop doing the activity that you think caused the injury

- Tell your parents or guardian or your doctor if any of these happens:

    - You have pain that is very bad, gets worse, or lasts more than a few days

    - There is swelling where you got hurt

    - The pain gets in the way of your activities or sleep

    - Your injury is causing numbness

- Follow your doctor's instructions on how to care for your injury and deal with any pain

- Rest for as long as your doctor says and don't play again until your doctor gives you the okay, or you will risk not getting

Part Three

Other Pain-Related Injuries and Disorders

Chapter 21

Burns

Facts about Burns

What Is a Burn?

A burn is tissue damage caused by heat, chemicals, electricity, sunlight or nuclear radiation. The most common burns are those caused by scalds, building fires and flammable liquids and gases.

- **First-degree burns** affect only the outer layer (the epidermis) of the skin.

- **Second-degree burns** damage the epidermis and the layer beneath it (the dermis).

- **Third-degree burns** involve damage or complete destruction of the skin to its full depth and damage to underlying tissues.

How Does the Body React to a Severe Burn?

The swelling and blistering characteristic of burns is caused by the loss of fluid from damaged blood vessels. In severe cases, such fluid

This chapter contains text excerpted from the following sources: Text under the heading "Facts about Burns" is excerpted from "Burns Fact Sheet," National Institute of General Medical Sciences (NIGMS), April 6, 2016; Text under the heading "Burn Pain" is excerpted from "Burn Triage and Treatment—Thermal Injuries," Chemical Hazards Emergency Medical Management (CHEMM), U.S. Department of Health and Human Services (HHS), April 29, 2017.

loss can cause shock. Burns often lead to infection, due to damage to the skin's protective barrier.

How Are Burns Treated?

Over half of burn patients in the United States are treated in specialized burn centers, and most hospitals have trauma teams that care exclusively for patients with traumatic injuries that may accompany burns.

In many cases, topical antibiotics (skin creams or ointments) are used to prevent infection. For third-degree burns and some second-degree ones, immediate blood transfusion and/or extra fluids are needed to maintain blood pressure. Grafting with natural or artificial materials speeds the post-burn healing process.

What Is Skin Grafting?

There are two types of skin grafts. An autologous skin graft transfers skin from one part of the body to another while an allograft transfers skin from another person, sometimes even a cadaver. Scientists typically take cells from the epidermal layer of skin and then grow them into large sheets of cells in the laboratory. They do not yet know how to grow the lower, dermal layer of skin in the lab. For this reason, surgeons, after removing burned skin, first cover the area with an artificial material and then add the cell sheets on top. This procedure helps encourage the growth of new skin.

What Is the Prognosis for Severe Burn Victims?

A few decades ago, burns covering half the body were often fatal. Now, thanks to research, many people with burns covering 90 percent of their bodies can survive, although they often have permanent impairments and scars.

Burn Pain

- After a chemical mass casualty incident, trauma with or without burns is expected to be common.

- Burn therapy adds significant logistical requirements and complexity to the medical response in a chemical mass casualty incident.

- Burns complicating physical injury and/or chemical injury decrease the likelihood of survival.

- Healthcare providers with burn expertise are needed to optimize burn care.

Diagnosis of Burns

- A burn is the partial or complete destruction of skin caused by some form of energy, usually thermal energy.
- Burn severity is dictated by:
  - Percent total body surface area (TBSA) involvement
  - Burns >20–25% TBSA require IV fluid resuscitation
  - Burns >30–40% TBSA may be fatal without treatment
- In adults: "Rule of Nines" is used as a rough indicator of percent TBSA

Table 21.1. Rule of Nines for Establishing Extent of Body Surface Burned

Anatomic Surface	% of total body surface
Head and neck	9%
Anterior trunk	18%
Posterior trunk	18%
Arms, including hands	9% each
Legs, including feet	18% each
Genitalia	1%

- **In children,** adjust percents because they have proportionally larger heads (up to 20%) and smaller legs (13% in infants) than adults
- Lund—Browder diagrams improve the accuracy of the percent TBSA for children.
  - Palmar hand surface is approximately 1percent TBSA
  - Depth of burn injury (deeper burns are more severe)
- Superficial burns (first-degree and superficial second-degree burns)
- Deep burns (deep second-degree to fourth-degree burns)
- Age

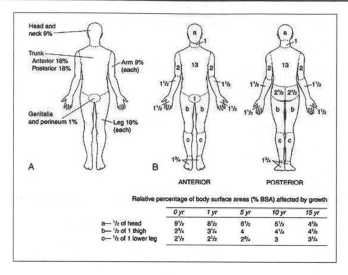

Figure 21.1. *Estimating Percent Total Body Surface Area in Children Affected by Burns*

(A) Rule of "nines"
(B) Lund-Browder diagram for estimating extent of burns

- Mortality for any given burn size increases with age
- Smoke inhalation injury
- Delay in resuscitation
- Need for escharotomies and fasciotomies
- Use of alcohol or drugs (especially methamphetamine)

Treatment

- All burn patients should initially be treated with the principles of Advanced Burn and/or Trauma Life Support
  - The ABC's (airway, breathing, circulation) of trauma take precedent over caring for the burn
  - Search for other signs of trauma
- Airway
  - Extensive burns may lead to massive edema
  - Obstruction may result from upper airway swelling

- Risk of upper airway obstruction increases with
- Signs of airway obstruction
- Tracheostomies not needed during resuscitation period
- Remember: Intubation can lead to complications, so do not intubate if not needed
- Breathing
  - Hypoxia
  - Carbon monoxide (CO)
  - Smoke inhalation injury
- Circulation
  - Obtain Intravenous (IV) access anywhere possible
  - Resuscitation in burn shock (first 24 hours)
  - Complications of over-resuscitation
- Wound Care
  - During initial or emergent care, wound care is of secondary importance
  - Advanced Burn Life Support recommendations
  - Skin grafting
- Medications
  - All pain meds should be given IV
  - Tetanus prophylaxis should be given as appropriate
  - Prophylactic antibiotics are contraindicated

Special Burns

- General information
  - Often require specialized care
  - Calling a verified burn center is advised
- Electrical injuries
  - Extent of injury may not be apparent
  - Cardiac arrhythmias may occur

- Myoglobinuria may be present
- Compartment syndromes are common
- Long-term neuro-psychiatric problems may result
- Chemical Burns
  - Brush off powder
  - Prolonged irrigation required
  - Do not seek antidote
  - Special chemical burns require contacting a verified burn center

Chapter 22

Cancer Pain

General Information about Cancer Pain

Pain is one of the most common symptoms in cancer patients. Pain can be caused by cancer, treatment for cancer, or a combination of factors. Tumors, surgery, intravenous chemotherapy, radiation therapy, targeted therapy, supportive care therapies such as bisphosphonates, and diagnostic procedures may cause you pain.

Younger patients are more likely to have cancer pain and pain flares than older patients. Patients with advanced cancer have more severe pain, and many cancer survivors have pain that continues after cancer treatment ends.

This chapter is about ways to control cancer pain in adults.

Pain control can improve your quality of life.

Pain can be controlled in most patients who have cancer. Although cancer pain cannot always be relieved completely, there are ways to lessen pain in most patients. Pain control can improve your quality of life all through your cancer treatment and after it ends.

Pain can be managed before, during, and after diagnostic and treatment procedures.

Many diagnostic and treatment procedures are painful. It helps to start pain control before the procedure begins. Some drugs may be

---

This chapter includes text excerpted from "Cancer Pain (PDQ®)—Patient Version," National Cancer Institute (NCI), September 23, 2016.

267

used to help you feel calm or fall asleep. Treatments such as imagery or relaxation can also help control pain and anxiety related to treatment. Knowing what will happen during the procedure and having a relative or friend stay with you may also help lower anxiety.

Different cancer treatments may cause specific types of pain.

Patients may have different types of pain depending on the treatments they receive, including:

- Spasms, stinging, and itching caused by intravenous chemotherapy.

- Mucositis (sores or inflammation in the mouth or other parts of the digestive system) caused by chemotherapy or targeted therapy.

- Skin pain, rash, or hand-foot syndrome (redness, tingling, or burning in the palms of the hands and/or the soles of feet) caused by chemotherapy or targeted therapy.

- Pain in joints and muscles throughout the body caused by paclitaxel or aromatase inhibitor therapy.

- Osteonecrosis of the jaw caused by bisphosphonates given for cancer that has spread to the bone.

- Pain syndromes caused by radiation, including mucositis, pain flares, and dermatitis.

Cancer pain may affect quality of life and ability to function even after treatment ends.

Pain that is severe or continues after cancer treatment ends increases the risk of anxiety and depression. Patients may be disabled by their pain, unable to work, or feel that they are losing support once their care moves from their oncology team back to their primary care team. Feelings of anxiety and depression can worsen cancer pain and make it harder to control.

Each patient needs a personal plan to control cancer pain.

Each person's diagnosis, cancer stage, response to pain, and personal likes and dislikes are different. For this reason, each patient needs a personal plan to control cancer pain. You, your family, and your healthcare team can work together to manage your pain. As part of your pain control plan, your healthcare provider can give you and your family members written instructions to control your pain at home. Find out who you should call if you have questions.

Assessment of Cancer Pain

You and your healthcare team work together to assess cancer pain.

It's important that the cause of the pain is found early and treated quickly. Your healthcare team will help you measure pain levels often, including at the following times:

- After starting cancer treatment
- When there is new pain
- After starting any type of pain treatment

To learn about your pain, the healthcare team will ask you to describe the pain with the following questions:

- When did the pain start?
- How long does the pain last?
- Where is the pain? You will be asked to show exactly where the pain is on your body or on a drawing of a body.
- How strong is the pain?
- Have there been changes in where or when the pain occurs?
- What makes the pain better or worse?
- Is the pain worse during certain times of the day or night?
- Is there breakthrough pain (intense pain that flares up quickly even when pain control medicine is being used)?
- Do you have symptoms, such as trouble sleeping, fatigue, depression, or anxiety?
- Does pain get in the way of activities of daily life, such as eating, bathing, or moving around?

Your healthcare team will also take into account:

- Past and current pain treatments
- Prognosis (chance of recovery)
- Other conditions you may have, such as kidney, liver, or heart disease
- Past and current use of nicotine, alcohol, or sleeping pills
- Personal or family history of substance abuse

- Personal history of childhood sexual abuse
- Your own choices

This information will be used to decide how to help relieve your pain. This may include drugs or other treatments. In some cases, patients are referred to pain specialists or palliative care specialists. Your healthcare team will work with you to decide whether the benefits of treatment outweigh any risks and how much improvement you should expect. After pain control is started, the doctor will continue to assess how well it is working for you and make changes if needed.

A family member or caregiver may be asked to give answers for a patient who has a problem with speech, language, or understanding.

Physical and neurological exams will be done to help plan pain control.

The following exams will be done:

- Physical exam and history.
- Neurological exam.

Your healthcare team will also assess your psychological, social, and spiritual needs.

Using Drugs to Control Cancer Pain

Your doctor will prescribe drugs to help relieve your pain. These drugs need to be taken at scheduled times to keep a constant level of the drug in the body to help keep the pain from coming back. Drugs may be taken by mouth or given in other ways, such as by infusion or injection.

Your doctor may prescribe extra doses of a drug that can be taken as needed for pain that occurs between scheduled doses of the drug. The doctor will adjust the drug dose for your needs.

A scale from 0 to 10 is used to measure how severe the pain is and decide which pain medicine to use. On this scale:

- 0 means no pain.
- 1 to 3 means mild pain.
- 4 to 6 means moderate pain.
- 7 to 10 means severe pain.

Acetaminophen and nonsteroidal anti-inflammatory drugs (NSAIDs) may be used to relieve mild pain.

Acetaminophen and NSAIDs help relieve mild pain. They may be given with opioids for moderate to severe pain.

Pain relievers of this type include:

- Acetaminophen

- Celecoxib

- Diclofenac

- Ibuprofen

- Ketoprofen

- Ketorolac

Patients, especially older patients, who are taking acetaminophen or NSAIDs need to be closely watched for side effects.

Opioids are used to relieve moderate to severe pain.

Opioids work very well to relieve moderate to severe pain. Some patients with cancer pain stop getting pain relief from opioids if they take them for a long time. This is called tolerance. Larger doses or a different opioid may be needed if your body stops responding to the same dose. Tolerance of an opioid is a physical dependence on it. This is not the same as addiction (psychological dependence).

Since 1999, there have been four times the number of prescriptions written for opioids and four times the number of deaths caused by drug overdose in the United States. Although most patients who are prescribed opioids for cancer pain use them safely, a small percentage of patients may become addicted to opioids. Your doctor will carefully prescribe and monitor your opioid doses so that you are treated for pain safely.

There are several types of opioids:

- Buprenorphine

- Codeine

- Diamorphine

- Fentanyl

- Hydrocodone

- Hydromorphone

- Methadone

- Morphine (the most commonly used opioid for cancer pain)

- Oxycodone

- Oxymorphone

- Tapentadol

- Tramadol

The doctor will prescribe drugs and the times they should be taken in order to best control your pain. Also, it is important that patients and family caregivers know how to safely use, store, and dispose of opioids.

Most patients with cancer pain will need to receive opioids on a regular schedule.

Receiving opioids on a regular schedule helps relieve the pain and keeps it from getting worse. The amount of time between doses depends on which opioid you are using. The correct dose is the amount of opioid that controls your pain with the fewest side effects. The dose will be slowly adjusted until there is a good balance between pain relief and side effects. If opioid tolerance does occur, the dose may be increased or a different opioid may be needed.

Opioids may be given in different ways.

Opioids may be given by the following ways:

- Mouth

- Rectum

- Skin patches

- Nose spray

- Intravenous (IV) line

- Subcutaneous injection

- Intraspinal injection

Other drugs may be added to help treat your pain.

Other drugs may be given while you are taking opioids for pain relief. These are drugs that help the opioids work better, treat symptoms, and relieve certain types of pain. The following types of drugs may be used:

- Antidepressants

- Anticonvulsants

- Local anesthetics

- Corticosteroids

- Stimulants

- Bisphosphonates and denosumab

There are big differences in how patients respond to these drugs. Side effects are common and should be reported to your doctor.

Bisphosphonates (pamidronate and zoledronic acid) are drugs that are sometimes used when cancer has spread to the bones. They are given as an intravenous infusion and combined with other treatments to decrease pain and reduce risk of broken bones. However, bisphosphonates sometimes cause severe side effects. Talk to your doctor if you have severe muscle or bone pain. Bisphosphonate therapy may need to be stopped.

The use of bisphosphonates is also linked to the risk of bisphosphonate-associated osteonecrosis (BON).

Denosumab is another drug that may be used when cancer has spread to the bones. It is given as a subcutaneous injection and may help prevent and relieve pain. It is not used in certain patients, such as patients with myeloma.

Chapter 23

Chest Pain

Chapter Contents

Section 23.1

Signs and Symptoms of a Heart Attack

This section includes text excerpted from "Heart Attack," National Heart, Lung, and Blood Institute (NHLBI), January 27, 2015.

What Is a Heart Attack?

A heart attack happens when the flow of oxygen-rich blood to a section of heart muscle suddenly becomes blocked and the heart can't get oxygen. If blood flow isn't restored quickly, the section of heart muscle begins to die.

Heart attack treatment works best when it's given right after symptoms occur. If you think you or someone else is having a heart attack, even if you're not sure, call 9–1–1 right away.

What Are the Symptoms of a Heart Attack?

Not all heart attacks begin with the sudden, crushing chest pain that often is shown on TV or in the movies. In one study, for example, one-third of the patients who had heart attacks had no chest pain. These patients were more likely to be older, female, or diabetic.

The symptoms of a heart attack can vary from person to person. Some people can have few symptoms and are surprised to learn they've had a heart attack. If you've already had a heart attack, your symptoms may not be the same for another one. It is important for you to know the most common symptoms of a heart attack and also remember these facts:

- Heart attacks can start slowly and cause only mild pain or discomfort. Symptoms can be mild or more intense and sudden. Symptoms also may come and go over several hours.

- People who have high blood sugar (diabetes) may have no symptoms or very mild ones.

- The most common symptom, in both men and women, is chest pain or discomfort.

- Women are somewhat more likely to have shortness of breath, nausea and vomiting, unusual tiredness (sometimes for days), and pain in the back, shoulders, and jaw.

Some people don't have symptoms at all. Heart attacks that occur without any symptoms or with very mild symptoms are called silent heart attacks.

Most Common Symptoms

The most common warning symptoms of a heart attack for both men and women are:

- Chest pain or discomfort
- Upper body discomfort
- Shortness of breath

The symptoms of angina can be similar to the symptoms of a heart attack. Angina is chest pain that occurs in people who have coronary heart disease, usually when they're active. Angina pain usually lasts for only a few minutes and goes away with rest.

Chest pain or discomfort that doesn't go away or changes from its usual pattern (for example, occurs more often or while you're resting) can be a sign of a heart attack.

All chest pain should be checked by a doctor.

Other Common Signs and Symptoms

Pay attention to these other possible symptoms of a heart attack:

- Breaking out in a cold sweat
- Feeling unusually tired for no reason, sometimes for days (especially if you are a woman)
- Nausea (feeling sick to the stomach) and vomiting
- Light-headedness or sudden dizziness
- Any sudden, new symptoms or a change in the pattern of symptoms you already have (for example, if your symptoms become stronger or last longer than usual)

Not everyone having a heart attack has typical symptoms. If you've already had a heart attack, your symptoms may not be the same for another one. However, some people may have a pattern of symptoms that recur.

The more signs and symptoms you have, the more likely it is that you're having a heart attack.

Quick Action Can Save Your Life

The signs and symptoms of a heart attack can develop suddenly. However, they also can develop slowly—sometimes within hours, days, or weeks of a heart attack.

Any time you think you might be having heart attack symptoms or a heart attack, don't ignore it or feel embarrassed to call for help. Call 9–1–1 for emergency medical care, even if you are not sure whether you're having a heart attack.

Section 23.2

Angina

This section includes text excerpted from "Angina,"
National Heart, Lung, and Blood Institute (NHLBI),
June 1, 2011. Reviewed June 2017.

What Is Angina?

Angina is chest pain or discomfort that occurs if an area of your heart muscle doesn't get enough oxygen-rich blood.

Angina may feel like pressure or squeezing in your chest. The pain also can occur in your shoulders, arms, neck, jaw, or back. Angina pain may even feel like indigestion.

Angina isn't a disease; it's a symptom of an underlying heart problem. Angina usually is a symptom of coronary heart disease (CHD).

CHD is the most common type of heart disease in adults. It occurs if a waxy substance called plaque builds up on the inner walls of your coronary arteries. These arteries carry oxygen-rich blood to your heart.

Plaque

Plaque narrows and stiffens the coronary arteries. This reduces the flow of oxygen-rich blood to the heart muscle, causing chest pain. Plaque buildup also makes it more likely that blood clots will form in your arteries. Blood clots can partially or completely block blood flow, which can cause a heart attack.

Angina also can be a symptom of coronary microvascular disease (MVD). This is heart disease that affects the heart's smallest coronary arteries. In coronary MVD, plaque doesn't create blockages in the arteries like it does in CHD.

Studies have shown that coronary MVD is more likely to affect women than men. Coronary MVD also is called cardiac syndrome X and nonobstructive CHD.

Types of Angina

The major types of angina are stable, unstable, variant (Prinzmetal's), and microvascular. Knowing how the types differ is important. This is because they have different symptoms and require different treatments.

Stable Angina

Stable angina is the most common type of angina. It occurs when the heart is working harder than usual. Stable angina has a regular pattern. ("Pattern" refers to how often the angina occurs, how severe it is, and what factors trigger it.)

If you have stable angina, you can learn its pattern and predict when the pain will occur. The pain usually goes away a few minutes after you rest or take your angina medicine.

Stable angina isn't a heart attack, but it suggests that a heart attack is more likely to happen in the future.

Unstable Angina

Unstable angina doesn't follow a pattern. It may occur more often and be more severe than stable angina. Unstable angina also can occur with or without physical exertion, and rest or medicine may not relieve the pain.

Unstable angina is very dangerous and requires emergency treatment. This type of angina is a sign that a heart attack may happen soon.

Variant (Prinzmetal's) Angina

Variant angina is rare. A spasm in a coronary artery causes this type of angina. Variant angina usually occurs while you're at rest, and the pain can be severe. It usually happens between midnight and early morning. Medicine can relieve this type of angina.

Microvascular Angina

Microvascular angina can be more severe and last longer than other types of angina. Medicine may not relieve this type of angina.

What Causes Angina?

Underlying Causes

Angina usually is a symptom of coronary heart disease (CHD). This means that the underlying causes of angina generally are the same as the underlying causes of CHD.

Research suggests that CHD starts when certain factors damage the inner layers of the coronary arteries. These factors include:

- Smoking

- High amounts of certain fats and cholesterol in the blood

- High blood pressure

- High amounts of sugar in the blood due to insulin resistance or diabetes

Plaque may begin to build up where the arteries are damaged. When plaque builds up in the arteries, the condition is called atherosclerosis.

Plaque narrows or blocks the arteries, reducing blood flow to the heart muscle. Some plaque is hard and stable and causes the arteries to become narrow and stiff. This can greatly reduce blood flow to the heart and cause angina.

Other plaque is soft and more likely to rupture (break open) and cause blood clots. Blood clots can partially or totally block the coronary arteries and cause angina or a heart attack.

Immediate Causes

Many factors can trigger angina pain, depending on the type of angina you have.

Stable Angina

Physical exertion is the most common trigger of stable angina. Severely narrowed arteries may allow enough blood to reach the heart when the demand for oxygen is low, such as when you're sitting.

However, with physical exertion—like walking up a hill or climbing stairs—the heart works harder and needs more oxygen.

Other triggers of stable angina include:

• Emotional stress

• Exposure to very hot or cold temperatures

• Heavy meals

• Smoking

Unstable Angina

Blood clots that partially or totally block an artery cause unstable angina.

If plaque in an artery ruptures, blood clots may form. This creates a blockage. A clot may grow large enough to completely block the artery and cause a heart attack.

Blood clots may form, partially dissolve, and later form again. Angina can occur each time a clot blocks an artery.

Variant Angina

A spasm in a coronary artery causes variant angina. The spasm causes the walls of the artery to tighten and narrow. Blood flow to the heart slows or stops. Variant angina can occur in people who have CHD and in those who don't.

The coronary arteries can spasm as a result of:

• Exposure to cold

• Emotional stress

• Medicines that tighten or narrow blood vessels

• Smoking

• Cocaine use

Microvascular Angina

This type of angina may be a symptom of coronary microvascular disease (MVD). Coronary MVD is heart disease that affects the heart's smallest coronary arteries.

Reduced blood flow in the small coronary arteries may cause microvascular angina. Plaque in the arteries, artery spasms, or damaged or diseased artery walls can reduce blood flow through the small coronary arteries.

Who Is at Risk for Angina?

Angina is a symptom of an underlying heart problem. It's usually a symptom of coronary heart disease (CHD), but it also can be a symptom of coronary microvascular disease (MVD). So, if you're at risk for CHD or coronary MVD, you're also at risk for angina.

The major risk factors for CHD and coronary MVD include:

- Unhealthy cholesterol levels.
- High blood pressure.
- Smoking.
- Insulin resistance or diabetes.
- Overweight or obesity.
- Metabolic syndrome.
- Lack of physical activity.
- Unhealthy diet.
- Older age. (The risk increases for men after 45 years of age and for women after 55 years of age.)
- Family history of early heart disease.

People sometimes think that because men have more heart attacks than women, men also suffer from angina more often. In fact, overall, angina occurs equally among men and women.

Microvascular angina, however, occurs more often in women. About 70 percent of the cases of microvascular angina occur in women around the time of menopause.

Unstable angina occurs more often in older adults. Variant angina is rare; it accounts for only about 2 out of 100 cases of angina. People who have variant angina often are younger than those who have other forms of angina.

What Are the Signs and Symptoms of Angina?

Pain and discomfort are the main symptoms of angina. Angina often is described as pressure, squeezing, burning, or tightness in the chest. The pain or discomfort usually starts behind the breastbone.

Pain from angina also can occur in the arms, shoulders, neck, jaw, throat, or back. The pain may feel like indigestion. Some people say that angina pain is hard to describe or that they can't tell exactly where the pain is coming from.

Signs and symptoms such as nausea (feeling sick to your stomach), fatigue (tiredness), shortness of breath, sweating, light-headedness, and weakness also may occur.

Women are more likely to feel discomfort in the neck, jaw, throat, abdomen, or back. Shortness of breath is more common in older people and those who have diabetes. Weakness, dizziness, and confusion can mask the signs and symptoms of angina in elderly people.

Symptoms also vary based on the type of angina you have.

Because angina has so many possible symptoms and causes, all chest pain should be checked by a doctor. Chest pain that lasts longer than a few minutes and isn't relieved by rest or angina medicine may be a sign of a heart attack. Call 9–1–1 right away.

Stable Angina

The pain or discomfort:

- Occurs when the heart must work harder, usually during physical exertion

- Doesn't come as a surprise, and episodes of pain tend to be alike

- Usually lasts a short time (5 minutes or less)

- Is relieved by rest or medicine

- May feel like gas or indigestion

- May feel like chest pain that spreads to the arms, back, or other areas

Unstable Angina

The pain or discomfort:

- Often occurs at rest, while sleeping at night, or with little physical exertion

- Comes as a surprise

- Is more severe and lasts longer than stable angina (as long as 30 minutes)

- Usually isn't relieved by rest or medicine

- May get worse over time
- May mean that a heart attack will happen soon

Variant Angina

The pain or discomfort:

- Usually occurs at rest and during the night or early morning hours
- Tends to be severe
- Is relieved by medicine

Microvascular Angina

The pain or discomfort:

- May be more severe and last longer than other types of angina pain
- May occur with shortness of breath, sleep problems, fatigue, and lack of energy
- Often is first noticed during routine daily activities and times of mental stress

How Is Angina Diagnosed?

The most important issues to address when you go to the doctor with chest pain are:

- What's causing the chest pain
- Whether you're having or are about to have a heart attack

Angina is a symptom of an underlying heart problem, usually coronary heart disease (CHD). The type of angina pain you have can be a sign of how severe the CHD is and whether it's likely to cause a heart attack.

If you have chest pain, your doctor will want to find out whether it's angina. He or she also will want to know whether the angina is stable or unstable. If it's unstable, you may need emergency medical treatment to try to prevent a heart attack.

To diagnose chest pain as stable or unstable angina, your doctor will do a physical exam, ask about your symptoms, and ask about your risk factors for and your family history of CHD or other heart diseases.

Your doctor also may ask questions about your symptoms, such as:

- What brings on the pain or discomfort and what relieves it?
- What does the pain or discomfort feel like (for example, heaviness or tightness)?
- How often does the pain occur?
- Where do you feel the pain or discomfort?
- How severe is the pain or discomfort?
- How long does the pain or discomfort last?

Diagnostic Tests and Procedures

If your doctor thinks that you have unstable angina or that your angina is related to a serious heart condition, he or she may recommend one or more tests.

- EKG (Electrocardiogram)
- Stress Testing
- Chest X-ray
- Coronary Angiography and Cardiac Catheterization
- Computed Tomography Angiography
- Blood Tests

How Is Angina Treated?

Treatments for angina include lifestyle changes, medicines, medical procedures, cardiac rehabilitation (rehab), and other therapies. The main goals of treatment are to:

- Reduce pain and discomfort and how often it occurs
- Prevent or lower your risk for heart attack and death by treating your underlying heart condition

Lifestyle changes and medicines may be the only treatments needed if your symptoms are mild and aren't getting worse. If lifestyle changes and medicines don't control angina, you may need medical procedures or cardiac rehab.

Unstable angina is an emergency condition that requires treatment in a hospital.

Lifestyle Changes

Making lifestyle changes can help prevent episodes of angina. You can:

- Slow down or take rest breaks if physical exertion triggers angina.

- Avoid large meals and rich foods that leave you feeling stuffed if heavy meals trigger angina.

- Try to avoid situations that make you upset or stressed if emotional stress triggers angina. Learn ways to handle stress that can't be avoided.

You also can make lifestyle changes that help lower your risk for coronary heart disease. One of the most important changes is to quit smoking. Smoking can damage and tighten blood vessels and raise your risk for CHD. Talk with your doctor about programs and products that can help you quit. Also, try to avoid secondhand smoke.

Medicines

Nitrates are the medicines most commonly used to treat angina. They relax and widen blood vessels. This allows more blood to flow to the heart, while reducing the heart's workload.

Nitroglycerin is the most commonly used nitrate for angina. Nitroglycerin that dissolves under your tongue or between your cheek and gum is used to relieve angina episodes.

Nitroglycerin pills and skin patches are used to prevent angina episodes. However, pills and skin patches act too slowly to relieve pain during an angina attack.

Other medicines also are used to treat angina, such as beta blockers, calcium channel blockers, ACE inhibitors, oral antiplatelet medicines, or anticoagulants (blood thinners). These medicines can help:

- Lower blood pressure and cholesterol levels

- Slow the heart rate

- Relax blood vessels

- Reduce strain on the heart

- Prevent blood clots from forming

People who have stable angina may be advised to get annual flu shots.

Medical Procedures

If lifestyle changes and medicines don't control angina, you may need a medical procedure to treat the underlying heart disease. Both angioplasty and coronary artery bypass grafting (CABG) are commonly used to treat heart disease.

Angioplasty opens blocked or narrowed coronary arteries. During angioplasty, a thin tube with a balloon or other device on the end is threaded through a blood vessel to the narrowed or blocked coronary artery.

Once in place, the balloon is inflated to push the plaque outward against the wall of the artery. This widens the artery and restores blood flow.

Angioplasty can improve blood flow to your heart and relieve chest pain. A small mesh tube called a stent usually is placed in the artery to help keep it open after the procedure.

During CABG, healthy arteries or veins taken from other areas in your body are used to bypass (that is, go around) your narrowed coronary arteries. Bypass surgery can improve blood flow to your heart, relieve chest pain, and possibly prevent a heart attack.

You will work with your doctor to decide which treatment is better for you.

Enhanced External Counterpulsation Therapy

Enhanced external counterpulsation (EECP) therapy is helpful for some people who have angina. Large cuffs, similar to blood pressure cuffs, are put on your legs. The cuffs are inflated and deflated in sync with your heartbeat.

EECP therapy improves the flow of oxygen-rich blood to your heart muscle and helps relieve angina. You typically get 35 one hour treatment sessions over a span of 7 weeks.

How Can Angina Be Prevented?

You can prevent or lower your risk for angina and heart disease by making lifestyle changes and treating related conditions.

Making Lifestyle Changes

Healthy lifestyle choices can help prevent or delay angina and heart disease. To adopt a healthy lifestyle, you can:

- Quit smoking and avoid secondhand smoke

- Avoid angina triggers

- Follow a healthy diet

- Be physically active

- Maintain a healthy weight

- Learn ways to handle stress and relax

- Take your medicines as your doctor prescribes

Treating Related Conditions

You also can help prevent or delay angina and heart disease by treating related conditions, such as high blood cholesterol, high blood pressure, diabetes, and overweight or obesity.

If you have one or more of these conditions, talk with your doctor about how to control them. Follow your treatment plan and take all of your medicines as your doctor prescribes.

Section 23.3

Tietze Syndrome

This section includes text excerpted from "Tietze Syndrome," Genetic and Rare Diseases Information Center (GARD), National Center for Advancing Translational Sciences (NCATS), February 13, 2017.

Tietze syndrome is an inflammatory condition characterized by chest pain and swelling of the cartilage around the ribs. Specifically, people with Tietze syndrome have swelling of the cartilage that joins the upper ribs to the breastbone. This is called the costochondral junction. Signs and symptoms of this condition usually develop in people who are under the age of 40. Symptoms include mild to severe chest pain that may extend into the arms and shoulders. The chest, shoulders, and arms may also have redness and warmth. In some cases, Tietze syndrome may resolve on its own without treatment, while other people experience patterns of pain followed by some relief of pain. Management for pain includes options such as minimizing physical activity, applying heat or ice as directed by your doctor, and taking pain medications and/or nonsteroidal anti-inflammatory drugs. Your doctor may also recommend seeing a chiropractor.

Of note, this syndrome is different from Tietz syndrome, which is characterized by profound hearing loss from birth, fair skin, and light-colored hair.

Symptoms of Tietze Syndrome

The signs and symptoms of Tietze syndrome usually develop before age 40. The most common symptom is mild to severe chest pain that may extend into the arms and shoulders. The onset of pain can be sudden or gradual and may worsen with coughing, sneezing, exercise, or quick movements such as opening or closing doors.

Tietze syndrome is characterized by swelling of the cartilage of the ribs, specifically one of the three ribs that are closest to the head. Most cases of Tietze syndrome have symptoms of pain on one side of the body only (unilateral) and affect only one rib. The affected joint is typically tender and swollen. While the pain associated with Tietze syndrome usually subsides after several weeks or months, the swelling may persist. Some people affected by Tietze syndrome have patterns of relapse and remission, meaning they experience periods of pain and periods when the pain subsides.

Causes of Tietze Syndrome

The exact underlying cause of Tietze syndrome is currently unknown. Some researchers have speculated that small injuries to the chest wall may contribute to the development of the condition. These small are known as microtraumas and are too small to cause damage that is noticeable from the outside, but they may cause damage or swelling to the ribs. These microtraumas could be caused by a sudden event such as a car accident or surgery or due to chronic small traumas such as those that might be caused by frequent coughing or vomiting.

Inheritance of Tietze Syndrome

Tietze syndrome is not thought to be inherited. Most cases occur sporadically in people with no family history of the condition.

Diagnosis of Tietze Syndrome

Tietze syndrome is a diagnosis of exclusion. This means that a diagnosis is made in people with chest pain and swelling of the cartilage that joins the upper ribs to the breastbone (costochondral junction).

First, however, other conditions with similar signs and symptoms must be ruled out. A thorough physical exam and various tests may be necessary to exclude other conditions. These tests may include an electrocardiogram to rule out any heart problems, as well as X-rays and computerized tomography (CT) scans. Magnetic resonance imaging (MRI) can show thickening and enlargement of the affected cartilage.

Treatment of Tietze Syndrome

In some individuals, the pain associated with Tietze syndrome resolves on its own without any treatment. Management options for others may include avoidance of strenuous activity, applying heat or ice as directed by your doctor, taking pain medications, and/or nonsteroidal anti-inflammatory drugs. Some people benefit from corticosteroid or lidocaine injections if the pain does not respond to any other treatment.

Prognosis of Tietze Syndrome

The long-term outlook for people with Tietze syndrome is generally good. Most people are not severely affected by this condition and life expectancy is normal.

Chapter 24

Dental and Facial Pain

Chapter Contents

291

Section 24.1

Burning Mouth Syndrome

This section includes text excerpted from
"Burning Mouth Syndrome," Genetic and Rare Diseases
Information Center (GARD), National Center for Advancing
Translational Sciences (NCATS), March 28, 2016.

Burning mouth syndrome (BMS) is characterized by long-lasting burning sensations of the mouth. The pain may affect the tongue, gums, lips, palate, throat, or the entire mouth. Burning mouth syndrome may be primary or secondary. Experts believe that the primary form may be caused by damage to the nerves that control pain and taste. The secondary form is caused by an underlying medical condition. In many cases, the underlying cause in unknown. Treatment depends on the symptoms present and aims to control them.

What Are the Symptoms of Burning Mouth Syndrome?

Symptoms of burning mouth syndrome may include severe burning or tingling in the mouth which may persist or come and go over the course of months to years. The tongue is usually affected, but the pain may also be in the lips, gums, palate, throat or whole mouth. The burning sensation may be absent in the morning and increase over the course of the day, start first thing in the morning and last all day, or come and go all day long. For many, the pain is reduced when eating or drinking. Other symptoms may include a sensation of dry mouth with increased thirst, a bitter or metallic taste, or loss of taste.

What Causes Burning Mouth Syndrome?

Burning mouth syndrome can be primary or secondary. Some research suggests that primary burning mouth syndrome is caused by damage to the nerves that control pain and taste. Secondary burning mouth syndrome is usually caused by an underlying medical condition.

Some of the problems that have been linked to secondary burning mouth syndrome include:

- **Dry mouth,** which can be caused by various medications or underlying health problems

- **Other oral conditions**, such as fungal infections, oral lichen planus, or geographic tongue

- **Nutritional deficiencies**, such as lack of iron, zinc, folic acid, thiamin, riboflavin, pyridoxine, and cobalamin

- **Dentures**, especially if they don't fit well and irritate the mouth

- **Allergies or reactions to foods**, additives, dyes or dental work

- **Certain medications**, in particular those for high blood pressure

- **Oral habits** such as tooth grinding, tongue thrusting, or biting of the tongue

- **Endocrine disorders**, such as diabetes or hypothyroidism

- **Excessive mouth irritation** which may result from over-brushing, use of abrasive toothpastes, overuse of mouth-washes, or drinking too many acidic drinks

- **Psychological factors**, such as anxiety, depression, or stress

For many people, the underlying cause of burning mouth syndrome cannot be identified.

How Might Burning Mouth Syndrome Be Treated?

If the underlying cause of burning mouth syndrome is determined, treatment is aimed at the triggering factor(s). If no cause can be found, treatment can be challenging. The following are potential therapies for burning mouth syndrome; it is strongly recommended that you work with your healthcare provider in determining which therapy is right for you.

- A lozenge-type form of the anticonvulsant medication clonazepam (Klonopin)

- Oral thrush medications

- Medications that block nerve pan

- Certain antidepressants

- B vitamins

- Cognitive behavioral therapy

- Special oral rinses or mouth washes

- Saliva replacement products

- Capsaicin

In addition to these medications, the following measures may be helpful in reducing symptoms of burning mouth syndrome:

- Sip water frequently

- Suck on ice chips

- Chew sugarless gum

- Avoid irritating substances like tobacco, hot or spicy foods, alcoholic beverages, mouthwashes that contain alcohol, and products high in acid, like citrus fruits and juices, as well as cinnamon or mint.

Section 24.2

Tooth Pain

Toothache

Causes of Toothaches

Toothaches are primarily caused by tooth decay, which may initially result in pain when eating sweet, cold, or hot food. Decay can irritate the tooth's pulp—the inner core of teeth that contains nerves and connective tissue—stimulating the nerves and resulting in pain. Other causes of toothache include infection, bleeding gums, tooth trauma, grinding teeth, abnormal bite, gum disease, and the emergence of new teeth (in babies and young children). Sinus problems, ear infections, temporomandibular joint disorders (TMJ/TMD), and tension in the facial muscles could also cause toothaches, generally accompanied by headaches. In some cases, pain surrounding the teeth and jaws could indicate an underlying heart disorder, such as angina.

Symptoms of a Toothache

Since toothache pain can be caused by a number of dental and medical conditions, the symptoms can only be diagnosed after a complete evaluation by a dentist. You may notice pus in the region of a toothache as a result of an abscess that is caused by an infection. An abscess could also be the result of gum disease, usually characterized by inflamed tissues and bleeding gums. Consult a dentist if you observe the following symptoms:

- Fever
- Difficulty breathing or swallowing
- Swelling in the region of a tooth
- Discharge of foul-tasting fluid
- Continuous pain

Alleviating Pain in an Emergency

It is important to consult a dentist for a toothache, since leaving the condition untreated might lead to serious complications later.

If you are unable to consult a dentist right away, the self-care procedure below may help provide temporary relief:

- Use warm water to rinse your mouth.
- Floss gently to remove food particles that are stuck in your teeth.
- Take on over-the-counter medication, such as ibuprofen or acetaminophen, for pain relief.
- Do not apply aspirin directly to the affected tooth, since this may burn the gum tissue.
- Apply an over-the-counter antiseptic with benzocaine to the tooth or gums for pain relief. Clove oil (eugenol) applied to the gums may also help numb the pain. Rub the oil directly on the surface or soak a cotton swab with the oil and apply it to the tooth.
- Apply cold compresses to the cheek to reduce pain and swelling.

How a Dentist Helps

A dentist will determine the location and cause of the tooth pain with an oral examination. He or she will look for redness, swelling, and other visible indications of the cause. And an X-ray exam will help the dentist confirm an impacted tooth, decay, bone disorder, or other problems.

Depending on the underlying cause, antibiotics and pain relievers are typically prescribed to improve the healing of the toothache.

An advanced infection at the time of examination may require extraction of the tooth or root-canal surgery, which involves removal of the infected pulp from within the teeth.

Preventing Tooth Pain

The best way to prevent tooth pain is to practice regular oral hygiene. Failure to brush and floss after meals significantly increases the risk of developing cavities and the resulting toothaches. Use the following tips to help prevent tooth pain:

- Brush at least twice a day, after meals and snacks.
- Floss daily to help prevent gum disease.
- Visit a dentist regularly for professional cleaning and an oral examination.

Hypersensitive Teeth

Causes of Sensitivity

If you experience a sharp, temporary pain on consuming hot coffee or ice cream, when breathing through the mouth, or when brushing or flossing, you may have a condition known as "sensitive teeth." Sensitive teeth can be caused by tooth decay, cracks in teeth, worn tooth enamel, exposed tooth roots, receding gums, periodontal disease, and overly aggressive brushing.

Symptoms of Sensitivity

The crowns of the teeth are covered by a strong protective layer of enamel. Below the gum line is a layer known as the cementum that covers the teeth and protects the root. Another layer called dentin covers the teeth underneath the enamel and the cementum. Dentin is less dense than enamel and cementum and has tubules that reach the core of the teeth. When the layers covering the dentin wear off, the tubules are exposed, allowing sensitivity to occur when hot or cold food stimulate the cells and nerves within the teeth. Periodontal disease—disease of the gums—may also lead to hyper-sensitive teeth. If left untreated, periodontal disease can result in the separation of gum tissue from the tooth leaving pockets for bacteria to invade. The layers of the tooth can then erode leaving the root exposed. Regular dental checkups are highly recommended for the prevention, detection, and early treatment of periodontal disease and other problems.

Treatment of Sensitivity

An evaluation by a dentist is essential to diagnose hypersensitivity and rule out other causes of tooth pain. Based on circumstances, a dentist might recommend the following:

- Desensitizing toothpaste
- Fluoride
- Bonding
- Surgical gum graft
- Root canal

Preventing Teeth Sensitivity

Proper oral hygiene is essential to avoid teeth sensitivity. Brush twice per day using a soft-bristled toothbrush and fluoridated toothpaste. Floss on a daily basis. Do not use extremely abrasive toothpaste, and avoid aggressive and excessive brushing and flossing. Talk to your dentist about a mouth guard if you grind your teeth. Tooth-grinding can fracture teeth and lead to sensitivity. Limit the intake of acidic foods and drinks, such as carbonated beverages, citrus fruits, yogurt, and wine. They can erode enamel over time and cause sensitivity. Use a straw to consume acidic liquids to prevent contact with teeth. After consuming acidic food and drinks, neutralize acidity levels in your mouth by drinking milk or water.

Do not brush immediately after consuming acidic substances because the acid softens the enamel, which could erode easily when brushing.

Cracked Teeth

Under the outer layer of enamel that surrounds the teeth, there is a hard layer of dentin. The dentin covers an inner core that is made of pulp. The pulp contains tissue, blood vessels, and nerves. When a tooth is cracked, chewing irritates the pulp and this causes pain. The pulp may become damaged to the extent that it does not heal completely. Extensive cracks may also lead to infection of the pulp, which can spread to the bone and gums. It can sometimes be difficult to breathe cold air or consume hot or cold food with a cracked tooth. Bite on a clean piece of moist gauze to relieve the pain until you reach the dentist's office. Do not apply aspirin to tooth surfaces to relieve pain. It could cause burns.

Symptoms

Cracked teeth often cause erratic pain when chewing, when releasing pressure after biting, or when teeth are exposed to extremes in temperature. The pain may be intermittent, so a dentist may have difficulty determining which tooth is affected. It may be wise to consult an endodontist, a specialist in treating dental pulp, if you experience the symptoms of a cracked tooth.

Treatment

The treatment for cracked teeth depends on the location and the type of damage that has occurred. Do not delay seeing a dentist. With proper treatment cracked teeth can often be repaired to restore normal function.

Craze lines. Tiny cracks on the outer enamel of the teeth generally don't require treatment. They are very common and do not usually cause pain.

Chipped teeth. Chipped teeth are a common result of dental injuries. Chips can often be reattached or bonded with a tooth-colored filling. A crown can also be set over the tooth, if necessary.

Fractured cusp. The surface of a tooth may break off—often around a filling—and result in a fractured cusp. The fracture does not damage the pulp in most cases and does not usually cause pain. Treatments for the condition generally include fillings and crowns.

Vertical crack. In a vertically cracked tooth, the crack extends from the chewing surface down to the root. The tooth may not be broken, but the crack can eventually spread. Early diagnosis is necessary in order to save the tooth in such cases. If the crack does not extend to the pulp, root-canal surgery can save the tooth, but if the crack extends below the gum line, the tooth will likely need to be extracted.

Split tooth. A cracked tooth may progress in time into a split tooth, one that has separate segments that can divide into two portions. A split tooth generally cannot be saved fully, but proper endodontic treatment may be able to save part of it. An examination to evaluate the extent of damage will determine how much of the tooth can be saved.

Vertical root fracture. This is a fracture on the tooth that extends from the root upwards to the chewing surface. Symptoms and signs are usually minimal and might not be immediately noticeable. Such fractures are most often detected when the bone and gum near the site get infected. Treatment often involve extraction of the tooth, but endodontic treatment may help in retaining a portion of the tooth.

Healing

Broken teeth do not heal like broken bone. Cracked teeth may worsen and break off in spite of treatment, resulting in loss of teeth. A crown could provide maximum protection but is not appropriate in all cases. The specific kind of treatment you receive is important, because with proper intervention cracked teeth can be repaired to provide years of normal chewing function. Consult an endodontist to benefit from the best intervention in your case.

Prevention

You may not be able to prevent cracked teeth entirely, but here are some steps you can take to help make your teeth less vulnerable to cracks:

- Do not chew on very hard food substances, like ice or unpopped popcorn kernels. And don't make a habit of chewing on hard objects, such as pens.
- Try not to clench or grind your teeth.
- If you clench or grind your teeth while sleeping, talk to your dentist about a retainer or a mouth guard.
- When playing contact sports, wear a mouth guard or protective mask.

Tooth Abscess

A tooth abscess is a pus deposit caused by bacterial infection. Abscesses can occur in any region of the tooth for a number of different reasons. A periodontal abscess usually occurs in the gums next to a decayed root. Periapical abscesses form at the tip of a tooth's root, usually due to an untreated cavity or previous dental work. A dentist will drain the pus and treat the infection with medication. In order to save the tooth, a root-canal procedure might be necessary, but in some cases the tooth may need to be extracted. It is risky to leave a tooth abscess untreated, since it can lead to life-threatening complications.

Symptoms

Some of the symptoms of a tooth abscess include:

* Severe and persistent throbbing pain radiating to the neck or ear.

* Sensitivity to heat and cold.

* Sensitivity to pressure when biting or chewing.

* Fever, chills, nausea, or vomiting.

* Swelling in the face or cheek.

* Tender and swollen lymph nodes in the face or neck.

* Foul smelling and tasting salty fluid in the mouth.

When to Consult a Dentist

When the above symptoms occur, you must consult a dentist immediately. If you have swelling in the face accompanied by fever and you cannot reach a dentist, go to an emergency room. Difficulty in breathing or swallowing indicates that the infection is advanced and has spread further into the jaws and other regions of the body.

Risk Factors

The risk of developing a tooth abscess is significantly increased with poor oral hygiene. Failing to brush and floss regularly can not only result in tooth decay and gum disease, but may also invite bacteria that could lead to abscesses and their serious complications. The risk of abscesses is also increased by a high-sugar diet. The regular consumption of sweets and sugary carbonated beverages can result in cavities that might later develop into abscesses.

Complications

Although a rupture in a tooth abscess may reduce pain significantly, it is essential to seek medical treatment. The pus may not drain completely, or the infection may spread to other areas of the body, like the neck or the head. Sepsis—a life-threatening condition—may develop if an abscess is left untreated and allowed to proliferate. And a weakened immune system could spread the infection from a tooth abscess even more quickly.

Diagnosis

- **Dental examination.** A dentist will first make a thorough oral examination to confirm a tooth abscess.
- **Tapping the teeth.** An abscess is usually present at the tip of the root, and a slight tap will induce pain.
- **X-ray.** An X-ray will confirm the presence of an abscess and allow the dentist to evaluate the spread of the infection.
- **CT scan.** If the abscess has spread, a CT scan will help the dentist determine the extent of infection.

Treatment

These are some of the procedures a dentist will likely follow to treat a tooth abscess:

- **Drain the abscess.** The dentist will make an incision in the abscess, drain the pus, then wash the area with saline.
- **Root canal.** A root canal can treat infection and help save a tooth. The dentist drills into the tooth and removes the pulp. The empty chamber is then filled inert material and sealed. Finally, a crown may be set on the tooth for protection.
- **Tooth extraction.** If the tooth cannot be saved, the dentist will extract the tooth and treat the abscess by draining it and treating the infection.
- **Prescribing antibiotics.** An infection that is limited to the area of the abscess may not require antibiotics, but a dentist will

recommend antibiotics if the infection has spread to adjoining areas. Antibiotics will also be prescribed if you have a weakened immune system.

Phantom Tooth Pain

Phantom pain—also called atypical facial pain, neuropathic orofacial pain, or atypical odontalgia—presents as pain in a tooth or teeth without a specific cause. It usually begins after an extraction or following an endodontic procedure, and in time the pain can spread to other parts of the face. The pain is termed atypical because it is dissimilar to normal tooth pain. Typical pain comes and goes and is aggravated by biting or chewing or by touch and pressure. It can be attributed to identifiable causes, such as decay, periodontal disease, or injury. Treatment usually relieves the pain. Phantom pain, on the other hand, is a throbbing and constant pain at the site of an extraction or root canal that is not affected by hot or cold food substances or by biting or chewing. Local anesthetics and other pain treatments may or may not provide relief, and the intensity of pain may vary from mild to severe. This presents an inexplicable situation to the dentist who might attempt more treatment that provides no symptomatic improvement.

Causes

Since the causes of phantom tooth pain remain unclear, it is termed "idiopathic." It is more common in women than in men, and it tends to occur more often in middle-aged and older people. Research has found a link between anxiety and depression and phantom tooth pain, but the association remains unclear. Phantom tooth pain is a dysfunction or short-circuiting of the nerves that carry sensations from the teeth and jaw to the brain. Molecular or biochemical changes have been observed in areas of the brain that process pain, which could be the cause of the phantom pain.

Treatment

Dental treatment usually doesn't alleviate phantom tooth pain. It may lessen the severity, but it often returns. This is because the pain is a result of a dysfunction of the brain and nerves that process pain.

Phantom tooth pain is treated using a variety of medications, most commonly tricyclic antidepressants, such as amitriptyline, which in this case are prescribed for their pain-relieving properties, rather than their antidepressant benefits. Medicines prescribed for chronic pain conditions, such as gabapentin, baclofen, and duloxetine, are also often prescribed. This treatment reduces the pain but may not eliminate it completely. Phantom tooth pain may or may not be a permanent condition, but in some cases the symptoms disappear after a length of time or with prolonged treatment. Sometimes the pain persists and may require lifelong medication. Phantom tooth pain is a rare condition, and some dentists may not be familiar with its diagnosis and treatment. It is best to consult a dentist with an advanced specialization, such as oral medicine or orofacial pain.

References

1. "Sensitive Teeth: Causes and Treatment," American Dental Association, December 2003.

2. Carr, Alan. "What Causes Sensitive Teeth, and How Can I Treat Them?" Mayo Clinic, December 6, 2014.

3. "What Causes a Toothache?" Delta Dental, June 2010.

4. "Tooth Abscess," Mayo Clinic, February 16, 2016.

5. Falace, D. "Atypical Odontalgia," American Academy of Oral Medicine, January 22, 2015.

6. "Cracked Teeth," American Association of Endodontists, n.d.

Section 24.3

Temporomandibular Joint Disorders

This section includes text excerpted from "TMJ Disorders," National Institute of Dental and Craniofacial Research (NIDCR), April 2015.

Temporomandibular joint and muscle disorders, commonly called "TMJ," are a group of conditions that cause pain and dysfunction in the jaw joint and the muscles that control jaw movement. Healthcare professionals don't know for certain how many people have TMJ disorders, but some estimates suggest that over 10 million Americans are affected. The condition appears to be more common in women than men.

For most people, pain in the area of the jaw joint or muscles does not signal a serious problem. Generally, discomfort from these conditions is occasional and temporary, often occurring in cycles. The pain eventually goes away with little or no treatment. Some people, however, develop significant, long-term symptoms.

If you have questions about TMJ disorders, you are not alone. Researchers, too, are looking for answers to what causes these conditions and what the best treatments are. Until the healthcare professionals have scientific evidence for safe and effective treatments, it's important to avoid, when possible, procedures that can cause permanent changes in your bite or jaw. This section provides information you should know if you have been told by a dentist or physician that you have a TMJ disorder.

What Is the Temporomandibular Joint?

The temporomandibular joint connects the lower jaw, called the mandible, to the bone at the side of the head—the temporal bone. If you place your fingers just in front of your ears and open your mouth, you can feel the joints. Because these joints are flexible, the jaw can move smoothly up and down and side to side, enabling us to talk, chew and yawn. Muscles attached to and surrounding the jaw joint control its position and movement.

When we open our mouths, the rounded ends of the lower jaw, called condyles, glide along the joint socket of the temporal bone. The condyles slide back to their original position when we close our mouths. To keep this motion smooth, a soft disc lies between the condyle and the temporal bone. This disc absorbs shocks to the jaw joint from chewing and other movements.

The temporomandibular joint is different from the body's other joints. The combination of hinge and sliding motions makes this joint among the most complicated in the body. Also, the tissues that make up the temporomandibular joint differ from other load-bearing joints, like the knee or hip. Because of its complex movement and unique makeup, the jaw joint and its controlling muscles can pose a tremendous challenge to both patients and healthcare providers when problems arise.

What Are TMJ Disorders?

Disorders of the jaw joint and chewing muscles—and how people respond to them—vary widely. Researchers generally agree that the conditions fall into three main categories:

1. Myofascial pain involves discomfort or pain in the muscles that control jaw function.

2. Internal derangement of the joint involves a displaced disc, dislocated jaw, or injury to the condyle.

3. Arthritis refers to a group of degenerative/inflammatory joint disorders that can affect the temporomandibular joint.

A person may have one or more of these conditions at the same time. Some people have other health problems that co-exist with TMJ disorders, such as chronic fatigue syndrome, sleep disturbances or fibromyalgia, a painful condition that affects muscles and other soft tissues throughout the body. These disorders share some common symptoms, which suggests that they may share similar underlying mechanisms of disease. However, it is not known whether they have a common cause.

Rheumatic disease, such as arthritis, may also affect the temporomandibular joint as a secondary condition. Rheumatic diseases refer to a large group of disorders that cause pain, inflammation, and stiffness in the joints, muscles, and bone. Arthritis and some TMJ disorders involve inflammation of the tissues that line the joints. The exact relationship between these conditions is not known.

How jaw joint and muscle disorders progress is not clear. Symptoms worsen and ease over time, but what causes these changes is not known. Most people have relatively mild forms of the disorder. Their symptoms improve significantly, or disappear spontaneously, within weeks or months. For others, the condition causes long-term, persistent and debilitating pain.

What Causes TMJ Disorders?

Trauma to the jaw or temporomandibular joint plays a role in some TMJ disorders. But for most jaw joint and muscle problems, scientists don't know the causes. Because the condition is more common in women than in men, scientists are exploring a possible link between female hormones and TMJ disorders.

For many people, symptoms seem to start without obvious reason. Research disputes the popular belief that a bad bite or orthodontic braces can trigger TMJ disorders.

There is no scientific proof that sounds—such as clicking—in the jaw joint lead to serious problems. In fact, jaw sounds are common in the general population. Jaw noises alone, without pain or limited jaw movement, do not indicate a TMJ disorder and do not warrant treatment.

What Are the Signs and Symptoms?

A variety of symptoms may be linked to TMJ disorders. Pain, particularly in the chewing muscles and/or jaw joint, is the most common symptom. Other likely symptoms include:

- radiating pain in the face, jaw, or neck,

- jaw muscle stiffness,

- limited movement or locking of the jaw,

- painful clicking, popping or grating in the jaw joint when opening or closing the mouth,

- a change in the way the upper and lower teeth fit together.

How Are TMJ Disorders Diagnosed?

There is no widely accepted, standard test now available to correctly diagnose TMJ disorders. Because the exact causes and symptoms are not clear, identifying these disorders can be difficult and confusing. Currently, healthcare providers note the patient's description of symptoms, take a detailed medical and dental history, and examine problem areas, including the head, neck, face, and jaw. Imaging studies may also be recommended.

You may want to consult your doctor to rule out other known causes of pain. Facial pain can be a symptom of many conditions, such as sinus or ear infections, various types of headaches, and facial neuralgias (nerve-related facial pain). Ruling out these problems first helps in identifying TMJ disorders.

How Are TMJ Disorders Treated?

Because more studies are needed on the safety and effectiveness of most treatments for jaw joint and muscle disorders, experts strongly recommend using the most conservative, reversible treatments possible. Conservative treatments do not invade the tissues of the face, jaw, or joint, or involve surgery. Reversible treatments do not cause permanent changes in the structure or position of the jaw or teeth. Even when TMJ disorders have become persistent, most patients still do not need aggressive types of treatment.

Conservative Treatments

Because the most common jaw joint and muscle problems are temporary and do not get worse, simple treatment may be all that is necessary to relieve discomfort.

Self-Care Practices

There are steps you can take that may be helpful in easing symptoms, such as:

- eating soft foods,

- applying ice packs,

- avoiding extreme jaw movements (such as wide yawning, loud singing, and gum chewing),

- learning techniques for relaxing and reducing stress,

- practicing gentle jaw stretching and relaxing exercises that may help increase jaw movement. Your healthcare provider or a physical therapist can recommend exercises if appropriate for your particular condition.

Pain Medications

For many people with TMJ disorders, short-term use of over-the-counter pain medicines or nonsteroidal anti-inflammatory drugs (NSAIDs), such as ibuprofen, may provide temporary relief from jaw discomfort. When necessary, your dentist or physician can prescribe stronger pain or anti-inflammatory medications, muscle relaxants, or antidepressants to help ease symptoms.

Stabilization Splints

Your physician or dentist may recommend an oral appliance, also called a stabilization splint or bite guard, which is a plastic guard that fits over the upper or lower teeth. Stabilization splints are the most widely used treatments for TMJ disorders. Studies of their effectiveness in providing pain relief, however, have been inconclusive. If a stabilization splint is recommended, it should be used only for a short time and should not cause permanent changes in the bite. If a splint causes or increases pain, or affects your bite, stop using it and see your healthcare provider.

The conservative, reversible treatments described are useful for temporary relief of pain and they are not cures for TMJ disorders. If symptoms continue over time, come back often, or worsen, tell your doctor.

Botox

Botox® (botulinum toxin type A) is a drug made from the same bacterium that causes food poisoning. Used in small doses, Botox injections can actually help alleviate some health problems and have been approved by the U.S. Food and Drug Administration (FDA) for certain disorders. However, Botox is currently not approved by the FDA for use in TMJ disorders.

Results from recent clinical studies are inconclusive regarding the effectiveness of Botox for treatment of chronic TMJ disorders. Additional research is underway to learn how Botox specifically affects jaw muscles and their nerves. The findings will help determine if this drug may be useful in treating TMJ disorders.

Irreversible Treatments

Irreversible treatments that have not been proven to be effective— and may make the problem worse—include orthodontics to change the bite; crown and bridge work to balance the bite; grinding down teeth to bring the bite into balance, called "occlusal adjustment"; and repositioning splints, also called orthotics, which permanently alter the bite.

Surgery

Other types of treatments, such as surgical procedures, invade the tissues. Surgical treatments are controversial, often irreversible, and should be avoided where possible. There have been no long-term clinical trials to study the safety and effectiveness of surgical treatments for TMJ disorders. Nor are there standards to identify people who would most likely benefit from surgery. Failure to respond to conservative treatments, for example, does not automatically mean that surgery is necessary. If surgery is recommended, be sure to have the doctor explain to you, in words you can understand, the reason for the treatment, the risks involved, and other types of treatment that may be available.

Implants

Surgical replacement of jaw joints with artificial implants may cause severe pain and permanent jaw damage. Some of these devices may fail to function properly or may break apart in the jaw over time. If you have already had temporomandibular joint surgery, be very cautious about considering additional operations. Persons undergoing multiple surgeries on the jaw joint generally have a poor outlook for normal, pain-free joint function. Before undergoing any surgery on the jaw joint, it is extremely important to get other independent opinions and to fully understand the risks.

The U.S. Food and Drug Administration (FDA) monitors the safety and effectiveness of medical devices implanted in the body, including artificial jaw joint implants. Patients and their healthcare providers can report serious problems with TMJ implants to the FDA through MedWatch at www.fda.gov/medwatch or telephone toll-free at 1-800-332-1088.

Section 24.4

Trigeminal Neuralgia

This section includes text excerpted from "Trigeminal Neuralgia Fact Sheet," National Institute of Neurological Disorders and Stroke (NINDS), June 2013. Reviewed June 2017.

Trigeminal neuralgia (TN), also called tic douloureux, is a chronic pain condition that affects the trigeminal or 5th cranial nerve, one of the most widely distributed nerves in the head. TN is a form of neuropathic pain (pain associated with nerve injury or nerve lesion.) The typical or "classic" form of the disorder (called "Type 1" or TN1) causes extreme, sporadic, sudden burning or shock-like facial pain that lasts anywhere from a few seconds to as long as two minutes per episode. These attacks can occur in quick succession, in volleys lasting as long as two hours. The "atypical" form of the disorder (called "Type 2" or TN2), is characterized by constant aching, burning, stabbing pain of somewhat lower intensity than Type 1. Both forms of pain may occur in the same person, sometimes at the same time. The intensity of pain can be physically and mentally incapacitating.

The trigeminal nerve is one of 12 pairs of nerves that are attached to the brain. The nerve has three branches that conduct sensations from the upper, middle, and lower portions of the face, as well as the oral cavity, to the brain. The ophthalmic, or upper, branch supplies sensation to most of the scalp, forehead, and front of the head. The maxillary, or middle, branch stimulates the cheek, upper jaw, top lip, teeth and gums, and to the side of the nose. The mandibular, or lower, branch supplies nerves to the lower jaw, teeth and gums, and bottom lip. More than one nerve branch can be affected by the disorder. Rarely, both sides of the face may be affected at different times in an individual, or even more rarely at the same time (called bilateral TN).

What Causes Trigeminal Neuralgia (TN)?

TN is associated with a variety of conditions. TN can be caused by a blood vessel pressing on the trigeminal nerve as it exits the brainstem. This compression causes the wearing away or damage to the protective coating around the nerve (the myelin sheath). TN symptoms can also occur in people with multiple sclerosis, a disease that causes deterioration of the trigeminal nerve's myelin sheath. Rarely, symptoms of TN may be caused by nerve compression from a tumor, or a tangle of arteries and veins called an arteriovenous malformation. Injury to the trigeminal nerve (perhaps the result of sinus surgery, oral surgery, stroke, or facial trauma) may also produce neuropathic facial pain.

What Are the Symptoms of TN?

Pain varies, depending on the type of TN, and may range from sudden, severe, and stabbing to a more constant, aching, burning sensation. The intense flashes of pain can be triggered by vibration or contact with the cheek (such as when shaving, washing the face, or applying makeup), brushing teeth, eating, drinking, talking, or being exposed to the wind. The pain may affect a small area of the face or may spread. Bouts of pain rarely occur at night, when the affected individual is sleeping.

TN is typified by attacks that stop for a period of time and then return, but the condition can be progressive. The attacks often worsen over time, with fewer and shorter pain-free periods before they recur. Eventually, the pain-free intervals disappear and medication to control the pain becomes less effective. The disorder is not fatal, but can be debilitating. Due to the intensity of the pain, some individuals may avoid daily activities or social contacts because they fear an impending attack.

Who Is Affected?

Trigeminal neuralgia occurs most often in people over age 50, although it can occur at any age, including infancy. The possibility of TN being caused by multiple sclerosis increases when it occurs in young adults. The incidence of new cases is approximately 12 per 100,000 people per year; the disorder is more common in women than in men.

How Is TN Diagnosed?

TN diagnosis is based primarily on the person's history and description of symptoms, along with results from physical and neurological examinations. Other disorders that cause facial pain should be ruled out before TN is diagnosed. Some disorders that cause facial pain include post-herpetic neuralgia (nerve pain following an outbreak of shingles), cluster headaches, and temporomandibular joint disorder (TMJ, which causes pain and dysfunction in the jaw joint and muscles that control jaw movement). Because of overlapping symptoms and the large number of conditions that can cause facial pain, obtaining a correct diagnosis is difficult, but finding the cause of the pain is important as the treatments for different types of pain may differ.

Most people with TN eventually will undergo a magnetic resonance imaging (MRI) scan to rule out a tumor or multiple sclerosis as the cause of their pain. This scan may or may not clearly show a blood vessel compressing the nerve. Special MRI imaging procedures can reveal the presence and severity of compression of the nerve by a blood vessel.

A diagnosis of classic trigeminal neuralgia may be supported by an individual's positive response to a short course of an antiseizure medication. Diagnosis of TN2 is more complex and difficult, but tends to be supported by a positive response to low doses of tricyclic antidepressant medications (such as amitriptyline and nortriptyline), similar to other neuropathic pain diagnoses.

311

How Is TN Treated?

Treatment options include medicines, surgery, and complementary approaches.

Medications

Anticonvulsant medicines—used to block nerve firing—are generally effective in treating TN1 but often less effective in TN2. These drugs include carbamazepine, oxcarbazepine, topiramate, gabapentin, pregabalin, clonazepam, phenytoin, lamotrigine, and valproic acid.

Surgery

A rhizotomy (rhizolysis) is a procedure in which nerve fibers are damaged to block pain. A rhizotomy for TN always causes some degree of sensory loss and facial numbness. Several forms of rhizotomy are available to treat trigeminal neuralgia:

- Balloon compression

- Glycerol injection

- Radiofrequency thermal lesioning

- Stereotactic radiosurgery

- Microvascular decompression (MVD)

A neurectomy (also called partial nerve section), which involves cutting part of the nerve, may be performed near the entrance point of the nerve at the brainstem during an attempted microvascular decompression if no vessel is found to be pressing on the trigeminal nerve. Neurectomies also may be performed by cutting superficial branches of the trigeminal nerve in the face. When done during microvascular decompression, a neurectomy will cause more long-lasting numbness in the area of the face that is supplied by the nerve or nerve branch that is cut. However, when the operation is performed in the face, the nerve may grow back and in time sensation may return. With neurectomy, there is risk of creating anesthesia dolorosa.

Surgical treatment for TN2 is usually more problematic than for TN1, particularly where vascular compression is not detected in brain imaging prior to a proposed procedure. Many neurosurgeons advise against the use of MVD or rhizotomy in individuals for whom TN2 symptoms predominate over TN1, unless vascular compression has been confirmed. MVD for TN2 is also less successful than for TN1.

Complementary Approaches

Some individuals manage trigeminal neuralgia using complementary techniques, usually in combination with drug treatment. These therapies offer varying degrees of success. Some people find that low-impact exercise, yoga, creative visualization, aroma therapy, or meditation may be useful in promoting well-being. Other options include acupuncture, upper cervical chiropractic, biofeedback, vitamin therapy, and nutritional therapy. Some people report modest pain relief after injections of botulinum toxin to block activity of sensory nerves.

Chronic pain from TN is frequently very isolating and depressing for the individual. Conversely, depression and sleep disturbance may render individuals more vulnerable to pain and suffering. Some individuals benefit from supportive counseling or therapy by a psychiatrist or psychologist. However, there is no evidence that TN is psychogenic in origin or caused by depression, and persons with TN require effective medical or surgical treatment for their pain.

Chapter 25

Complex Regional Pain Syndrome

Complex regional pain syndrome (CRPS) is a chronic (lasting greater than six months) pain condition that most often affects one limb (arm, leg, hand, or foot) usually after an injury. CRPS is believed to be caused by damage to, or malfunction of, the peripheral and central nervous systems. The central nervous system is composed of the brain and spinal cord; the peripheral nervous system involves nerve signaling from the brain and spinal cord to the rest of the body. CRPS is characterized by prolonged or excessive pain and changes in skin color, temperature, and/or swelling in the affected area.

CRPS is divided into two types: CRPS-I and CRPS-II. Individuals without a confirmed nerve injury are classified as having CRPS-I (previously known as reflex sympathetic dystrophy syndrome). CRPS-II (previously known as causalgia) is when there is an associated, confirmed nerve injury. As some research has identified evidence of nerve injury in CRPS-I, it is unclear if this disorders will always be divided into two types. Nonetheless, the treatment is similar.

CRPS symptoms vary in severity and duration, although some cases are mild and eventually go away. In more severe cases, individuals may not recover and may have long-term disability.

This chapter includes text excerpted from "Complex Regional Pain Syndrome Fact Sheet," National Institute of Neurological Disorders and Stroke (NINDS), January 2017.

Who Can Get Complex Regional Pain Syndrome (CRPS)?

Although it is more common in women, CRPS can occur in anyone at any age, with a peak at age 40. CRPS is rare in the elderly. Very few children under age 10 and almost no children under age 5 are affected.

What Are the Symptoms of CRPS?

The key symptom is prolonged severe pain that may be constant. It has been described as "burning," "pins and needles" sensation, or as if someone were squeezing the affected limb. The pain may spread to the entire arm or leg, even though the injury might have only involved a finger or toe. In rare cases, pain can sometimes even travel to the opposite extremity. There is often increased sensitivity in the affected area, known as allodynia, in which normal contact with the skin is experienced as very painful.

People with CRPS also experience changes in skin temperature, skin color, or swelling of the affected limb. This is due to abnormal microcirculation caused by damage to the nerves controlling blood flow and temperature. As a result, an affected arm or leg may feel warmer or cooler compared to the opposite limb. The skin on the affected limb may change color, becoming blotchy, blue, purple, pale, or red.

Other common features of CRPS include:

- changes in skin texture on the affected area; it may appear shiny and thin

- abnormal sweating pattern in the affected area or surrounding areas

- changes in nail and hair growth patterns

- stiffness in affected joints

- problems coordinating muscle movement, with decreased ability to move the affected body part

- abnormal movement in the affected limb, most often fixed abnormal posture (called dystonia) but also tremors in or jerking of the limb.

What Causes CRPS?

It is unclear why some individuals develop CRPS while others with similar trauma do not. In more than 90 percent of cases, the condition is triggered by a clear history of trauma or injury. The most common triggers are fractures, sprains/strains, soft tissue injury (such as burns, cuts, or bruises), limb immobilization (such as being in a cast), surgery, or even minor medical procedures such as needle stick. CRPS represents an abnormal response that magnifies the effects of the injury. Some people respond excessively to a trigger that causes no problem for other people, such as what is observed in people who have food allergies.

Peripheral nerve abnormalities found in individuals with CRPS usually involve the small unmyelinated and thinly myelinated sensory nerve fibers (axons) that carry pain messages and signals to blood vessels. (Myelin is a mixture of proteins and fat-like substances that surround and insulate some nerve fibers.) Because small fibers in the nerves communicate with blood vessels, injuries to the fibers may trigger the many different symptoms of CRPS. Molecules secreted from the ends of hyperactive small nerve fibers are thought to contribute to inflammation and blood vessel abnormalities. These peripheral nerve abnormalities in turn trigger damage in the spinal cord and brain.

Blood vessels in the affected limb may dilate (open wider) or leak fluid into the surrounding tissue, causing red, swollen skin. The dilation and constriction of small blood vessels is controlled by small nerve fiber axons as well as chemical messengers in the blood. The underlying muscles and deeper tissues can become starved of oxygen and nutrients, which causes muscle and joint pain as well as damage. The blood vessels may over-constrict (clamp down), causing old, white, or bluish skin.

CRPS also affects the immune system. High levels of inflammatory chemicals (cytokines) have been found in the tissues of people with CRPS. These contribute to the redness, swelling, and warmth reported by many patients. CRPS is more common in individuals with other inflammatory and autoimmune conditions such as asthma.

Limited data suggest that CRPS also may be influenced by genetics. Rare family clusters of CRPS have been reported. Familial CRPS may be more severe with earlier onset, greater dystonia, and more than one limb being affected.

Occasionally CRPS develops without any known injury. In these cases, an infection, a blood vessel problem, or entrapment of the nerves may have caused an internal injury. A physician will perform a thorough examination in order to identify a cause.

In many cases, CRPS results from a variety of causes. In such instances, treatments are directed at all of the contributing factors.

How Is CRPS Diagnosed?

Currently there is no specific test that can confirm CRPS. Its diagnosis is based on a person's medical history, and signs and symptoms that match the definition. Since other conditions can cause similar symptoms, careful examination is important. As most people improve gradually over time, the diagnosis may be more difficult later in the course of the disorder.

Testing also may be used to help rule out other conditions, such as arthritis, Lyme disease, generalized muscle diseases, a clotted vein, or small fiber polyneuropathies, because these require different treatment. The distinguishing feature of CRPS is that of an injury to the affected area. Such individuals should be carefully assessed so that an alternative treatable disorder is not overlooked.

Magnetic resonance imaging or triple-phase bone scans may be requested to help confirm a diagnosis. While CRPS is often associated with excess bone resorption, a process in which certain cells break down the bone and release calcium into the blood, this finding may be observed in other illnesses as well.

What Is the Prognosis?

The outcome of CRPS is highly variable. Younger persons, children, and teenagers tend to have better outcomes. While older people can have good outcomes, there are some individuals who experience severe pain and disability despite treatment. Anecdotal evidence suggests early treatment, particularly rehabilitation, is helpful in limiting the disorder, a concept that has not yet been proven in clinical studies. More research is needed to understand the causes of CRPS, how it progresses, and the role of early treatment.

How Is CRPS Treated?

The following therapies are often used:

- Rehabilitation and physical therapy

- Psychotherapy

- Medications

  - Bisphosphonates, such as high dose alendronate or intravenous pamidronate.

  - Non-steroidal anti-inflammatory drugs to treat moderate pain, including over-the-counter aspirin, ibuprofen, and naproxen.

- Corticosteroids that treat inflammation/swelling and edema, such as prednisolone and methylprednisolone (used mostly in the early stages of CRPS).

- Drugs initially developed to treat seizures or depression but now shown to be effective for neuropathic pain, such as gabapentin, pregabalin, amitriptyline, nortriptyline, and duloxetine.

- Botulinum toxin injections.

- Opioids such as oxycontin, morphine, hydrocodone, fentanyl, and Vicodin. These drugs must be prescribed and monitored under close supervision of a physician, as these drugs may be addictive.

- N-methyl-D-aspartate (NMDA) receptor antagonists such as dextromethorphan and ketamine.

- Topical local anesthetic creams and patches such as lidocaine.

- All drugs or combination of drugs can have various side effects such as drowsiness, dizziness, increased heartbeat, and impaired memory. Inform a healthcare professional of any changes once drug therapy begins.

- Sympathetic nerve block

- Surgical sympathectomy

- Spinal cord stimulation

- Other types of neural stimulation

- Intrathecal drug pumps

  - Intravenous immunoglobulin (IVIG)

  - Ketamine

  - Graded motor imagery

Several alternative therapies have been used to treat other painful conditions. Options include behavior modification, acupuncture, relaxation techniques (such as biofeedback, progressive muscle relaxation, and guided motion therapy), and chiropractic treatment.

Chapter 26

Deep Vein Thrombosis and Pulmonary Embolism (DVT/PE)

Deep vein thrombosis and pulmonary embolism (DVT/PE) are often underdiagnosed and serious, but preventable medical conditions.

Deep vein thrombosis (DVT) is a medical condition that occurs when a blood clot forms in a deep vein. These clots usually develop in the lower leg, thigh, or pelvis, but they can also occur in the arm.

It is important to know about DVT because it can happen to anybody and can cause serious illness, disability, and in some cases, death. The good news is that DVT is preventable and treatable if discovered early.

Complications of Deep Vein Thrombosis (DVT)

The most serious complication of DVT happens when a part of the clot breaks off and travels through the bloodstream to the lungs, causing a blockage called pulmonary embolism (PE). If the clot is small, and with appropriate treatment, people can recover from PE. However, there could be some damage to the lungs. If the clot is large, it can stop blood from reaching the lungs and is fatal.

This chapter includes text excerpted from "Venous Thromboembolism (Blood Clots)," Centers for Disease Control and Prevention (CDC), April 6, 2017.

In addition, nearly one-third of people who have a DVT will have long-term complications caused by the damage the clot does to the valves in the vein called post-thrombotic syndrome (PTS). People with PTS have symptoms such as swelling, pain, discoloration, and in severe cases, scaling or ulcers in the affected part of the body. In some cases, the symptoms can be so severe that a person becomes disabled.

For some people, DVT and PE can become a chronic illness; about 30 percent of people who have had a DVT or PE are at risk for another episode.

Risk Factors for DVT

Almost anyone can have a DVT. However, certain factors can increase the chance of having this condition. The chance increases even more for someone who has more than one of these factors at the same time.

Following is a list of factors that increase the risk of developing DVT:

- Injury to a vein, often caused by:

  - Fractures,

  - Severe muscle injury, or

  - Major surgery (particularly involving the abdomen, pelvis, hip, or legs).

- Slow blood flow, often caused by:

  - Confinement to bed (e.g., due to a medical condition or after surgery);

  - Limited movement (e.g., a cast on a leg to help heal an injured bone);

  - Sitting for a long time, especially with crossed legs; or

  - Paralysis.

- Increased estrogen, often caused by:

  - Birth control pills

  - Hormone replacement therapy, sometimes used after menopause

  - Pregnancy, for up to 6 weeks after giving birth

- Certain chronic medical illnesses, such as:
  - Heart disease
  - Lung disease
  - Cancer and its treatment
  - Inflammatory bowel disease (Crohn's disease or ulcerative colitis)
- Other factors that increase the risk of DVT include:
  - Previous DVT or PE
  - Family history of DVT or PE
  - Age (risk increases as age increases)
  - Obesity
  - A catheter located in a central vein
  - Inherited clotting disorders

Preventing DVT

The following tips can help prevent DVT:

- Move around as soon as possible after having been confined to bed, such as after surgery, illness, or injury.
- If you're at risk for DVT, talk to your doctor about:
  - Graduated compression stockings (sometimes called "medical compression stockings")
  - Medication (anticoagulants) to prevent DVT.
- When sitting for long periods of time, such as when traveling for more than four hours:
  - Get up and walk around every 2 to 3 hours.
  - Exercise your legs while you're sitting by:
    - Raising and lowering your heels while keeping your toes on the floor.
    - Raising and lowering your toes while keeping your heels on the floor.
    - Tightening and releasing your leg muscles.
  - Wear loose-fitting clothes.

- You can reduce your risk by maintaining a healthy weight, avoiding a sedentary lifestyle, and following your doctor's recommendations based on your individual risk factors.

Symptoms of DVT and PE

Know the signs. Know your risk. Seek care. Everybody should know the signs and symptoms of DVT/PE, their risk for DVT/PE, to talk to their healthcare provider about their risk, and to seek care immediately if they have any sign or symptom of DVT/PE.

DVT

About half of people with DVT have no symptoms at all. The following are the most common symptoms of DVT that occur in the affected part of the body:

- Swelling

- Pain

- Tenderness

- Redness of the skin

If you have any of these symptoms, you should see your doctor as soon as possible.

Pulmonary Embolism (PE)

You can have a PE without any symptoms of a DVT.
Signs and symptoms of PE can include:

- Difficulty in breathing.

- Faster than normal or irregular heartbeat.

- Chest pain or discomfort, which usually worsens with a deep breath or coughing.

- Coughing up blood.

- Very low blood pressure, lightheadedness, or fainting

If you have any of these symptoms, you should seek medical help immediately.

Diagnosis of DVT and PE

The diagnosis of DVT or PE requires special tests that can only be performed by a doctor. That is why it is important for you to seek medical care if you experience any of the symptoms of DVT or PE.

Treatments for DVT and PE

Treatments for DVT

Medication is used to prevent and treat DVT. Compression stockings (also called graduated compression stockings) are sometimes recommended to prevent DVT and relieve pain and swelling. These might need to be worn for 2 years or more after having DVT. In severe cases, the clot might need to be removed surgically.

Treatments for PE

Immediate medical attention is necessary to treat PE. In cases of severe, life-threatening PE, there are medicines called thrombolytics that can dissolve the clot. Other medicines, called anticoagulants, may be prescribed to prevent more clots from forming. Some people may need to be on medication long-term to prevent future blood clots.

Chapter 27

Ear Pain

What Is an Ear Infection?

Ear infections can affect the ear canal or the middle ear. Acute otitis externa (AOE) is the scientific name for an infection of the ear canal, which is also called swimmer's ear.

Middle ear infections are called *Otitis Media*, and there are two types of middle ear infections:

- Otitis Media with Effusion (OME) occurs when fluid builds up in the middle ear without pain, pus, fever, or other signs and symptoms of infection.

- Acute Otitis Media (AOM) occurs when fluid builds up in the middle ear and is often caused by bacteria, but can also be caused by viruses.

This chapter contains text excerpted from the following sources: Text under the heading "What Is an Ear Infection?" is excerpted from "Preventing and Treating Ear Infections," Centers for Disease Control and Prevention (CDC), June 17, 2017; Text beginning with the heading "Otitis Media with Effusion" is excerpted from "Ear Infection," Centers for Disease Control and Prevention (CDC), April 17, 2015; Text under the heading "What Is Acute Otitis Externa (Swimmer's Ear)?" is excerpted from "Water, Sanitation and Environmentally-Related Hygiene," Centers for Disease Control and Prevention (CDC), March 11, 2015.

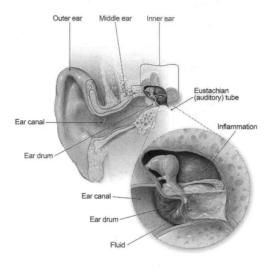

Figure 27.1. *Fluid Buildup in Middle Ear*

Otitis Media with Effusion

Otitis media with effusion, or OME, is a buildup of fluid in the middle ear without signs and symptoms of infection (pain, redness of the eardrum, pus, fever). The most common reasons for this fluid buildup include:

- allergies

- changes in air pressure due to travel or elevation changes

- drinking while laying on your back

- irritants such as cigarette smoke

- previous respiratory infections

OME almost always goes away on its own and will not benefit from antibiotics. After a respiratory tract infection has gone away, fluid may remain inside the ear and take a month or longer to go away. Sometimes this fluid can become infected, leading to acute otitis media (AOM). OME is more common than AOM.

Acute Otitis Media

Acute otitis media, or AOM, is the type of ear infection that affects the inside of the ear and can be painful. AOM is often caused by bacteria, but can also be caused by viruses. The bacteria that usually cause AOM are *Streptococcus pneumoniae*, *Haemophilus influenzae*, and *Moraxella catarrhalis*. The viruses that most commonly cause AOM are respiratory syncytial virus (RSV), rhinoviruses, influenza viruses, and adenoviruses.

AOM may improve with antibiotics, but they are not always necessary since not all AOM is caused by bacteria.

Risk Factors

There are many things that can increase your risk for OME or AOM, including:

- age (children younger than 2 years are at higher risk)
- daycare attendance
- drinking from a bottle while laying down
- exposure to air pollution or secondhand smoke
- season (ear infections are more common during fall and winter)

Signs and Symptoms

Children with OME do not act sick and will not have any obvious symptoms, although temporary problems with hearing may be present. Symptoms more commonly associated with AOM include:

- difficulty balancing
- excessive crying
- fever
- fluid draining from ears
- headache
- irritability, especially with infants and toddlers
- problems with hearing
- pulling at ears, especially with children
- sleep disturbances

When to Seek Medical Care

See a healthcare professional if you or your child has any of the following:

- temperature higher than 100.4 °F

- discharge of blood or pus from the ears

- symptoms that have not improved or have gotten worse after being diagnosed with an ear infection

If your child is younger than three months of age and has a fever, it's important to always call your healthcare professional right away.

Diagnosis and Treatment

Ear infections can be diagnosed with a special instrument called an otoscope, which is used to look inside the ear at the eardrum. Your healthcare professional can also perform a special test using the otoscope to see if fluid has collected behind the eardrum. If OME is present, fluid may be visible, but there will be no signs of infection. If there are signs of infection, then AOM may be present.

Your healthcare professional will consider several factors when determining if antibiotics are needed for an ear infection: age, illness severity, certainty a bacterial infection is present, and options for follow-up. Since ear infections will often get better on their own without antibiotic treatment, your healthcare professional may decide to wait a few days before prescribing antibiotics. When an ear infection is caused by a virus, antibiotic treatment will not help it get better and may even cause harm in both children and adults.

If symptoms continue to last for more than one month for OME or 2 days for AOM, you should schedule a follow-up appointment with your healthcare professional.

Symptom Relief

Rest, over-the-counter (OTC) medicines and other self-care methods may help you or your child feel better. Remember, always use OTC products as directed. Many OTC products are not recommended for children of certain ages.

Prevention

There are steps you can take to help prevent getting an ear infection, including:

- avoid smoking and exposure to secondhand smoke

- bottle feed your baby in the upright position

- breastfeed your baby for 12 months or more if possible

- keep you and your child up to date with recommended immunizations

What Is Acute Otitis Externa (Swimmer's Ear)?

Swimmer's ear is a common problem that can cause pain and discomfort for children and swimmers of all ages. In the United States, swimmer's ear results in an estimated 2.4 million healthcare visits every year and nearly half a billion dollars in healthcare costs.

Swimmer's ear is an infection of the outer ear canal. Symptoms of swimmer's ear usually appear within a few days of swimming and include:

- Itchiness inside the ear.

- Redness and swelling of the ear.

- Pain when the infected ear is tugged or when pressure is placed on the ear.

- Pus draining from the infected ear.

Although all age groups are affected by swimmer's ear, it is more common in children and can be extremely painful.

How is Swimmer's Ear Spread at Recreational Water Venues?

Swimmer's ear can occur when water stays in the ear canal for long periods of time, providing the perfect environment for germs to grow and infect the skin. Germs found in pools and at other recreational water venues are one of the most common causes of swimmer's ear.

Swimmer's ear cannot be spread from one person to another.

If you think you have swimmer's ear, consult your healthcare provider. Swimmer's ear can be treated with antibiotic ear drops.

Is There a Difference between a Childhood Middle Ear Infection and Swimmer's Ear?

Yes. Swimmer's ear is not the same as the common childhood middle ear infection. If you can wiggle the outer ear without pain or discomfort then your ear condition is probably not swimmer's ear.

How Do I Protect Myself and My Family?

To reduce the risk of swimmer's ear:

DO keep your ears as dry as possible.

- Use a bathing cap, ear plugs, or custom-fitted swim molds when swimming.

DO dry your ears thoroughly after swimming or showering.

- Use a towel to dry your ears well.
- Tilt your head to hold each ear facing down to allow water to escape the ear canal.
- Pull your earlobe in different directions while your ear is faced down to help water drain out.
- If you still have water left in your ears, consider using a hair dryer to move air within the ear canal.
  - Put the dryer on the lowest heat and speed/fan setting.
  - Hold the dryer several inches from your ear.

DON'T put objects in your ear canal (including cotton-tip swabs, pencils, paperclips, or fingers).

DON'T try to remove ear wax. Ear wax helps protect your ear canal from infection.

- If you think that your ear canal is blocked by ear wax, consult your healthcare provider.

CONSULT your healthcare provider about using ear drops after swimming.

- **Drops should not be used** by people with ear tubes, damaged ear drums, outer ear infections, or ear drainage (pus or liquid coming from the ear).

CONSULT your healthcare provider if you have ear pain, discomfort, or drainage from your ears.

ASK your pool/hot tub operator if disinfectant and pH levels are checked at least twice per day—hot tubs and pools with proper disinfectant and pH levels are less likely to spread germs.

USE pool test strips to check the pool or hot tub yourself for adequate disinfectant and pH levels.

Chapter 28

Gastrointestinal Pain

Chapter Contents

Section 28.1

Abdominal Adhesions

This section includes text excerpted from "Abdominal Adhesions,"
National Institute of Diabetes and Digestive and Kidney
Diseases (NIDDK), September 2013. Reviewed June 2017.

Abdominal adhesions are bands of fibrous tissue that can form
between abdominal tissues and organs. Normally, internal tissues and
organs have slippery surfaces, preventing them from sticking together
as the body moves. However, abdominal adhesions cause tissues and
organs in the abdominal cavity to stick together.

What Is the Abdominal Cavity?

The abdominal cavity is the internal area of the body between the
chest and hips that contains the lower part of the esophagus, stomach,
small intestine, and large intestine. The esophagus carries food and
liquids from the mouth to the stomach, which slowly pumps them into
the small and large intestines. Abdominal adhesions can kink, twist, or
pull the small and large intestines out of place, causing an intestinal
obstruction. Intestinal obstruction, also called a bowel obstruction,
results in the partial or complete blockage of movement of food or stool
through the intestines.

What Causes Abdominal Adhesions?

Abdominal surgery is the most frequent cause of abdominal adhesions. Surgery-related causes include:

- cuts involving internal organs

- handling of internal organs

- drying out of internal organs and tissues

- contact of internal tissues with foreign materials, such as gauze,
  surgical gloves, and stitches

- blood or blood clots that were not rinsed away during surgery

Abdominal adhesions can also result from inflammation not related to surgery, including:

- appendix rupture
- radiation treatment
- gynecological infections
- abdominal infections

Rarely, abdominal adhesions form without apparent cause.

How Common Are Abdominal Adhesions and Who Is at Risk?

Of patients who undergo abdominal surgery, 93 percent develop abdominal adhesions. Surgery in the lower abdomen and pelvis, including bowel and gynecological operations, carries an even greater chance of abdominal adhesions. Abdominal adhesions can become larger and tighter as time passes, sometimes causing problems years after surgery.

What Are the Symptoms of Abdominal Adhesions?

In most cases, abdominal adhesions do not cause symptoms. When symptoms are present, chronic abdominal pain is the most common.

What Are the Complications of Abdominal Adhesions?

Abdominal adhesions can cause intestinal obstruction and female infertility—the inability to become pregnant after a year of trying.

Abdominal adhesions can lead to female infertility by preventing fertilized eggs from reaching the uterus, where fetal development takes place. Women with abdominal adhesions in or around their fallopian tubes have an increased chance of ectopic pregnancy—a fertilized egg growing outside the uterus. Abdominal adhesions inside the uterus may result in repeated miscarriages—a pregnancy failure before 20 weeks.

Seek Help for Emergency Symptoms

A complete intestinal obstruction is life threatening and requires immediate medical attention and often surgery. Symptoms of an intestinal obstruction include:

- severe abdominal pain or cramping

- nausea

- vomiting

- bloating

- loud bowel sounds

- abdominal swelling

- the inability to have a bowel movement or pass gas

- constipation—a condition in which a person has fewer than three bowel movements a week; the bowel movements may be painful

A person with these symptoms should seek medical attention immediately.

How Are Abdominal Adhesions and Intestinal Obstructions Diagnosed?

Abdominal adhesions cannot be detected by tests or seen through imaging techniques such as X-rays or ultrasound. Most abdominal adhesions are found during surgery performed to examine the abdomen. However, abdominal X-rays, a lower gastrointestinal (GI) series, and computerized tomography (CT) scans can diagnose intestinal obstructions.

- Abdominal X-rays

- A lower GI series

- CT scans

How Are Abdominal Adhesions and Intestinal Obstructions Treated?

Abdominal adhesions that do not cause symptoms generally do not require treatment. Surgery is the only way to treat abdominal adhesions that cause pain, intestinal obstruction, or fertility problems. More surgery, however, carries the risk of additional abdominal adhesions. People should speak with their healthcare provider about the best way to treat their abdominal adhesions.

Complete intestinal obstructions usually require immediate surgery to clear the blockage. Most partial intestinal obstructions can be managed without surgery.

How Can Abdominal Adhesions Be Prevented?

Abdominal adhesions are difficult to prevent; however, certain surgical techniques can minimize abdominal adhesions.

Laparoscopic surgery decreases the potential for abdominal adhesions because several tiny incisions are made in the lower abdomen instead of one large incision. The surgeon inserts a laparoscope—a thin tube with a tiny video camera attached—into one of the small incisions. The camera sends a magnified image from inside the body to a video monitor. Patients will usually receive general anesthesia during this surgery.

If laparoscopic surgery is not possible and a large abdominal incision is required, at the end of surgery a special film-like material can be inserted between organs or between the organs and the abdominal incision. The film-like material, which looks similar to wax paper and is absorbed by the body in about a week, hydrates organs to help prevent abdominal adhesions.

Other steps taken during surgery to reduce abdominal adhesions include:

- using starch- and latex-free gloves
- handling tissues and organs gently
- shortening surgery time
- using moistened drapes and swabs
- occasionally applying saline solution

Eating, Diet, and Nutrition

Researchers have not found that eating, diet, and nutrition play a role in causing or preventing abdominal adhesions. A person with a partial intestinal obstruction may relieve symptoms with a liquid or low-fiber diet, which is more easily broken down into smaller particles by the digestive system.

Section 28.2

Appendicitis

This section includes text excerpted from "Appendicitis,"
National Institute of Diabetes and Digestive and Kidney
Diseases (NIDDK), November 2014.

Definition and Facts

What Is Appendicitis?

Appendicitis is inflammation of your appendix.

How Common Is Appendicitis?

In the United States, appendicitis is the most common cause of acute abdominal pain requiring surgery. Over 5 percent of the population develops appendicitis at some point.

Who Is More Likely to Develop Appendicitis?

Appendicitis most commonly occurs in the teens and twenties but may occur at any age.

What Are the Complications of Appendicitis?

If appendicitis is not treated, it may lead to complications. The complications of a ruptured appendix are:

- peritonitis, which can be a dangerous condition. Peritonitis happens if your appendix bursts and infection spreads in your abdomen. If you have peritonitis, you may be very ill and have:
  - fever
  - nausea
  - severe tenderness in your abdomen
  - vomiting
- an abscess of the appendix called an appendiceal abscess.

Symptoms and Causes

What Are the Symptoms of Appendicitis?

The most common symptom of appendicitis is pain in your abdomen. If you have appendicitis, you'll most often have pain in your abdomen that:

- begins near your belly button and then moves lower and to your right
- gets worse in a matter of hours
- gets worse when you move around, take deep breaths, cough, or sneeze
- is severe and often described as different from any pain you've felt before
- occurs suddenly and may even wake you up if you're sleeping
- occurs before other symptoms

Other symptoms of appendicitis may include:

- loss of appetite
- nausea
- vomiting
- constipation or diarrhea
- an inability to pass gas
- a low-grade fever
- swelling in your abdomen
- the feeling that having a bowel movement will relieve discomfort

Symptoms can be different for each person and can seem like the following conditions that also cause pain in the abdomen:

- abdominal adhesions
- constipation
- inflammatory bowel disease, which includes Crohn's disease and ulcerative colitis, long-lasting disorders that cause irritation and ulcers in the gastrointestinal (GI) tract
- intestinal obstruction
- pelvic inflammatory disease

What Causes Appendicitis?

Appendicitis can have more than one cause, and in many cases the cause is not clear. Possible causes include:

- Blockage of the opening inside the appendix
- enlarged tissue in the wall of your appendix, caused by infection in the GI tract or elsewhere in your body
- inflammatory bowel disease
- stool, parasites, or growths that can clog your appendiceal lumen
- trauma to your abdomen

When Should I Seek a Doctor's Help?

Appendicitis is a medical emergency that requires immediate care. See a healthcare professional or go to the emergency room right away if you think you or a child has appendicitis. A doctor can help treat the appendicitis and reduce symptoms and the chance of complications.

Diagnosis

How Do Doctors Diagnose Appendicitis?

Most often, healthcare professionals suspect the diagnosis of appendicitis based on your symptoms, your medical history, and a physical exam. A doctor can confirm the diagnosis with an ultrasound, X-ray, or magnetic resonance imaging (MRI) exam.

- Medical History
- Physical Exam
- Lab Tests
  - Blood tests
  - Urinalysis
  - Pregnancy test
  - Imaging Tests
- Abdominal ultrasound
- Magnetic resonance imaging (MRI)
- CT scan

Treatment

How Do Doctors Treat Appendicitis?

Doctors typically treat appendicitis with surgery to remove the appendix. Surgeons perform the surgery in a hospital with general anesthesia. Your doctor will recommend surgery if you have continuous abdominal pain and fever, or signs of a burst appendix and infection. Prompt surgery decreases the chance that your appendix will burst.

Healthcare professionals call the surgery to remove the appendix an appendectomy. A surgeon performs the surgery using one of the following methods:

- Laparoscopic surgery
- Laparotomy

After surgery, most patients completely recover from appendicitis and don't need to make changes to their diet, exercise, or lifestyle. Surgeons recommend that you limit physical activity for the first 10 to 14 days after a laparotomy and for the first 3 to 5 days after laparoscopic surgery.

What If the Surgeon Finds a Normal Appendix?

In some cases, a surgeon finds a normal appendix during surgery. In this case, many surgeons will remove it to eliminate the future possibility of appendicitis. Sometimes surgeons find a different problem, which they may correct during surgery.

Can Doctors Treat Appendicitis without Surgery?

Some cases of mild appendicitis may be cured with antibiotics alone. All patients suspected of having appendicitis are treated with antibiotics before surgery, and some patients may improve completely before surgery is performed.

How Do Doctors Treat Complications of a Burst Appendix?

Treating the complications of a burst appendix will depend on the type of complication. In most cases of peritonitis, a surgeon will remove your appendix immediately with surgery. The surgeon will use laparotomy to clean the inside of your abdomen to prevent infection and then remove your appendix. Without prompt treatment, peritonitis can cause death.

A surgeon may drain the pus from an appendiceal abscess during surgery or, more commonly, before surgery. To drain an abscess, the surgeon places a tube in the abscess through the abdominal wall. You leave the drainage tube in place for about 2 weeks while you take antibiotics to treat infection. When the infection and inflammation are under control, about 6 to 8 weeks later, surgeons operate to remove what remains of the burst appendix.

Eating, Diet, and Nutrition

How Can Your Diet Help Prevent or Relieve Appendicitis?

Researchers have not found that eating, diet, and nutrition cause or prevent appendicitis.

Section 28.3

Crohn's Disease

This section includes text excerpted from "Crohn's Disease," National Institute of Diabetes and Digestive and Kidney Diseases (NIDDK), November 2016.

Definition and Facts

What Is Crohn's Disease?

Crohn's disease is a chronic disease that causes inflammation and irritation in your digestive tract. Most commonly, Crohn's affects your small intestine and the beginning of your large intestine. However, the disease can affect any part of your digestive tract, from your mouth to your anus. Learn more about your digestive system and how it works.

Crohn's disease is an inflammatory bowel disease (IBD). Ulcerative colitis and microscopic colitis are other common types of IBD.

Crohn's disease most often begins gradually and can become worse over time. You may have periods of remission that can last for weeks or years.

Who Is More Likely to Develop Crohn's Disease?

Crohn's disease can develop in people of any age and is more likely to develop in people:

- between the ages of 20 and 29

- who have a family member, most often a sibling or parent, with IBD

- who smoke cigarettes

What Other Health Problems Do People with Crohn's Disease Have?

If you have Crohn's disease in your large intestine, you may be more likely to develop colon cancer. If you receive ongoing treatment for Crohn's disease and stay in remission, you may reduce your chances of developing colon cancer.

Talk with your doctor about how often you should get screened for colon cancer. Screening is testing for diseases when you have no symptoms. Screening for colon cancer can include colonoscopy with biopsies. Although screening does not reduce your chances of developing colon cancer, it may help to find cancer at an early stage and improve the chance of curing the cancer.

Symptoms and Causes

What Are the Symptoms of Crohn's Disease?

The most common symptoms of Crohn's disease are:

- diarrhea

- cramping and pain in your abdomen

- weight loss

Other symptoms include:

- anemia

- eye redness or pain

- feeling tired

- fever

- joint pain or soreness

- nausea or loss of appetite

- skin changes that involve red, tender bumps under the skin

Your symptoms may vary depending on the location and severity of your inflammation.

Some research suggests that stress, including the stress of living with Crohn's disease, can make symptoms worse. Also, some people may find that certain foods can trigger or worsen their symptoms.

What Causes Crohn's Disease?

Doctors aren't sure what causes Crohn's disease. Experts think the following factors may play a role in causing Crohn's disease.

- Autoimmune reaction

- Genes

- Other factors:

  - Smoking

  - Nonsteroidal anti-inflammatory drugs (NSAIDs)

  - High-fat diet

Diagnosis

How Do Doctors Diagnose Crohn's Disease?

Doctors typically use a combination of tests to diagnose Crohn's disease. Your doctor will also ask you about your medical history—including medicines you are taking—and your family history and will perform a physical exam.

- Physical Exam

- Diagnostic Tests

  - lab tests

  - upper gastrointestinal (GI) series

  - computed tomography (CT) scan

  - intestinal endoscopy

Your doctor may also perform tests to rule out other diseases, such as ulcerative colitis, diverticular disease, or cancer, that cause symptoms similar to those of Crohn's disease.

What Tests Do Doctors Use to Diagnose Crohn's Disease?

Your doctor may perform the following tests to help diagnose Crohn's disease:
Lab Tests

- Blood tests.

  - Red blood cells

  - White blood cells

- Stool tests

- Intestinal endoscopy

  - push enteroscopy

  - single- or double-balloon enteroscopy

  - spiral enteroscopy

- Capsule endoscopy

- Upper GI series

- CT scan

Treatment

How Do Doctors Treat Crohn's Disease?

Doctors treat Crohn's disease with medicines, bowel rest, and surgery.
No single treatment works for everyone with Crohn's disease. The goals of treatment are to decrease the inflammation in your intestines, to prevent flare-ups of your symptoms, and to keep you in remission.

- Medicines

  - Aminosalicylates

  - Corticosteroids

  - Immunomodulators

  - Biologic therapies

  - Other medicines

    - acetaminophen

- antibiotics
- loperamide
- Bowel Rest
- Surgery
- Small bowel resection
  - laparoscopic
  - open surgery
- Subtotal colectomy
  - laparoscopic colectomy
  - open surgery
- Proctocolectomy and ileostomy

Eating, Diet, and Nutrition

How Can My Diet Help the Symptoms of Crohn's Disease?

Changing your diet can help reduce symptoms. Talk with your doctor about specific dietary recommendations and changes.

Your doctor may recommend nutritional supplements and vitamins if you do not absorb enough nutrients. For safety reasons, talk with your doctor before using dietary supplements, such as vitamins, or any complementary or alternative medicines or medical practices.

Section 28.4

Diverticulosis and Diverticulitis

This section includes text excerpted from "Diverticular
Disease," National Institute of Diabetes and Digestive and
Kidney Diseases (NIDDK), May 2016.

Definition and Facts

What Is Diverticulosis?

Diverticulosis is a condition that occurs when small pouches, or
sacs, form and push outward through weak spots in the wall of your
colon. These pouches are most common in the lower part of your colon,
called the sigmoid colon. One pouch is called a diverticulum. Multiple
pouches are called diverticula. Most people with diverticulosis do not
have symptoms or problems.

When diverticulosis does cause symptoms or problems, doctors
call this diverticular disease. For some people, diverticulosis causes
symptoms such as changes in bowel movement patterns or pain in the
abdomen. Diverticulosis may also cause problems such as diverticular
bleeding and diverticulitis.

Diverticular Bleeding

Diverticular bleeding occurs when a small blood vessel within the
wall of a pouch, or diverticulum, bursts.

Diverticulitis

Diverticulitis occurs when you have diverticulosis and one or a few
of the pouches in the wall of your colon become inflamed. Diverticulitis
can lead to serious complications.

What Are the Complications of Diverticulitis?

Diverticulitis can come on suddenly and cause other problems, such
as the following:

347

- **Abscess.** An abscess is a painful, swollen, infected, and pus-filled area just outside your colon wall that may make you ill with nausea, vomiting, fever, and severe tenderness in your abdomen.

- **Perforation.** A perforation is a small tear or hole in a pouch in your colon.

- **Peritonitis.** Peritonitis is inflammation or infection of the lining of your abdomen. Pus and stool that leak through a perforation can cause peritonitis.

- **Fistula.** A fistula is an abnormal passage, or tunnel, between two organs or between an organ and the outside of your body. The most common types of fistula with diverticulitis occur between the colon and the bladder or between the colon and the vagina in women.

- **Intestinal obstruction.** An intestinal obstruction is a partial or total blockage of the movement of food or stool through your intestines.

How Common Are Diverticulosis and Diverticulitis?

Diverticulosis is quite common, especially as people age. Research suggests that about 35 percent of U.S. adults age 50 years or younger have diverticulosis, while about 58 percent of those older than age 60 have diverticulosis. Most people with diverticulosis will never develop symptoms or problems.

Experts used to think that 10 to 25 percent of people with diverticulosis would develop diverticulitis. However, research suggests that the percentage who develop diverticulitis may be much lower—less than 5 percent.

In the United States, about 200,000 people are hospitalized for diverticulitis each year. About 70,000 people are hospitalized for diverticular bleeding each year.

Who Is More Likely to Have Diverticulosis and Diverticulitis?

People are more likely to develop diverticulosis and diverticulitis as they age.

Among people ages 50 and older, women are more likely than men to develop diverticulitis. However, among people younger than age 50, men are more likely to develop diverticulitis.

Symptoms and Causes

What Are the Symptoms of Diverticulosis?

Most people with diverticulosis do not have symptoms. If your diverticulosis causes symptoms, they may include:

- bloating

- constipation or diarrhea

- cramping or pain in your lower abdomen

Other conditions, such as irritable bowel syndrome and peptic ulcers, cause similar symptoms, so these symptoms may not mean you have diverticulosis. If you have these symptoms, see your doctor.

If you have diverticulosis and develop diverticular bleeding or diverticulitis, these conditions also cause symptoms.

What Are the Symptoms of Diverticular Bleeding?

In most cases, when you have diverticular bleeding, you will suddenly have a large amount of red or maroon-colored blood in your stool.

Diverticular bleeding may also cause dizziness or lightheadedness, or weakness. See your doctor right away if you have any of these symptoms.

What Are the Symptoms of Diverticulitis?

When you have diverticulitis, the inflamed pouches most often cause pain in the lower left side of your abdomen. The pain is usually severe and comes on suddenly, though it can also be mild and get worse over several days. The intensity of the pain can change over time.

Diverticulitis may also cause:

- constipation or diarrhea

- fevers and chills

- nausea or vomiting

What Causes Diverticulosis and Diverticulitis?

Experts are not sure what causes diverticulosis and diverticulitis. Researchers are studying several factors that may play a role in causing these conditions.

Fiber

For more than 50 years, experts thought that following a low-fiber diet led to diverticulosis. However, research has found that a low-fiber diet may not play a role. This study also found that a high-fiber diet with more frequent bowel movements may be linked with a greater chance of having diverticulosis. Talk with your doctor about how much fiber you should include in your diet.

Genes

Some studies suggest that genes may make some people more likely to develop diverticulosis and diverticulitis. Experts are still studying the role genes play in causing these conditions.

Other Factors

Studies have found links between diverticular disease—diverticulosis that causes symptoms or problems such as diverticular bleeding or diverticulitis—and the following factors:

- Certain medicines—including nonsteroidal anti-inflammatory drugs (NSAIDs), such as aspirin, and steroids

- Lack of exercise

- Obesity

- Smoking

Diverticulitis may begin when bacteria or stool get caught in a pouch in your colon. A decrease in healthy bacteria and an increase in disease-causing bacteria in your colon may also lead to diverticulitis.

Diagnosis

How Do Doctors Diagnose Diverticulosis and Diverticulitis?

If your doctor suspects you may have diverticulosis or diverticulitis, your doctor may use your medical history, a physical exam, and tests to diagnose these conditions.

Doctors may also diagnose diverticulosis if they notice pouches in the colon wall while performing tests, such as routine X-rays or colonoscopy, for other reasons.

Medical History

Your doctor will ask about your medical history, including your

- bowel movement patterns
- diet
- health
- medicines
- symptoms

Physical Exam

Your doctor will perform a physical exam, which may include a digital rectal exam. During a digital rectal exam, your doctor will have you bend over a table or lie on your side while holding your knees close to your chest. After putting on a glove, the doctor will slide a lubricated finger into your anus to check for pain, bleeding, hemorrhoids, or other problems.

What Tests Do Doctors Use to Diagnose Diverticulosis and Diverticulitis?

Your doctor may use the following tests to help diagnose diverticulosis and diverticulitis:

- Blood test
- CT scan
- Lower GI series
- Colonoscopy

Treatment

How Do Doctors Treat Diverticulosis?

The goal of treating diverticulosis is to prevent the pouches from causing symptoms or problems. Your doctor may recommend the following treatments.

- High-fiber Diet
- Fiber supplements
- Medicines
- Probiotics

How Do Doctors Treat Diverticular Bleeding?

Diverticular bleeding is rare. If you have bleeding, it can be severe. In some people, the bleeding may stop by itself and may not require treatment. However, if you have bleeding from your rectum—even a small amount—you should see a doctor right away.

To find the site of the bleeding and stop it, a doctor may perform a colonoscopy. Your doctor may also use a computerized tomography (CT) scan or an angiogram to find the bleeding site. An angiogram is a special kind of X-ray in which your doctor threads a thin, flexible tube through a large artery, often from your groin, to the bleeding area.

Colon Resection

If your bleeding does not stop, a surgeon may perform abdominal surgery with a colon resection. In a colon resection, the surgeon removes the affected part of your colon and joins the remaining ends of your colon together. You will receive general anesthesia for this procedure.

In some cases, during a colon resection, it may not be safe for the surgeon to rejoin the ends of your colon right away. In this case, the surgeon performs a temporary colostomy. Several months later, in a second surgery, the surgeon rejoins the ends of your colon and closes the opening in your abdomen.

How Do Doctors Treat Diverticulitis?

If you have diverticulitis with mild symptoms and no other problems, a doctor may recommend that you rest, take oral antibiotics, and follow a liquid diet for a period of time. If your symptoms ease after a few days, the doctor will recommend gradually adding solid foods back into your diet.

Severe cases of diverticulitis that come on quickly and cause complications will likely require a hospital stay and involve intravenous (IV) antibiotics. A few days without food or drink will help your colon rest.

If the period without food or drink is longer than a few days, your doctor may give you an IV liquid food mixture. The mixture contains:

- carbohydrates
- proteins
- fats
- vitamins
- minerals

How Do Doctors Treat Complications of Diverticulitis?

Your doctor may recommend the following to treat complications of diverticulitis:

Abscess. Your doctor may need to drain an abscess if it is large or does not clear up with antibiotics.

Perforation. If you have a perforation, you will likely need surgery to repair the tear or hole. Additional surgery may be needed to remove a small part of your colon if the surgeon cannot repair the perforation.

Peritonitis. Peritonitis requires immediate surgery to clean your abdominal cavity. You may need a colon resection at a later date after a course of antibiotics. You may also need a blood transfusion if you have lost a lot of blood. Without prompt treatment, peritonitis can be fatal.

Fistula. Surgeons can correct a fistula by performing a colon resection and removing the fistula.

Intestinal obstruction. If your large intestine is completely blocked, you will need emergency surgery, with possible colon resection. Partial blockage is not an emergency, so you can schedule the surgery or other corrective procedures.

Diet and Nutrition

What Should I Eat If I Have Diverticulosis or Diverticulitis?

If you have diverticulosis or if you have had diverticulitis in the past, your doctor may recommend eating more foods that are high in fiber.

The *Dietary Guidelines for Americans*, 2015–2020, recommends a dietary fiber intake of 14 grams per 1,000 calories consumed. For example, for a 2,000-calorie diet, the fiber recommendation is 28 grams per day.

Section 28.5

Gallstones

This section includes text excerpted from "Gallstones," National
Institute of Diabetes and Digestive and Kidney Diseases (NIDDK),
November 2013. Reviewed June 2017.

Gallstones are hard particles that develop in the gallbladder. The
gallbladder is a small, pear-shaped organ located in the upper right
abdomen—the area between the chest and hips—below the liver.

Gallstones can range in size from a grain of sand to a golf ball.
The gallbladder can develop a single large gallstone, hundreds of tiny
stones, or both small and large stones. Gallstones can cause sudden
pain in the upper right abdomen. This pain, called a gallbladder attack
or biliary colic, occurs when gallstones block the ducts of the biliary
tract.

What Is the Biliary Tract?

The biliary tract consists of the gallbladder and the bile ducts. The
bile ducts carry bile and other digestive enzymes from the liver and
pancreas to the duodenum—the first part of the small intestine.

The liver produces bile—a fluid that carries toxins and waste products
out of the body and helps the body digest fats and the fat-soluble vitamins A, D, E, and K. Bile mostly consists of cholesterol, bile salts, and
bilirubin. Bilirubin, a reddish-yellow substance, forms when hemoglobin
from red blood cells breaks down. Most bilirubin is excreted through bile.

The bile ducts of the biliary tract include the hepatic ducts, the common bile duct, the pancreatic duct, and the cystic duct. The gallbladder
stores bile. Eating signals the gallbladder to contract and empty bile
through the cystic duct and common bile duct into the duodenum to
mix with food.

What Causes Gallstones?

Imbalances in the substances that make up bile cause gallstones.
Gallstones may form if bile contains too much cholesterol, too much

bilirubin, or not enough bile salts. Scientists do not fully understand why these imbalances occur. Gallstones also may form if the gallbladder does not empty completely or often enough.

The two types of gallstones are cholesterol and pigment stones:

1. Cholesterol stones, usually yellow-green in color, consist primarily of hardened cholesterol. In the United States, more than 80 percent of gallstones are cholesterol stones.

2. Pigment stones, dark in color, are made of bilirubin.

Who Is at Risk for Gallstones?

Certain people have a higher risk of developing gallstones than others:

- Women are more likely to develop gallstones than men. Extra estrogen can increase cholesterol levels in bile and decrease gallbladder contractions, which may cause gallstones to form. Women may have extra estrogen due to pregnancy, hormone replacement therapy, or birth control pills.

- People over age 40 are more likely to develop gallstones than younger people.

- People with a family history of gallstones have a higher risk.

- American Indians have genetic factors that increase the amount of cholesterol in their bile. In fact, American Indians have the highest rate of gallstones in the United States—almost 65 percent of women and 30 percent of men have gallstones.

- Mexican Americans are at higher risk of developing gallstones.

Other factors that affect a person's risk of gallstones include:

- **Obesity.** People who are obese, especially women, have increased risk of developing gallstones. Obesity increases the amount of cholesterol in bile, which can cause stone formation.

- **Rapid weight loss.** As the body breaks down fat during prolonged fasting and rapid weight loss, the liver secretes extra cholesterol into bile. Rapid weight loss can also prevent the gallbladder from emptying properly. Low-calorie diets and bariatric surgery—surgery that limits the amount of food a person can eat or digest—lead to rapid weight loss and increased risk of gallstones.

- **Diet.** Research suggests diets high in calories and refined carbo-hydrates and low in fiber increase the risk of gallstones. Refined carbohydrates are grains processed to remove bran and germ, which contain nutrients and fiber. Examples of refined carbohy-drates include white bread and white rice.

- **Certain intestinal diseases.** Diseases that affect normal absorption of nutrients, such as Crohn's disease, are associated with gallstones.

- **Metabolic syndrome, diabetes, and insulin resistance.** These conditions increase the risk of gallstones. Metabolic syn-drome also increases the risk of gallstone complications. Meta-bolic syndrome is a group of traits and medical conditions linked to being overweight or obese that puts people at risk for heart disease and type 2 diabetes.

Pigment stones tend to develop in people who have:

- **cirrhosis**—a condition in which the liver slowly deteriorates and malfunctions due to chronic, or long lasting, injury

- **infections** in the bile ducts

- **severe hemolytic anemias**—conditions in which red blood cells are continuously broken down, such as sickle cell anemia

What Are the Symptoms and Complications of Gallstones?

Many people with gallstones do not have symptoms. Gallstones that do not cause symptoms are called asymptomatic, or silent, gallstones. Silent gallstones do not interfere with the function of the gallbladder, liver, or pancreas.

If gallstones block the bile ducts, pressure increases in the gall-bladder, causing a gallbladder attack. The pain usually lasts from 1 to several hours. Gallbladder attacks often follow heavy meals, and they usually occur in the evening or during the night.

Gallbladder attacks usually stop when gallstones move and no longer block the bile ducts. However, if any of the bile ducts remain blocked for more than a few hours, complications can occur. Complica-tions include inflammation, or swelling, of the gallbladder and severe damage or infection of the gallbladder, bile ducts, or liver.

A gallstone that becomes lodged in the common bile duct near the duodenum and blocks the pancreatic duct can cause gallstone pancreatitis—inflammation of the pancreas.

Left untreated, blockages of the bile ducts or pancreatic duct can be fatal.

How Are Gallstones Diagnosed?

A healthcare provider will usually order an ultrasound exam to diagnose gallstones. Other imaging tests may also be used.

- Ultrasound exam

- Computerized tomography (CT) scan

- Magnetic resonance imaging (MRI)

- Cholescintigraphy

- Endoscopic retrograde cholangiopancreatography (ERCP)

Healthcare providers also use blood tests to look for signs of infection or inflammation of the bile ducts, gallbladder, pancreas, or liver. A blood test involves drawing blood at a healthcare provider's office or commercial facility and sending the sample to a lab for analysis.

Gallstone symptoms may be similar to those of other conditions, such as appendicitis, ulcers, pancreatitis, and gastroesophageal reflux disease.

Sometimes, silent gallstones are found when a person does not have any symptoms. For example, a healthcare provider may notice gallstones when performing ultrasound for a different reason.

How Are Gallstones Treated?

If gallstones are not causing symptoms, treatment is usually not needed. However, if a person has a gallbladder attack or other symptoms, a healthcare provider will usually recommend treatment. A person may be referred to a gastroenterologist—a doctor who specializes in digestive diseases—for treatment. If a person has had one gallbladder attack, more episodes will likely follow.

The usual treatment for gallstones is surgery to remove the gallbladder. If a person cannot undergo surgery, nonsurgical treatments may be used to dissolve cholesterol gallstones. A healthcare provider may use ERCP to remove stones in people who cannot undergo surgery or to remove stones from the common bile duct in people who are about to have gallbladder removal surgery.

Surgery

Surgeons perform two types of cholecystectomy:

1. Laparoscopic cholecystectomy

2. Open cholecystectomy

Nonsurgical Treatments

Two types of nonsurgical treatments can be used to dissolve cholesterol gallstones:

1. Oral dissolution therapy

2. Shock wave lithotripsy

Eating, Diet, and Nutrition

Factors related to eating, diet, and nutrition that increase the risk of gallstones include:

- obesity

- rapid weight loss

- diets high in calories and refined carbohydrates and low in fiber

People can decrease their risk of gallstones by maintaining a healthy weight through proper diet and nutrition.

Ursodiol can help prevent gallstones in people who rapidly lose weight through low-calorie diets or bariatric surgery. People should talk with their healthcare provider or dietitian about what diet is right for them.

Section 28.6

Gas in the Digestive Tract

This section includes text excerpted from "Gas in the Digestive Tract," National Institute of Diabetes and Digestive and Kidney Diseases (NIDDK), July 2016.

Definition and Facts

What Is Gas?

Gas is air in your digestive tract. Gas leaves your body through your mouth when you burp or through your anus when you pass gas.

Flatulence is excess gas in your stomach or intestines that can cause bloating and flatus. Flatus, gas that leaves your body through your anus, can contain small amounts of sulfur. Flatus that contains more sulfur has more of an odor.

How Common Is Gas?

Everyone has gas. People may think that they burp or pass gas too often and that they have too much gas. Having too much gas is uncommon.

Who Is More Likely to Get Gas?

Certain conditions may cause you to have more gas or to have more symptoms when you have a normal amount of gas in your digestive tract. People who swallow more air or eat certain foods may be more likely to have more gas.

Symptoms and Causes

What Are the Symptoms of Gas?

The most common gas symptoms include burping, passing gas, bloating, and pain or discomfort in your abdomen. Gas symptoms vary from person to person.

Burping

Burping, or belching, once in awhile, especially during and after meals, is normal. If you burp a lot, you may be swallowing too much air and releasing it before the air enters your stomach.

Passing Gas

Passing gas around 13 to 21 times a day is normal.

Bloating

Bloating is a feeling of fullness or swelling in your abdomen. Bloating most often occurs during or after a meal.

Pain or Discomfort in Your Abdomen

You may feel pain or discomfort in your abdomen when gas does not move through your intestines normally.

When Should I Talk with a Doctor about My Gas Symptoms?

You should talk with your doctor if:

- gas symptoms bother you
- your symptoms change suddenly
- you have other symptoms with gas—such as constipation, diarrhea, or weight loss

What Causes Gas?

Gas normally enters your digestive tract when you swallow air and when bacteria in your large intestine break down certain undigested foods. You may have more gas in your digestive tract if you swallow more air or eat certain foods.

Swallowed Air

Everyone swallows a small amount of air when eating and drinking. You swallow more air when you:

- chew gum
- drink carbonated, or fizzy, drinks

- eat or drink too fast

- smoke

- suck on hard candy

- wear loose-fitting dentures

Swallowed air that doesn't leave your stomach by burping moves into your intestines and passes through your anus.

Bacteria in Your Large Intestine

Your stomach and small intestine don't fully digest some of the carbohydrates—sugars, starches, and fiber—in the food you eat. Undigested carbohydrates will pass to your large intestine, which contains bacteria. These bacteria break down undigested carbohydrates and create gas in the process.

What Foods, Drinks, or Products Cause Gas?

A variety of foods, drinks, and products can cause gas. See the following table for examples.

Table 28.1. Examples of Foods, Drinks, and Products That Can Cause Gas

Foods		
Vegetables	**Fruits**	**Milk Products**
Asparagus	Apples	Cheese
Artichokes	Peaches	Ice cream
Black beans	Pears	Yogurt
Broccoli	**Whole Grains**	**Packaged Foods with**
Brussels Sprouts	Bran	**Lactose**
Cabbage	Whole wheat	Bread
Cauliflower		Cereal
Kidney beans		Salad dressing
Mushrooms		
Navy beans		
Onions		
Pinto beans		
Drinks		
Apple juice	Carbonated drinks	Fruit drinks (such as fruit
Pear juice	Drinks with High-fructose	punch)
	Corn syrup	Milk

Table 28.1. Continued

Products
Sugar-free Products with Sorbitol, Mannitol, or Xylitol Candies Gum
Dietary Supplements and Additives Certain types of fiber, such as inulin and fructo-oligosaccharide, that may be added to processed foods to replace fat or sugar fiber supplements

What Conditions Cause Excess Gas or Increase Gas Symptoms?

Some conditions can cause you to have more gas than usual or have more symptoms when you have gas. These conditions include the following:

Small intestinal bacterial overgrowth. Small intestinal bacterial overgrowth is an increase in the number of bacteria or a change in the type of bacteria in your small intestine. These bacteria can produce extra gas and may also cause diarrhea and weight loss. Small intestinal bacterial overgrowth is most often a complication of other conditions.

IBS. Irritable bowel syndrome (IBS) is a group of symptoms—including pain or discomfort in your abdomen and changes in your bowel movement patterns—that occur together. IBS can affect how gas moves through your intestines. You may also feel bloated due to increased sensitivity to normal amounts of gas.

GERD. Gastroesophageal reflux disease (GERD) is a chronic condition that occurs when stomach contents flow back up into your esophagus. People with GERD may burp a lot to relieve discomfort.

Problems in digesting carbohydrates. Problems in digesting carbohydrates that can lead to gas and bloating include:

- **lactose intolerance,** a condition in which you have digestive symptoms such as bloating, gas, or diarrhea after eating or drinking milk or milk products.

- **dietary fructose intolerance,** a condition in which you have digestive symptoms such as bloating, gas, or diarrhea after consuming foods that contain fructose.

- **celiac disease,** an immune disorder in which you cannot tolerate gluten, a protein found in wheat, rye, barley, and some products such as lip balm and cosmetics. If you have celiac disease, gluten damages the lining of your small intestine.

Conditions that affect how gas moves through your intestines. Conditions that affect how gas moves through your intestines can lead to problems with gas and bloating. These conditions include dumping syndrome, abdominal adhesions, abdominal hernias, and conditions that can cause an intestinal obstruction such as colon cancer or ovarian cancer.

Diagnosis

How Do Doctors Diagnose the Cause of Gas?

Doctors may diagnose the causes of excess gas or increased gas symptoms with a medical history and physical exam.

If your doctor thinks you may have a condition that causes excess gas or increases gas symptoms, he or she may order more tests.

Medical History

For a medical history, your doctor will ask about:

- your symptoms

- your eating habits

- prescription and over-the-counter medicines you take

- current and past medical conditions

Your doctor may ask you to keep a diary of the food you eat and when your gas symptoms occur. Your diary may show specific foods that are causing gas. Reviewing your diary may also help your doctor find out if you have more gas or are more sensitive to normal amounts of gas.

Physical Exam

During a physical exam, a doctor typically:

- checks for bloating or swelling in your abdomen

- listens to sounds within your abdomen using a stethoscope

- taps on your abdomen to check for tenderness or pain

Treatment

How Can I Reduce or Prevent Excess Gas?

To reduce or prevent excess gas and gas symptoms, your doctor may suggest the following:

- Swallow less air
- Quit smoking
- Change your diet
- Take medicines:
    - Alpha-galactosidase (Beano, Gas-Zyme 3x)
    - Simethicone (Gas-X, Mylanta Gas)
    - Lactase tablets and drops

Eating, Diet, and Nutrition

You may be able to reduce gas by avoiding or eating less of the foods that give you gas. You can keep a food diary to help figure out which foods give you gas and how much of the gas-producing foods you can handle.

You may try avoiding or limiting:

- carbonated, or fizzy, drinks
- fried and high-fat foods
- high-fiber foods for a few weeks and then slowly increasing your daily fiber intake
- sugar

Section 28.7

Gastroesophageal Reflux Disease (Heartburn)

This section includes text excerpted from "Acid Reflux (GER and GERD) in Adults," National Institute of Diabetes and Digestive and Kidney Diseases (NIDDK), November 2015.

Definition and Facts

What Is GER?

Gastroesophageal reflux (GER) happens when your stomach contents come back up into your esophagus.

Stomach acid that touches the lining of your esophagus can cause heartburn, also called acid indigestion.

Does GER Have Another Name?

Doctors also refer to GER as:

- Acid indigestion
- Acid reflux
- Acid regurgitation
- Heartburn
- Reflux

How Common Is GER?

Having GER once in awhile is common.

What Is GERD?

Gastroesophageal reflux disease (GERD) is a more serious and long-lasting form of GER.

What Is the Difference between GER and GERD?

GER that occurs more than twice a week for a few weeks could be GERD. GERD can lead to more serious health problems over time. If you think you have GERD, you should see your doctor.

How Common Is GERD?

GERD affects about 20 percent of the U.S. population.

Who Is More Likely to Have GERD?

Anyone can develop GERD, some for unknown reasons. You are more likely to have GERD if you are:

- overweight or obese
- a pregnant woman
- taking certain medicines
- a smoker or regularly exposed to secondhand smoke

What Are the Complications of GERD?

Without treatment, GERD can sometimes cause serious complications over time, such as:

Esophagitis. Esophagitis is inflammation in the esophagus. Adults who have chronic esophagitis over many years are more likely to develop precancerous changes in the esophagus.

Esophageal stricture. An esophageal stricture happens when your esophagus becomes too narrow. Esophageal strictures can lead to problems with swallowing.

Respiratory problems. With GERD you might breathe stomach acid into your lungs. The stomach acid can then irritate your throat and lungs, causing respiratory problems, such as:

- Asthma—a long-lasting disease in your lungs that makes you extra sensitive to things that you're allergic to
- Chest congestion, or extra fluid in your lungs
- A dry, long-lasting cough or a sore throat
- Hoarseness—the partial loss of your voice

- Laryngitis—the swelling of your voice box that can lead to a short-term loss of your voice

- Pneumonia—an infection in one or both of your lungs—that keeps coming back

- Wheezing—a high-pitched whistling sound when you breathe

Barrett esophagus. GERD can sometimes cause Barrett esophagus. A small number of people with Barrett esophagus develop a rare yet often deadly type of cancer of the esophagus.

If you have GERD, talk with your doctor about how to prevent or treat long-term problems.

Symptoms and Causes

What Are the Symptoms of GER and GERD?

If you have gastroesophageal reflux (GER), you may taste food or stomach acid in the back of your mouth.

The most common symptom of gastroesophageal reflux disease (GERD) is regular heartburn, a painful, burning feeling in the middle of your chest, behind your breastbone, and in the middle of your abdomen. Not all adults with GERD have heartburn.

Other common GERD symptoms include:

- bad breath

- nausea

- pain in your chest or the upper part of your abdomen

- problems swallowing or painful swallowing

- respiratory problems

- vomiting

- the wearing away of your teeth

Some symptoms of GERD come from its complications, including those that affect your lungs.

What Causes GER and GERD?

GER and GERD happen when your lower esophageal sphincter becomes weak or relaxes when it shouldn't, causing stomach contents to rise up into the esophagus. The lower esophageal sphincter becomes weak or relaxes due to certain things, such as:

- increased pressure on your abdomen from being overweight, obese, or pregnant

- certain medicines, including:

  - those that doctors use to treat asthma—a long-lasting disease in your lungs that makes you extra sensitive to things that you're allergic to

  - calcium channel blockers—medicines that treat high blood pressure

  - antihistamines—medicines that treat allergy symptoms

  - painkillers

  - sedatives—medicines that help put you to sleep

  - antidepressants—medicines that treat depression

- smoking, or inhaling secondhand smoke

A hiatal hernia can also cause GERD. Hiatal hernia is a condition in which the opening in your diaphragm lets the upper part of the stomach move up into your chest, which lowers the pressure in the esophageal sphincter.

When Should I Seek a Doctor's Help?

You should see a doctor if you have persistent GER symptoms that do not get better with over-the-counter medications or change in your diet.

Call a doctor right away if you:

- vomit large amounts

- have regular projectile, or forceful, vomiting

- vomit fluid that

- is green or yellow

- looks like coffee grounds

- contains blood

- have problems breathing after vomiting

- have pain in the mouth or throat when you eat
- have problems swallowing or painful swallowing

Diagnosis

How Do Doctors Diagnose GER?

In most cases, your doctor diagnoses gastroesophageal reflux (GER) by reviewing your symptoms and medical history. If your symptoms don't improve with lifestyle changes and medications, you may need testing.

How Do Doctors Diagnose GERD?

If your GER symptoms don't improve, if they come back frequently, or if you have trouble swallowing, your doctor may recommend testing you for gastroesophageal reflux disease (GERD).

Your doctor may refer you to a gastroenterologist to diagnose and treat GERD.

What Tests Do Doctors Use to Diagnose GERD?

Several tests can help a doctor diagnose GERD. Your doctor may order more than one test to make a diagnosis.

Upper Gastrointestinal (GI) Endoscopy and Biopsy

In an upper GI endoscopy, a gastroenterologist, surgeon, or other trained healthcare professional uses an endoscope to see inside your upper GI tract. This procedure takes place at a hospital or an outpatient center.

An intravenous (IV) needle will be placed in your arm to provide a sedative. Sedatives help you stay relaxed and comfortable during the procedure. In some cases, the procedure can be performed without sedation. You will be given a liquid anesthetic to gargle or spray anesthetic on the back of your throat. The doctor carefully feeds the endoscope down your esophagus and into your stomach and duodenum. A small camera mounted on the endoscope sends a video image to a monitor, allowing close examination of the lining of your upper GI tract. The endoscope pumps air into your stomach and duodenum, making them easier to see.

The doctor may perform a biopsy with the endoscope by taking a small piece of tissue from the lining of your esophagus. You won't feel the biopsy. A pathologist examines the tissue in a lab.

369

In most cases, the procedure only diagnoses GERD if you have moderate to severe symptoms.

Upper GI Series

An upper GI series looks at the shape of your upper GI tract.

An X-ray technician performs this procedure at a hospital or an outpatient center. A radiologist reads and reports on the X-ray images. You don't need anesthesia. A healthcare professional will tell you how to prepare for the procedure, including when to stop eating and drinking.

During the procedure, you will stand or sit in front of an X-ray machine and drink barium to coat the inner lining of your upper GI tract. The X-ray technician takes several X-rays as the barium moves through your GI tract. The upper GI series can't show GERD in your esophagus; rather, the barium shows up on the X-ray and can find problems related to GERD, such as:

- Hiatal hernias

- Esophageal strictures

- Ulcers

You may have bloating and nausea for a short time after the procedure. For several days afterward, you may have white or light-colored stools from the barium. A healthcare professional will give you instructions about eating, drinking, and taking your medicines after the procedure.

Esophageal pH and Impedance Monitoring

The most accurate procedure to detect acid reflux is esophageal pH and impedance monitoring. Esophageal pH and impedance monitoring measures the amount of acid in your esophagus while you do normal things, such as eating and sleeping.

A gastroenterologist performs this procedure at a hospital or an outpatient center as a part of an upper GI endoscopy. Most often, you can stay awake during the procedure.

A gastroenterologist will pass a thin tube through your nose or mouth into your stomach. The gastroenterologist will then pull the tube back into your esophagus and tape it to your cheek. The end of the tube in your esophagus measures when and how much acid comes up your esophagus. The other end of the tube attaches to a monitor outside your body that records the measurements.

You will wear a monitor for the next 24 hours. You will return to the hospital or outpatient center to have the tube removed.

This procedure is most useful to your doctor if you keep a diary of when, what, and how much food you eat and your GERD symptoms are after you eat. The gastroenterologist can see how your symptoms, certain foods, and certain times of day relate to one another. The procedure can also help show whether acid reflux triggers any respiratory symptoms.

Bravo Wireless Esophageal pH Monitoring

Bravo wireless esophageal pH monitoring also measures and records the pH in your esophagus to determine if you have GERD. A doctor temporarily attaches a small capsule to the wall of your esophagus during an upper endoscopy. The capsule measures pH levels in the esophagus and transmits information to a receiver. The receiver is about the size of a pager, which you wear on your belt or waistband.

You will follow your usual daily routine during monitoring, which usually lasts 48 hours. The receiver has several buttons on it that you will press to record symptoms of GERD such as heartburn. The nurse will tell you what symptoms to record. You will be asked to maintain a diary to record certain events such as when you start and stop eating and drinking, when you lie down, and when you get back up.

To prepare for the test talk to your doctor about medicines you are taking. He or she will tell you whether you can eat or drink before the procedure. After about seven to ten days the capsule will fall off the esophageal lining and pass through your digestive tract.

Esophageal Manometry

Esophageal manometry measures muscle contractions in your esophagus. A gastroenterologist may order this procedure if you're thinking about anti-reflux surgery.

The gastroenterologist can perform this procedure during an office visit. A healthcare professional will spray a liquid anesthetic on the back of your throat or ask you to gargle a liquid anesthetic.

The gastroenterologist passes a soft, thin tube through your nose and into your stomach. You swallow as the gastroenterologist pulls the tube slowly back into your esophagus. A computer measures and records the pressure of muscle contractions in different parts of your esophagus.

371

The procedure can show if your symptoms are due to a weak sphincter muscle. A doctor can also use the procedure to diagnose other esophagus problems that might have symptoms similar to heartburn. A healthcare professional will give you instructions about eating, drinking, and taking your medicines after the procedure.

Treatment

How Do You Control GER and GERD?

You may be able to control gastroesophageal reflux (GER) and gastroesophageal reflux disease (GERD) by:

- not eating or drinking items that may cause GER, such as greasy or spicy foods and alcoholic drinks

- not overeating

- not eating 2 to 3 hours before bedtime

- losing weight if you're overweight or obese

- quitting smoking and avoiding secondhand smoke

- taking over-the-counter medicines, such as Maalox, or Rolaids

How Do Doctors Treat GERD?

Depending on the severity of your symptoms, your doctor may recommend lifestyle changes, medicines, surgery, or a combination.

Lifestyle Changes

Making lifestyle changes can reduce your GER and GERD symptoms. You should:

- lose weight, if needed.

- wear loose-fitting clothing around your abdomen. Tight clothing can squeeze your stomach area and push acid up into your esophagus.

- stay upright for 3 hours after meals. Avoid reclining and slouching when sitting.

- sleep on a slight angle. Raise the head of your bed 6 to 8 inches by safely putting blocks under the bedposts. Just using extra pillows will not help.

- quit smoking and avoid secondhand smoke.

Over-the-Counter and Prescription Medicines

You can buy many GERD medicines without a prescription. However, if you have symptoms that will not go away, you should see your doctor.

All GERD medicines work in different ways. You may need a combination of GERD medicines to control your symptoms.

Antacids. Doctors often first recommend antacids to relieve heartburn and other mild GER and GERD symptoms. Antacids can have side effects, including diarrhea and constipation.

H2 blockers. H2 blockers decrease acid production. They provide short-term or on-demand relief for many people with GER and GERD symptoms. They can also help heal the esophagus, although not as well as other medicines. You can buy H2 blockers over-the-counter or your doctor can prescribe one.

Proton pump inhibitors (PPIs). PPIs lower the amount of acid your stomach makes. PPIs are better at treating GERD symptoms than H2 blockers. They can heal the esophageal lining in most people with GERD. Doctors often prescribe PPIs for long-term GERD treatment.

Prokinetics. Prokinetics help your stomach empty faster.

Antibiotics. Antibiotics, including erythromycin, can help your stomach empty faster. Erythromycin has fewer side effects than prokinetics; however, it can cause diarrhea.

Surgery

Your doctor may recommend surgery if your GERD symptoms don't improve with lifestyle changes or medicines. You're more likely to develop complications from surgery than from medicines.

Fundoplication is the most common surgery for GERD. In most cases, it leads to long-term reflux control.

A surgeon performs fundoplication using a laparoscope, a thin tube with a tiny video camera. During the operation, a surgeon sews the top of your stomach around your esophagus to add pressure to the lower end of your esophagus and reduce reflux. The surgeon performs the operation at a hospital. You receive general anesthesia and can leave the hospital in 1 to 3 days. Most people return to their usual daily activities in 2 to 3 weeks.

Endoscopic techniques, such as endoscopic sewing and radiofrequency, help control GERD in a small number of people. Endoscopic sewing uses small stitches to tighten your sphincter muscle. Radiofrequency creates heat lesions, or sores, that help tighten your sphincter muscle. A surgeon performs both operations using an endoscope at a hospital or an outpatient center, and you receive general anesthesia.

The results for endoscopic techniques may not be as good as those for fundoplication. Doctors don't use endoscopic techniques often.

Eating, Diet, and Nutrition

How Can Your Diet Help Prevent or Relieve GER or GERD?

You can prevent or relieve your symptoms from gastroesophageal reflux (GER) or gastroesophageal reflux disease (GERD) by changing your diet. You may need to avoid certain foods and drinks that make your symptoms worse. Other dietary changes that can help reduce your symptoms include:

- decreasing fatty foods

- eating small, frequent meals instead of three large meals

What Should I Avoid Eating If I Have GER or GERD?

Avoid eating or drinking the following items that may make GER or GERD worse:

- Chocolate

- Coffee

- Peppermint

- Greasy or spicy foods

- Tomatoes and tomato products

- Alcoholic drinks

What Can I Eat If I Have GER or GERD?

Eating healthy and balanced amounts of different types of foods is good for your overall health.

If you're overweight or obese, talk with your doctor or a dietitian about dietary changes that can help you lose weight and decrease your GERD symptoms.

Section 28.8

Irritable Bowel Syndrome

This section includes text excerpted from "Irritable Bowel Syndrome (IBS)," National Institute of Diabetes and Digestive and Kidney Diseases (NIDDK), February 2015.

Definition and Facts

What Is IBS?

Irritable bowel syndrome (IBS) is a group of symptoms—including pain or discomfort in your abdomen and changes in your bowel movement patterns—that occur together. Doctors call IBS a functional gastrointestinal (GI) disorder. Functional GI disorders happen when your GI tract behaves in an abnormal way without evidence of damage due to a disease.

Does IBS Have Another Name?

In the past, doctors called IBS colitis, mucous colitis, spastic colon, nervous colon, and spastic bowel. Experts changed the name to reflect the understanding that the disorder has both physical and mental causes and isn't a product of a person's imagination.

What Are the Four Types of IBS?

Doctors often classify IBS into one of four types based on your usual stool consistency. These types are important because they affect the types of treatment that are most likely to improve your symptoms.

The four types of IBS are:

- IBS with constipation, or IBS-C

- hard or lumpy stools at least 25 percent of the time

- loose or watery stools less than 25 percent of the time

- IBS with diarrhea, or IBS-D

  - loose or watery stools at least 25 percent of the time

  - hard or lumpy stools less than 25 percent of the time

- Mixed IBS, or IBS-M

  - hard or lumpy stools at least 25 percent of the time

  - loose or watery stools at least 25 percent of the time

- Unsubtyped IBS, or IBS-U

  - hard or lumpy stools less than 25 percent of the time

  - loose or watery stools less than 25 percent of the time

How Common Is IBS?

Studies estimate that IBS affects 10 to 15 percent of U.S. adults. However, only 5 to 7 percent of U.S. adults have received a diagnosis of IBS.

Who Is More Likely to Develop IBS?

IBS affects about twice as many women as men and most often occurs in people younger than age 45.

What Other Health Problems Do People with IBS Have?

People with IBS often suffer from other GI and non-GI conditions. GI conditions such as gastroesophageal reflux disease and dyspepsia are more common in people with IBS than the general population.

Non-GI conditions that people with IBS often have include:

- chronic fatigue syndrome

- chronic pelvic pain

- temporomandibular joint disorders

- depression

- anxiety

- somatoform disorders

Symptoms and Causes

What Are the Symptoms of IBS?

The most common symptoms of irritable bowel syndrome (IBS) include pain or discomfort in your abdomen and changes in how often you have bowel movements or how your stools look. The pain or discomfort of IBS may feel like cramping and have at least two of the following:

- Your pain or discomfort improves after a bowel movement.

- You notice a change in how often you have a bowel movement.

- You notice a change in the way your stools look.

IBS is a chronic disorder, meaning it lasts a long time, often years. However, the symptoms may come and go. You may have IBS if:

- You've had symptoms at least three times a month for the past 3 months.

- Your symptoms first started at least 6 months ago.

People with IBS may have diarrhea, constipation, or both. Some people with IBS have only diarrhea or only constipation. Some people have symptoms of both or have diarrhea sometimes and constipation other times. People often have symptoms soon after eating a meal.

Other symptoms of IBS are:

- bloating

- the feeling that you haven't finished a bowel movement

- whitish mucus in your stool

Women with IBS often have more symptoms during their menstrual periods.

While IBS can be painful, IBS doesn't lead to other health problems or damage your gastrointestinal (GI) tract.

What Causes IBS?

Doctors aren't sure what causes IBS. Experts think that a combination of problems can lead to IBS.

Physical Problems

- Brain-gut signal problems

- GI motility problems

- Pain sensitivity

- Infections

- Small intestinal bacterial overgrowth

- Neurotransmitters (Body chemicals)

- Genetics

- Food sensitivity

Mental Health Problems

Psychological, or mental health, problems such as panic disorder, anxiety, depression, and posttraumatic stress disorder are common in people with IBS. The link between mental health and IBS is unclear. GI disorders, including IBS, are sometimes present in people who have reported past physical or sexual abuse. Experts think people who have been abused tend to express psychological stress through physical symptoms.

If you have IBS, your colon may respond too much to even slight conflict or stress. Stress makes your mind more aware of the sensations in your colon. IBS symptoms can also increase your stress level.

Diagnosis

How Do Doctors Diagnose IBS?

Your doctor may be able to diagnose irritable bowel syndrome (IBS) based on a review of your medical history, symptoms, and physical exam. Your doctor may also order tests.

To diagnose IBS, your doctor will take a complete medical history and perform a physical exam.

Medical History

The medical history will include questions about:

- your symptoms

- family history of gastrointestinal (GI) tract disorders

- recent infections

- medicines

- stressful events related to the start of your symptoms

Your doctor will look for a certain pattern in your symptoms. Your doctor may diagnose IBS if:

- your symptoms started at least 6 months ago

- you've had pain or discomfort in your abdomen at least three times a month for the past 3 months

- your abdominal pain or discomfort has two or three of the following features:

  - Your pain or discomfort improves after a bowel movement.

  - You notice a change in how often you have a bowel movement.

  - You notice a change in the way your stools look.

Physical Exam

During a physical exam, your doctor usually:

- checks for abdominal bloating

- listens to sounds within your abdomen using a stethoscope

- taps on your abdomen checking for tenderness or pain

What Tests Do Doctors Use to Diagnose IBS?

In most cases, doctors don't need to perform tests to diagnose IBS. Your doctor may perform a blood test to check for other conditions or problems.

- Blood test

- Stool test

- Flexible sigmoidoscopy

- Colonoscopy

- Lower GI series

Treatment

How Do Doctors Treat IBS?

Though irritable bowel syndrome (IBS) doesn't have a cure, your doctor can manage the symptoms with a combination of diet, medicines, probiotics, and therapies for mental health problems. You may have to try a few treatments to see what works best for you. Your doctor can help you find the right treatment plan.

Changes in Eating, Diet, and Nutrition

Changes in eating, diet, and nutrition, such as following a FODMAP diet, can help treat your symptoms.

Medicines

Your doctor may recommend medicine to relieve your symptoms.

- Fiber supplements to relieve constipation when increasing fiber in your diet doesn't help.

- Laxatives to help with constipation. Laxatives work in different ways, and your doctor can recommend a laxative that's right for you.

- Loperamide to reduce diarrhea by slowing the movement of stool through your colon. Loperamide is an antidiarrheal that reduces diarrhea in people with IBS, though it doesn't reduce pain, bloating, or other symptoms.

- Antispasmodics, such as hyoscine, cimetropium, and pinaverium, help to control colon muscle spasms and reduce pain in your abdomen.

- Antidepressants, such as low doses of tricyclic antidepressants and selective serotonin reuptake inhibitors, to relieve IBS symptoms, including abdominal pain. In theory, because of their effect on colon transit, tricyclic antidepressants should be better for people with IBS with diarrhea, or IBS-D, and selective serotonin reuptake inhibitors should be better for people with IBS with constipation, or IBS-C, although studies haven't confirmed this theory. Tricyclic antidepressants work in people with IBS by reducing their sensitivity to pain in the gastrointestinal (GI) tract as well as normalizing their GI motility and secretion.

- Lubiprostone (Amitiza) for people who have IBS-C to improve abdominal pain or discomfort and constipation symptoms.

- Linaclotide (Linzess) for people who have IBS-C to relieve abdominal pain and increase how often you have bowel movements.

- The antibiotic rifaximin to reduce bloating by treating small intestinal bacterial overgrowth. However, experts are still debating and researching the use of antibiotics to treat IBS.

- Coated peppermint oil capsules to reduce IBS symptoms.

Follow your doctor's instructions when you use medicine to treat IBS. Talk with your doctor about possible side effects and what to do if you have them.

Some medicines can cause side effects. Ask your doctor and your pharmacist about side effects before taking any medicine.

Probiotics

Your doctor may also recommend probiotics. Probiotics are live microorganisms—tiny organisms that can be seen only with a microscope. These microorganisms, most often bacteria, are like the microorganisms that are normally present in your GI tract. Studies have found that taking large enough amounts of probiotics, specifically Bifidobacteria and certain probiotic combinations, can improve symptoms of IBS. However, researchers are still studying the use of probiotics to treat IBS.

You can find probiotics in dietary supplements, such as capsules, tablets, and powders, and in some foods, such as yogurt.

Discuss your use of complementary and alternative medical practices, including probiotics and dietary supplements, with your doctor.

Therapies for Mental Health Problems

Psychological therapies may improve your IBS symptoms.

Managing Stress

Learning to reduce stress can help improve IBS. With less stress, you may find you have less cramping and pain. You may also find it easier to manage your symptoms.

Some options for managing stress include:

- taking part in stress reduction and relaxation therapies such as meditation

- getting counseling and support

- taking part in regular exercise such as walking or yoga

- reducing stressful life situations as much as possible

- getting enough sleep

Talk Therapy

Talk therapy may reduce stress and improve your IBS symptoms. Two types of talk therapy that healthcare professionals use to treat IBS are cognitive behavioral therapy and psychodynamic, or interpersonal, therapy. Cognitive behavioral therapy focuses on your thoughts and actions. Psychodynamic therapy focuses on how your emotions affect your IBS symptoms. This type of therapy often involves relaxation and stress management techniques.

Gut-Directed Hypnotherapy

In gut-directed hypnotherapy, a therapist uses hypnosis to help you relax the muscles in the colon.

Mindfulness Training

Mindfulness training can teach you to focus your attention on sensations occurring at the moment and to avoid catastrophizing, or worrying about the meaning of those sensations.

Eating, Diet, and Nutrition

How Can My Diet Treat the Symptoms of IBS?

Eating smaller meals more often, or eating smaller portions, may help your irritable bowel syndrome (IBS) symptoms. Large meals can cause cramping and diarrhea if you have IBS.

Eating foods that are low in fat and high in carbohydrates, such as pasta, rice, whole-grain breads and cereals, fruits, and vegetables, may help.

Fiber may improve constipation symptoms caused by IBS because it makes stool soft and easier to pass. Fiber is a part of foods such as whole-grain breads and cereals, beans, fruits, and vegetables. The U.S. Department of Agriculture (USDA) and U.S. Department of Health and Human Services (HHS) state in its *Dietary Guidelines for Americans*, 2010 that adults should get 22 to 34 grams of fiber a day.

While fiber may help constipation, it may not reduce the abdominal discomfort or pain of IBS. In fact, some people with IBS may feel a bit more abdominal discomfort after adding more fiber to their diet. Add foods with fiber to your diet a little at a time to let your body get used to them. Too much fiber at once can cause gas, which can trigger symptoms in people with IBS. Adding fiber to your diet slowly, by 2 to 3 grams a day, may help prevent gas and bloating.

What Should I Avoid Eating to Ease IBS Symptoms?

Certain foods or drinks may make symptoms worse, such as:

- foods high in fat
- some milk products
- drinks with alcohol or caffeine
- drinks with large amounts of artificial sweeteners
- beans, cabbage, and other foods that may cause gas

To find out if certain foods trigger your symptoms, keep a diary and track:

- what you eat during the day
- what symptoms you have
- when symptoms occur

Take your notes to your doctor and talk about which foods seem to make your symptoms worse. You may need to avoid these foods or eat less of them.

Your doctor may recommend that you try a special diet—called low FODMAP or FODMAP—to reduce or avoid certain foods containing carbohydrates that are hard to digest. Examples of high FODMAP foods and products you may reduce or avoid include:

- fruits such as apples, apricots, blackberries, cherries, mango, nectarines, pears, plums, and watermelon, or juice containing any of these fruits

- canned fruit in natural fruit juice, or large quantities of fruit juice or dried fruit

- vegetables such as artichokes, asparagus, beans, cabbage, cauliflower, garlic and garlic salts, lentils, mushrooms, onions, and sugar snap or snow peas

- dairy products such as milk, milk products, soft cheeses, yogurt, custard, and ice cream

- wheat and rye products

- honey and foods with high-fructose corn syrup

- products, including candy and gum, with sweeteners ending in "–ol," such as:

  - sorbitol

  - mannitol

  - xylitol

  - maltitol

Section 28.9

Pancreatitis

This section includes text excerpted from "Pancreatitis," National Institute of Diabetes and Digestive and Kidney Diseases (NIDDK), August 2012. Reviewed June 2017.

Pancreatitis is inflammation of the pancreas. The pancreas is a large gland behind the stomach and close to the duodenum—the first part of the small intestine. The pancreas secretes digestive juices, or enzymes, into the duodenum through a tube called the pancreatic duct. Pancreatic enzymes join with bile—a liquid produced in the liver and stored in the gallbladder—to digest food. The pancreas also releases the hormones insulin and glucagon into the bloodstream. These hormones help the body regulate the glucose it takes from food for energy.

Normally, digestive enzymes secreted by the pancreas do not become active until they reach the small intestine. But when the pancreas is inflamed, the enzymes inside it attack and damage the tissues that produce them.

Pancreatitis can be acute or chronic. Either form is serious and can lead to complications. In severe cases, bleeding, infection, and permanent tissue damage may occur. Both forms of pancreatitis occur more often in men than women.

What Is Acute Pancreatitis?

Acute pancreatitis is inflammation of the pancreas that occurs suddenly and usually resolves in a few days with treatment. Acute pancreatitis can be a life-threatening illness with severe complications. Each year, about 210,000 people in the United States are admitted to the hospital with acute pancreatitis.1 The most common cause of acute pancreatitis is the presence of gallstones—small, pebble-like substances made of hardened bile—that cause inflammation in the pancreas as they pass through the common bile duct. Chronic, heavy alcohol use is also a common cause. Acute pancreatitis can occur within hours or as long as 2 days after consuming alcohol. Other causes of acute pancreatitis include abdominal trauma, medications, infections, tumors, and genetic abnormalities of the pancreas.

Symptoms

Acute pancreatitis usually begins with gradual or sudden pain in the upper abdomen that sometimes extends through the back. The pain may be mild at first and feel worse after eating. But the pain is often severe and may become constant and last for several days. A person with acute pancreatitis usually looks and feels very ill and needs immediate medical attention. Other symptoms may include:

- a swollen and tender abdomen

- nausea and vomiting

- fever

- a rapid pulse

Severe acute pancreatitis may cause dehydration and low blood pressure. The heart, lungs, or kidneys can fail. If bleeding occurs in the pancreas, shock and even death may follow.

Diagnosis

While asking about a person's medical history and conducting a thorough physical examination, the doctor will order a blood test to assist in the diagnosis. During acute pancreatitis, the blood contains at least three times the normal amount of amylase and lipase, digestive enzymes formed in the pancreas. Changes may also occur in other body chemicals such as glucose, calcium, magnesium, sodium, potassium, and bicarbonate. After the person's condition improves, the levels usually return to normal.

Diagnosing acute pancreatitis is often difficult because of the deep location of the pancreas. The doctor will likely order one or more of the following tests:

- Abdominal ultrasound

- Computerized tomography (CT) scan

- Endoscopic ultrasound (EUS)

- Magnetic resonance cholangiopancreatography (MRCP)

Treatment

Treatment for acute pancreatitis requires a few days' stay in the hospital for intravenous (IV) fluids, antibiotics, and medication to relieve pain. The person cannot eat or drink so the pancreas can rest. If vomiting occurs, a tube may be placed through the nose and into the stomach to remove fluid and air.

Unless complications arise, acute pancreatitis usually resolves in a few days. In severe cases, the person may require nasogastric feeding—a special liquid given in a long, thin tube inserted through the nose and throat and into the stomach—for several weeks while the pancreas heals.

Before leaving the hospital, the person will be advised not to smoke, drink alcoholic beverages, or eat fatty meals. In some cases, the cause of the pancreatitis is clear, but in others, more tests are needed after the person is discharged and the pancreas is healed.

Therapeutic Endoscopic Retrograde Cholangiopancreatography (ERCP) for Acute and Chronic Pancreatitis

ERCP is a specialized technique used to view the pancreas, gallbladder, and bile ducts and treat complications of acute and chronic pancreatitis—gallstones, narrowing or blockage of the pancreatic duct or bile ducts, leaks in the bile ducts, and pseudocysts—accumulations of fluid and tissue debris.

Soon after a person is admitted to the hospital with suspected narrowing of the pancreatic duct or bile ducts, a physician with specialized training performs ERCP.

After lightly sedating the patient and giving medication to numb the throat, the doctor inserts an endoscope—a long, flexible, lighted tube with a camera—through the mouth, throat, and stomach into the small intestine. The endoscope is connected to a computer and screen. The doctor guides the endoscope and injects a special dye into the pancreatic or bile ducts that helps the pancreas, gallbladder, and bile ducts appear on the screen while X-rays are taken.

The following procedures can be performed using ERCP:

- **Sphincterotomy**. Using a small wire on the endoscope, the doctor finds the muscle that surrounds the pancreatic duct or bile ducts and makes a tiny cut to enlarge the duct opening. When a pseudocyst is present, the duct is drained.

- **Gallstone removal**. The endoscope is used to remove pancreatic or bile duct stones with a tiny basket. Gallstone removal is sometimes performed along with a sphincterotomy.

- **Stent placement**. Using the endoscope, the doctor places a tiny piece of plastic or metal that looks like a straw in a narrowed pancreatic or bile duct to keep it open.

- **Balloon dilatation**. Some endoscopes have a small balloon that the doctor uses to dilate, or stretch, a narrowed pancreatic or bile duct. A temporary stent may be placed for a few months to keep the duct open.

People who undergo therapeutic ERCP are at slight risk for complications, including severe pancreatitis, infection, bowel perforation, or bleeding. Complications of ERCP are more common in people with acute or recurrent pancreatitis. A patient who experiences fever, trouble swallowing, or increased throat, chest, or abdominal pain after the procedure should notify a doctor immediately.

What Is Chronic Pancreatitis?

Chronic pancreatitis is inflammation of the pancreas that does not heal or improve—it gets worse over time and leads to permanent damage. Chronic pancreatitis, like acute pancreatitis, occurs when digestive enzymes attack the pancreas and nearby tissues, causing episodes of pain. Chronic pancreatitis often develops in people who are between the ages of 30 and 40.

The most common cause of chronic pancreatitis is many years of heavy alcohol use. The chronic form of pancreatitis can be triggered by one acute attack that damages the pancreatic duct. The damaged duct causes the pancreas to become inflamed. Scar tissue develops and the pancreas is slowly destroyed.

Other causes of chronic pancreatitis are:

- hereditary disorders of the pancreas

- cystic fibrosis—the most common inherited disorder leading to chronic pancreatitis

- hypercalcemia—high levels of calcium in the blood

- hyperlipidemia or hypertriglyceridemia—high levels of blood fats

- some medicines

- certain autoimmune conditions

Hereditary pancreatitis can present in a person younger than age 30, but it might not be diagnosed for several years. Episodes of abdominal pain and diarrhea lasting several days come and go over time and can progress to chronic pancreatitis. A diagnosis of hereditary pancreatitis is likely if the person has two or more family members with pancreatitis in more than one generation.

Symptoms

Most people with chronic pancreatitis experience upper abdominal pain, although some people have no pain at all. The pain may spread to the back, feel worse when eating or drinking, and become constant and disabling. In some cases, abdominal pain goes away as the condition worsens, most likely because the pancreas is no longer making digestive enzymes. Other symptoms include:

- nausea

- vomiting

- weight loss

- diarrhea

- oily stools

People with chronic pancreatitis often lose weight, even when their appetite and eating habits are normal. The weight loss occurs because the body does not secrete enough pancreatic enzymes to digest food, so nutrients are not absorbed normally. Poor digestion leads to malnutrition due to excretion of fat in the stool.

Diagnosis

Chronic pancreatitis is often confused with acute pancreatitis because the symptoms are similar. As with acute pancreatitis, the doctor will conduct a thorough medical history and physical examination. Blood tests may help the doctor know if the pancreas is still making enough digestive enzymes, but sometimes these enzymes appear normal even though the person has chronic pancreatitis.

In more advanced stages of pancreatitis, when malabsorption and diabetes can occur, the doctor may order blood, urine, and stool tests to help diagnose chronic pancreatitis and monitor its progression.

After ordering X-rays of the abdomen, the doctor will conduct one or more of the tests used to diagnose acute pancreatitis — abdominal ultrasound, CT scan, EUS, and MRCP.

Treatment

Treatment for chronic pancreatitis may require hospitalization for pain management, IV hydration, and nutritional support. Nasogastric feedings may be necessary for several weeks if the person continues to lose weight.

When a normal diet is resumed, the doctor may prescribe synthetic pancreatic enzymes if the pancreas does not secrete enough of its own. The enzymes should be taken with every meal to help the person digest food and regain some weight. The next step is to plan a nutritious diet that is low in fat and includes small, frequent meals. A dietitian can assist in developing a meal plan. Drinking plenty of fluids and limiting caffeinated beverages is also important.

People with chronic pancreatitis are strongly advised not to smoke or consume alcoholic beverages, even if the pancreatitis is mild or in the early stages.

Chapter 29

Gynecological Pain

Chapter Contents

Section 29.1

Childbirth and Pain

This section includes text excerpted from "Labor and Delivery,"
Eunice Kennedy Shriver National Institute of Child Health and
Human Development (NICHD), December 17, 2014.

When Does Labor Usually Start?

The due date is 40 weeks after the first day of the last menstrual
period, although sometimes it is determined by an ultrasound. For
most women, labor occurs sometime between week 37 and week 42 of
pregnancy. Labor that occurs before 37 weeks of pregnancy is considered premature, or preterm labor. Labor that occurs at 37 or 38 weeks
is now considered early term because babies born at that gestational
age are still immature.

Just as pregnancy is different for every woman, the start of labor,
the signs of labor, and the length of time it takes to go through labor will
vary from woman to woman and even from pregnancy to pregnancy.

Signs of Labor

Some signs that labor may be close (although, in fact, it still might
be weeks away) can include:

- **Lightening.** This term describes when the fetus "drops," or
  moves lower in the uterus. Not all fetuses drop before birth.
  Lightening gets its name from the feeling of lightness or relief
  that some women experience when the fetus moves away from
  the rib cage to the pelvic area. This allows some women to
  breathe easier and more deeply and to get relief from heartburn.

- **Increase in vaginal discharge.** Called "show" or "the bloody
  show," the discharge can be clear, pink, or slightly bloody. This
  occurs as the cervix begins to open (dilate) and can happen several days before labor or just as labor begins.

If a woman experiences any of the following signs of labor at any
point in pregnancy, she should contact her healthcare provider:

- Contractions every 10 minutes or more often

- Change in color of vaginal discharge

- Pain or pressure around the front of the pelvis or the rectum

- Low, dull backache

- Vaginal spotting or bleeding

- Abdominal cramps, with or without diarrhea

Sometimes, if the health of the mother or the fetus is at risk, a woman's healthcare provider will recommend inducing labor, using medically supervised methods, such as medication, to bring on labor.

Unless earlier delivery is medically necessary, waiting until at least 39 weeks before delivering gives mother and baby the best chance for healthy outcomes. During the last few weeks of pregnancy, the fetus's lungs, brain, and liver are still developing.

What Are the Stages of Labor?

Stage 1

The first stage of labor happens in two phases: early labor and active labor.

During **early labor:**

- The cervix starts to open or dilate.

- Strong and regular contractions last 30 to 60 seconds and come every 5 to 20 minutes.

- The woman may have a bloody show.

A woman may experience this phase for a few hours or days, especially if she is giving birth for the first time.

During **active labor:**

- Contractions become stronger, longer, and more painful.

- Contractions come closer together.

- The woman may not have much time to relax between contractions.

- The woman may feel pressure in her lower back.

- The cervix fully dilates to 10 centimeters.

Stage 2

During this stage, the cervix is fully dilated and ready for delivery. The woman will begin to push (or is sometimes told to "bear down") to allow the baby to move through the birth canal.

During **stage 2:**

- The woman may feel pressure on her rectum as the baby's head moves through the vagina.

- She may feel the urge to push, as if having a bowel movement.

- The baby's head starts to show (called "crowning").

- The healthcare provider guides the baby out of the vagina.

- Once the baby comes out, the healthcare provider cuts the umbilical cord, which connected mother and fetus during pregnancy.

This stage can last between 20 minutes and several hours. It usually lasts longer for first-time mothers.

Stage 3

During this stage, the placenta is delivered. The placenta is the organ that gave the fetus food and oxygen through the umbilical cord during the pregnancy.

During **stage 3:**

- Contractions begin 5 to 10 minutes after the baby is delivered.

- The woman may have chills or feel shaky.

It may take 5 to 30 minutes for the placenta to exit the vagina.

What Are the Options for Pain Relief during Labor and Delivery?

The amount of pain felt during labor and delivery is different for every woman. The level of pain can depend on many factors, including the size and position of the baby and the strength of contractions. Some women learn breathing and relaxation techniques to help them cope with the pain. These techniques can be used along with one or more pain-relieving drugs.

A woman should discuss the many aspects of labor with her healthcare provider well before labor begins to ensure that she understands all of the options, risks, and benefits of pain relief during labor and delivery. It might also be helpful to put all the decisions in writing to clarify the options chosen.

Types of Pain-Relieving Medications

Pain-relief drugs fall into two categories: analgesics and anesthetics. There are different forms of each.

Analgesics

Analgesics relieve pain without causing total loss of feeling or muscle movement. These drugs do not always stop pain completely, but they reduce it.

- **Systemic analgesics** affect the whole nervous system rather than a single area. They ease pain but do not cause the patient to go to sleep. Systemic analgesics are often used in early labor. They are not given right before delivery because they may slow the baby's breathing and reflexes. They are given in two ways:

  - Injected into a muscle or vein

  - Inhaled or breathed in with a mixture of oxygen. The woman holds a mask to her face, meaning she decides how much or how little analgesic is needed for pain relief.

- **Regional analgesics** relieve pain in one region of the body. In the United States, regional analgesia is the most common way to relieve pain during labor. Several types of regional analgesia can be given during labor:

  - Epidural analgesia, also called an epidural block or an epidural, causes loss of feeling in the lower body while the patient stays awake. The drug starts working about 10 to 20 minutes after it is given. A healthcare provider injects the drug near the spinal cord. A small tube (catheter) is placed through the needle. The needle is then withdrawn, but the tube stays in place. Small amounts of the drug can then be given through the catheter throughout labor without the need for another injection.

  - A spinal block is an injection of a much smaller amount of the drug into the sac of spinal fluid around the spine. The drug starts working right away, but it only lasts for 1 to 2 hours. Usually a spinal block is given only once during labor, to help with pain during delivery.

- A combined spinal-epidural block, also called a "walking epidural," gives the benefits of an epidural block and a spinal block. The spinal part relieves pain immediately. The epidural part allows drugs to be given throughout labor. Some women may be able to walk around after a combined spinal-epidural block.

Anesthetics

Anesthetics block all feeling, including pain.

- **General anesthesia** causes the patient to go to sleep. The patient does not feel pain while asleep.

- **Local anesthesia** removes all feeling, including pain, from a small part of the body while the patient stays awake. It does not lessen the pain of contractions. healthcare providers often use it when performing an episiotomy, a surgical cut made in the region between the vagina and anus to widen the vaginal opening for delivery, or when repairing vaginal tears that happen during birth.

What Is Natural Childbirth?

- Natural childbirth can refer to many different ways of giving birth without using pain medication, either in the home or at the hospital or birthing center.

Natural Forms of Pain Relief

Women who choose natural childbirth can use a number of natural ways to ease pain. These include:

- Emotional support
- Relaxation techniques
- A soothing atmosphere
- Moving and changing positions frequently
- Using a birthing ball
- Using soothing phrases and mental images
- Placing a heating pad or ice pack on the back or stomach

- Massage

- Taking a bath or shower

- Hypnosis

- Using soothing scents (aromatherapy)

- Acupuncture or acupressure

- Applying small doses of electrical stimulation to nerve fibers to activate the body's own pain-relieving substances (called transcutaneous electrical nerve stimulation, or TENS)

- Injecting sterile water into the lower back, which can relieve the intense discomfort and pain in the lower back known as back labor

A woman should discuss the many aspects of labor with her healthcare provider well before labor begins to ensure that she understands all of the options, risks, and benefits of pain relief during labor and delivery. It might also be helpful to put all the decisions in writing to clarify the options chosen.

Section 29.2

Dysmenorrhea

This section includes text excerpted from "Period Pain," U.S. National Library of Medicine (NLM), National Institutes of Health (NIH), November 15, 2016.

What Are Painful Periods?

Menstruation, or period, is normal vaginal bleeding that happens as part of a woman's monthly cycle. Many women have painful periods, also called dysmenorrhea. The pain is most often menstrual cramps, which are a throbbing, cramping pain in your lower abdomen. You may also have other symptoms, such as lower back pain, nausea, diarrhea, and headaches. Period pain is not the same as premenstrual syndrome (PMS). PMS causes many different symptoms, including weight gain, bloating, irritability, and fatigue. PMS often starts one to two weeks before your period starts.

What Causes Painful Periods?

There are two types of dysmenorrhea: primary and secondary. Each type has different causes.

Primary dysmenorrhea is the most common kind of period pain. It is period pain that is not caused by another condition. The cause is usually having too many prostaglandins, which are chemicals that your uterus makes. These chemicals make the muscles of your uterus tighten and relax, and this causes the cramps.

The pain can start a day or two before your period. It normally lasts for a few days, though in some women it can last longer.

You usually first start having period pain when you are younger, just after you begin getting periods. Often, as you get older, you have less pain. The pain may also get better after you have given birth.

Secondary dysmenorrhea often starts later in life. It is caused by conditions that affect your uterus or other reproductive organs, such as endometriosis and uterine fibroids. This kind of pain often gets worse over time. It may begin before your period starts, and continue after your period ends.

What Can I Do about Period Pain?

To help ease your period pain, you can try:

- Using a heating pad or hot water bottle on your lower abdomen
- Getting some exercise
- Taking a hot bath
- Doing relaxation techniques, including yoga and meditation

You might also try taking over-the-counter pain relievers such as nonsteroidal anti-inflammatory drugs (NSAIDs). NSAIDs include ibuprofen and naproxen. Besides relieving pain, NSAIDs reduce the amount of prostaglandins that your uterus makes, and lessen their effects. This helps to lessen the cramps. You can take NSAIDs when you first have symptoms, or when your period starts. You can keep taking them for a few days. You should not take NSAIDS if you have ulcers or other stomach problems, bleeding problems, or liver disease. You should also not take them if you are allergic to aspirin. Always check with your healthcare provider if you are not sure whether or not you should take NSAIDs.

It may also help to get enough rest and avoid using alcohol and tobacco.

When Should I Get Medical Help for My Period Pain?

For many women, some pain during your period is normal. However, you should contact your healthcare provider if:

- NSAIDs and self-care measures don't help, and the pain interferes with your life

- Your cramps suddenly get worse

- You are over 25 and you get severe cramps for the first time

- You have a fever with your period pain

- You have the pain even when you are not getting your period

How Is the Cause of Severe Period Pain Diagnosed?

To diagnose severe period pain, your healthcare provider will ask you about your medical history and do a pelvic exam. You may also have an ultrasound or other imaging test. If your healthcare provider thinks you have secondary dysmenorrhea, you might have laparoscopy. It is a surgery that that lets your healthcare provider look inside your body.

What Are Treatments for Severe Period Pain?

If your period pain is primary dysmenorrhea and you need medical treatment, your healthcare provider might suggest using hormonal birth control, such as the pill, patch, ring, or IUD. Another treatment option might be prescription pain relievers.

If you have secondary dysmenorrhea, your treatment depends upon the condition that is causing the problem. In some cases, you may need surgery.

Section 29.3

Endometriosis

This section includes text excerpted from "Endometriosis,"
Office on Women's Health (OWH), U.S. Department of
Health and Human Services (HHS), August 18, 2014.

Endometriosis happens when the lining of the uterus (womb) grows outside of the uterus. It may affect more than 11 percent of American women between 15 and 44. It is especially common among women in their 30s and 40s and may make it harder to get pregnant. Several different treatment options can help manage the symptoms and improve your chances of getting pregnant.

What Are the Symptoms of Endometriosis?

Symptoms of endometriosis can include:

- **Pain.** This is the most common symptom. Women with endometriosis may have many different kinds of pain. These include:

  - Very painful menstrual cramps. The pain may get worse over time.

  - Chronic (long-term) pain in the lower back and pelvis

  - Pain during or after sex. This is usually described as a "deep" pain and is different from pain felt at the entrance to the vagina when penetration begins.

  - Intestinal pain

  - Painful bowel movements or pain when urinating during menstrual periods. In rare cases, you may also find blood in your stool or urine.

- **Bleeding or spotting between menstrual periods.** This can be caused by something other than endometriosis. If it happens often, you should see your doctor.

- **Infertility,** or not being able to get pregnant.

- **Stomach (digestive) problems.** These include diarrhea, constipation, bloating, or nausea, especially during menstrual periods.

Why Does Endometriosis Cause Pain and Health Problems?

Endometriosis growths are benign (not cancerous). But they can still cause problems.

Endometriosis happens when tissue that is normally on the inside of your uterus or womb grows outside of your uterus or womb where it doesn't belong. Endometriosis growths bleed in the same way the lining inside of your uterus does every month—during your menstrual period. This can cause swelling and pain because the tissue grows and bleeds in an area where it cannot easily get out of your body.

The growths may also continue to expand and cause problems, such as:

- Blocking your fallopian tubes when growths cover or grow into your ovaries. Trapped blood in the ovaries can form cysts.

- Inflammation (swelling)

- Forming scar tissue and adhesions (type of tissue that can bind your organs together). This scar tissue may cause pelvic pain and make it hard for you to get pregnant.

- Problems in your intestines and bladder

How Common Is Endometriosis?

Endometriosis is a common health problem for women. Some women do not have symptoms and are never diagnosed, so it is difficult to know how many women have endometriosis. Researchers think that at least 11 percent of women, or more than 6 ½ million women in the United States, have endometriosis.

Who Gets Endometriosis?

Endometriosis can happen in any girl or woman who has menstrual periods, but it is more common in women in their 30s and 40s.

You might be more likely to get endometriosis if you have:

- Never had children

- Menstrual periods that last more than seven days

- Short menstrual cycles (27 days or fewer)
- A family member (mother, aunt, sister) with endometriosis
- A health problem that blocks the normal flow of menstrual blood from your body during your period

What Causes Endometriosis?

No one knows for sure what causes this disease. Researchers are studying possible causes:

- Problems with menstrual period flow
- Genetic factors
- Immune system problems
- Hormones
- Surgery

How Can I Prevent Endometriosis?

You can't prevent endometriosis. But you can reduce your chances of developing it by lowering the levels of the hormone estrogen in your body. Estrogen helps to thicken the lining of your uterus during your menstrual cycle.

To keep lower estrogen levels in your body, you can:

- **Talk to your doctor about hormonal birth control methods**, such as pills, patches or rings with lower doses of estrogen.

- **Exercise regularly** (more than 4 hours a week). This will also help you **keep a low percentage of body fat.** Regular exercise and a lower amount of body fat help decrease the amount of estrogen circulating through the body.

- **Avoid large amounts of alcohol.** Alcohol raises estrogen levels. No more than one drink per day is recommended for women who choose to drink alcohol.

- **Avoid large amount of drinks with caffeine.** Studies show that drinking more than one caffeinated drink a day, especially sodas and green tea, can raise estrogen levels.

How Is Endometriosis Diagnosed?

If you have symptoms of endometriosis, talk with your doctor. The doctor will talk to you about your symptoms and do or prescribe one or more of the following to find out if you have endometriosis:

- Pelvic exam

- Imaging test

- Magnetic resonance imaging (MRI)

- Medicine

- Hormonal birth control

- Gonadotropin-releasing hormone (GnRH) agonists

- If your pain gets better with hormonal medicine, you probably have endometriosis. But, these medicines work only as long as you take them. Once you stop taking them, your pain may come back.

- Laparoscopy

How Is Endometriosis Treated?

There is no cure for endometriosis, but treatments are available for the symptoms and problems it causes. Talk to your doctor about your treatment options.

Medicine

If you are not trying to get pregnant, hormonal birth control is generally the first step in treatment. This may include:

- Extended-cycle (you have only a few periods a year) or continuous cycle (you have no periods) birth control. These types of hormonal birth control are available in the pill or the shot and help stop bleeding and reduce or eliminate pain.

- Intrauterine device (IUD) to help reduce pain and bleeding. The hormonal IUD protects against pregnancy for up to 7 years. But the hormonal IUD may not help your pain and bleeding due to endometriosis for that long.

Hormonal treatment works only as long as it is taken and is best for women who do not have severe pain or symptoms.

If you are trying to get pregnant, your doctor may prescribe a gonadotropin-releasing hormone (GnRH) agonist. This medicine stops the body from making the hormones responsible for ovulation, the menstrual cycle, and the growth of endometriosis. This treatment causes a temporary menopause, but it also helps control the growth of endometriosis. Once you stop taking the medicine, your menstrual cycle returns, but you may have a better chance of getting pregnant.

Surgery

Surgery is usually chosen for severe symptoms, when hormones are not providing relief or if you are having fertility problems. During the operation, the surgeon can locate any areas of endometriosis and may remove the endometriosis patches. After surgery, hormone treatment is often restarted unless you are trying to get pregnant.

Other treatments you can try, alone or with any of the treatments listed above, include:

- **Pain medicine.** For mild symptoms, your doctor may suggest taking over-the-counter medicines for pain. These include ibuprofen (Advil and Motrin) or naproxen (Aleve).

- **Complementary and alternative medicine (CAM) therapies.** Some women report relief from pain with therapies such as acupuncture, chiropractic care, herbs like cinnamon twig or licorice root, or supplements, such as thiamine (vitamin B1), magnesium, or omega-3 fatty acids.

Does Endometriosis Go Away after Menopause?

For some women, the painful symptoms of endometriosis improve after menopause. As the body stops making the hormone estrogen, the growths shrink slowly. However, some women who take menopausal hormone therapy may still have symptoms of endometriosis.

If you are having symptoms of endometriosis after menopause, talk to your doctor about treatment options.

Section 29.4

Pelvic Inflammatory Disease

This section includes text excerpted from "Pelvic
Inflammatory Disease (PID)," Centers for Disease
Control and Prevention (CDC), January 25, 2017.

What Is Pelvic Inflammatory Disease?

Pelvic inflammatory disease (PID) is a clinical syndrome that
results from the ascension of microorganisms from the cervix and
vagina to the upper genital tract. PID can lead to infertility and permanent damage of a woman's reproductive organs.

How Do Women Get Pelvic Inflammatory Disease?

Women develop PID when certain bacteria, such as chlamydia or
gonorrhea, move upward from a woman's vagina or cervix into her
reproductive organs. PID is a serious complication of some sexually
transmitted diseases (STDs), especially chlamydia and gonorrhea.

What Causes Pelvic Inflammatory Disease?

A number of different microorganisms can cause or contribute to
PID. The sexually transmitted pathogens *Chlamydia trachomatis*
(CT) and *Neisseria gonorrhoeae* (NG) have been implicated in a third
to half of PID cases. However, endogenous microorganisms, including gram positive and negative anaerobic organisms and aerobic/
facultative gram positive and negative rods and cocci, found at high
levels in women with bacterial vaginosis, also have been implicated
in the pathogenesis of PID. Newer data suggest that *Mycoplasma
genitalium* may also play a role in PID and may be associated with
milder symptoms although one study failed to demonstrate a significant increase in PID following detection of *M. genitalium* in the lower
genital tract. Because of the polymicrobial nature of PID, broad-spectrum regimens that provide adequate coverage of likely pathogens
are recommended.

What Are the Signs and Symptoms of Pelvic Inflammatory Disease?

Women with PID present with a variety of clinical signs and symptoms that range from subtle and mild to severe. PID can go unrecognized by women and their healthcare providers when the symptoms are mild. Despite lack of symptoms, histologic evidence of endometritis has been demonstrated in women with subclinical PID. When present, signs and symptoms of PID are nonspecific, so other reproductive tract illnesses and diseases of both the urinary and the gastrointestinal tracts should be considered when evaluating a sexually active woman with lower abdominal pain. Pregnancy (including ectopic pregnancy) must also be excluded, as PID can occur concurrently with pregnancy.

When symptoms are present, the most common symptoms of PID are:

- Lower abdominal pain
- Mild pelvic pain
- Increased vaginal discharge
- Irregular menstrual bleeding
- Fever (>38° C)
- Pain with intercourse
- Painful and frequent urination
- Abdominal tenderness
- Pelvic organ tenderness
- Uterine tenderness
- Adnexal tenderness
- Cervical motion tenderness
- Inflammation

What are the complications of pelvic inflammatory disease?

Complications of PID include:

- Tubo-ovarian abscess (TOA)
- Tubal factor infertility

- Ectopic pregnancy

- Chronic pelvic pain

Recurrent episodes of PID and increased severity of tubal inflammation detected by laparoscopy are associated with greater risk of infertility following PID. However, even subclinical PID has been associated with infertility. This emphasizes the importance of following screening and treatment recommendations for chlamydia and gonorrhea to prevent PID when possible, and promptly and appropriately treating cases of PID that do occur.

Tubo-ovarian abscess (TOA) is a serious short-term complication of PID that is characterized by an inflammatory mass involving the fallopian tube, ovary, and, occasionally, other adjacent pelvic organs. The microbiology of TOAs is similar to PID and the diagnosis necessitates initial hospital admission. Treatment includes broad-spectrum antibiotics with or without a drainage procedure, with surgery often reserved for patients with suspected rupture or who fail to respond to antibiotics. Women infected with human immunodeficiency virus (HIV) may be at higher risk for TOA. Mortality from PID is less than 1 percent and is usually secondary to rupture of a TOA or to ectopic pregnancy.

How Is Pelvic Inflammatory Disease Diagnosed?

The wide variation in symptoms and signs associated with PID can make diagnosis challenging. No single historical, physical, or laboratory finding is both sensitive and specific for the diagnosis of PID. Clinicians should therefore maintain a low threshold for the diagnosis of PID, particularly in young, sexually active women.

Criteria have been developed for the diagnosis of PID.

Presumptive treatment for PID should be initiated in sexually active young women and other women at risk for sexually transmitted diseases (STDs) if they are experiencing pelvic or lower abdominal pain, if no cause for the illness other than PID can be identified, and if one or more of the following minimum clinical criteria are present on pelvic examination:

- cervical motion tenderness; or

- uterine tenderness; or

- adnexal tenderness.

The requirement that all three minimum criteria be present before the initiation of empiric treatment could result in insufficient sensitivity for the diagnosis of PID. After deciding whether to initiate empiric treatment, clinicians should also consider the risk profile for STDs.

More elaborate diagnostic evaluation frequently is needed because incorrect diagnosis and management of PID might cause unnecessary morbidity. For example, the presence of signs of lower-genital–tract inflammation (predominance of leukocytes in vaginal secretions, cervical exudates, or cervical friability), in addition to one of the three minimum criteria, increases the specificity of the diagnosis. One or more of the following additional criteria can be used to enhance the specificity of the minimum clinical criteria and support a diagnosis of PID:

- oral temperature >101°F (>38.3°C);

- abnormal cervical mucopurulent discharge or cervical friability;

- presence of abundant numbers of White blood cells (WBC) on saline microscopy of vaginal fluid;

- elevated erythrocyte sedimentation rate;

- elevated C-reactive protein; and

- laboratory documentation of cervical infection with *N. gonorrhoeae* or *C. trachomatis*.

Most women with PID have either mucopurulent cervical discharge or evidence of WBCs on a microscopic evaluation of a saline preparation of vaginal fluid (i.e., wet prep.) If the cervical discharge appears normal and no WBCs are observed on the wet prep of vaginal fluid, the diagnosis of PID is unlikely, and alternative causes of pain should be considered. A wet prep of vaginal fluid also can detect the presence of concomitant infections (e.g., BV and trichomoniasis).

The most specific criteria for diagnosing PID include:

- endometrial biopsy with histopathologic evidence of endometritis;

- transvaginal sonography or magnetic resonance imaging techniques showing thickened, fluid-filled tubes with or without free pelvic fluid or tubo-ovarian complex, or Doppler studies suggesting pelvic infection (e.g., tubal hyperemia); or

- laparoscopic findings consistent with PID.

A diagnostic evaluation that includes some of these more extensive procedures might be warranted in some cases. Endometrial biopsy is warranted in women undergoing laparoscopy who do not have visual evidence of salpingitis, because endometritis is the only sign of PID for some women.

A serologic test for human immunodeficiency virus (HIV) is also recommended. A pregnancy test should always be performed to exclude ectopic pregnancy and because PID can occur concurrently with pregnancy. When the diagnosis of PID is questionable, or when the illness is severe or not responding to therapy, further investigation may be warranted using other invasive procedures (endometrial biopsy, transvaginal ultrasonography, magnetic resonance imaging, or laparoscopy).

How Is Pelvic Inflammatory Disease Treated?

PID is treated with broad spectrum antibiotics to cover likely pathogens. Several types of antibiotics can cure PID. Antibiotic treatment does not, however, reverse any scarring that has already been caused by the infection. For this reason, it is critical that a woman receive care immediately if she has pelvic pain or other symptoms of PID. Prompt antibiotic treatment could prevent severe damage to the reproductive organs.

Recommended treatment regimens can be found in the *2015 STD Treatment Guidelines*. Healthcare providers should emphasize to their patients that although their symptoms may go away before the infection is cured, they should finish taking all of the prescribed medicine. Additionally, a woman's sex partner(s) should be treated to decrease the risk of re-infection, even if the partner(s) has no symptoms. Although sex partners may have no symptoms, they may still be infected with the organisms that can cause PID.

In certain cases, clinicians may recommend hospitalization to treat PID. This decision should be based on the judgment of the healthcare provider and the use of suggested criteria found in the *2015 STD Treatment Guidelines*. If a woman's symptoms continue, or if an abscess does not resolve, surgery may be needed.

Section 29.5

Uterine Fibroids

This section includes text excerpted from "Problem
Periods," Office on Women's Health (OWH), U.S. Department of
Health and Human Services (IIHS), January 15, 2015.

Fibroids are muscular tumors that grow in the wall of the uterus
(womb). Another medical term for fibroids is leiomyoma or just
"myoma." Fibroids are almost always benign (not cancerous). Fibroids
can grow as a single tumor, or there can be many of them in the uterus.
They can be as small as an apple seed or as big as a grapefruit. In
unusual cases they can become very large.

Why Should Women Know about Fibroids?

About 20 percent to 80 percent of women develop fibroids by the
time they reach age 50. Fibroids are most common in women in their
40s and early 50s. Not all women with fibroids have symptoms. Women
who do have symptoms often find fibroids hard to live with. Some have
pain and heavy menstrual bleeding. Fibroids also can put pressure
on the bladder, causing frequent urination, or the rectum, causing
rectal pressure. Should the fibroids get very large, they can cause the
abdomen (stomach area) to enlarge, making a woman look pregnant.

Who Gets Fibroids?

Factors that can increase a woman's risk of developing fibroids
includes:

- **Age.** Fibroids become more common as women age, especially
  during the 30s and 40s through menopause. After menopause,
  fibroids usually shrink.

- **Family history.** Having a family member with fibroids
  increases your risk. If a woman's mother had fibroids, her risk of
  having them is about three times higher than average.

- **Ethnic origin.** African-American women are more likely to
  develop fibroids than white women.

410

- **Obesity.** Women who are overweight are at higher risk for fibroids. For very heavy women, the risk is two to three times greater than average.

- **Eating habits.** Eating a lot of red meat (e.g., beef) and ham is linked with a higher risk of fibroids. Eating plenty of green vegetables seems to protect women from developing fibroids.

Where Can Fibroids Grow?

Most fibroids grow in the wall of the uterus. Doctors put them into three groups based on where they grow:

- **Submucosal** fibroids grow into the uterine cavity.

- **Intramural** fibroids grow within the wall of the uterus.

- **Subserosal** fibroids grow on the outside of the uterus.

Some fibroids grow on stalks that grow out from the surface of the uterus or into the cavity of the uterus. They might look like mushrooms. These are called **pedunculated** fibroids.

What Are Symptoms of Fibroids?

Most fibroids do not cause any symptoms, but some women with fibroids can have:

- Heavy bleeding (which can be heavy enough to cause anemia) or painful periods

- Feeling of fullness in the pelvic area (lower stomach area)

- Enlargement of the lower abdomen

- Frequent urination

- Pain during sex

- Lower back pain

- Complications during pregnancy and labor, including a six-time greater risk of cesarean section

- Reproductive problems, such as infertility, which is very rare

What Causes Fibroids?

No one knows for sure what causes fibroids. Researchers think that more than one factor could play a role. These factors could be:

- Hormonal (affected by estrogen and progesterone levels)

- Genetic (runs in families)

Because no one knows for sure what causes fibroids, researchers also don't know what causes them to grow or shrink. They do know that they are under hormonal control—both estrogen and progesterone. They grow rapidly during pregnancy, when hormone levels are high. They shrink when antihormone medication is used. They also stop growing or shrink once a woman reaches menopause.

Can Fibroids Turn into Cancer?

Fibroids are almost always benign (not cancerous). Rarely (less than one in 1,000) a cancerous fibroid will occur. This is called **leiomyosarcoma.** Doctors think that these cancers do not arise from an already-existing fibroid. Having fibroids does not increase the risk of developing a cancerous fibroid. Having fibroids also does not increase a woman's chances of getting other forms of cancer in the uterus.

What If I Become Pregnant and Have Fibroids?

Women who have fibroids are more likely to have problems during pregnancy and delivery. This doesn't mean there will be problems. Most women with fibroids have normal pregnancies. The most common problems seen in women with fibroids are:

- **Cesarean section.** The risk of needing a C-section is six times greater for women with fibroids.

- **Baby is breech.** The baby is not positioned well for vaginal delivery.

- Labor fails to progress.

- **Placental abruption.** The placenta breaks away from the wall of the uterus before delivery. When this happens, the fetus does not get enough oxygen.

- Preterm delivery.

Talk to your obstetrician if you have fibroids and become pregnant. All obstetricians have experience dealing with fibroids and pregnancy. Most women who have fibroids and become pregnant do not need to see an obstetrician (OB), who deals with high-risk pregnancies.

How Do I Know for Sure That I Have Fibroids?

Your doctor may find that you have fibroids when you see her or him for a regular pelvic exam to check your uterus, ovaries, and vagina. The doctor can feel the fibroid with her or his fingers during an ordinary pelvic exam, as a (usually painless) lump or mass on the uterus. Often, a doctor will describe how small or how large the fibroids are by comparing their size to the size your uterus would be if you were pregnant. For example, you may be told that your fibroids have made your uterus the size it would be if you were 16 weeks pregnant. Or the fibroid might be compared to fruits, nuts, or a ball, such as a grape or an orange, an acorn or a walnut, or a golf ball or a volleyball.

Your doctor can do imaging tests to confirm that you have fibroids. These are tests that create a "picture" of the inside of your body without surgery. These tests might include:

- Ultrasound

- Magnetic resonance imaging (MRI)

- X-rays

- CAT scan (CT)

- Hysterosalpingogram (HSG) or sonohysterogram

You might also need surgery to know for sure if you have fibroids. There are two types of surgery to do this:

- Laparoscopy

- Hysteroscopy

What Questions Should I Ask My Doctor If I Have Fibroids?

- How many fibroids do I have?

- What size is my fibroid(s)?

- Where is my fibroid(s) located (outer surface, inner surface, or in the wall of the uterus)?

- Can I expect fibroids to grow larger?

- How rapidly have they grown (if they were known about already)?

- How will I know if the fibroid(s) is growing larger?

- What problems can the fibroid(s) cause?

- What tests or imaging studies are best for keeping track of the growth of my fibroids?

- What are my treatment options if my fibroid(s) becomes a problem?

- What are your views on treating fibroids with a hysterectomy versus other types of treatments?

A second opinion is always a good idea if your doctor has not answered your questions completely or does not seem to be meeting your needs.

How Are Fibroids Treated?

Most women with fibroids do not have any symptoms. For women who do have symptoms, there are treatments that can help. Talk with your doctor about the best way to treat your fibroids. She or he will consider many things before helping you choose a treatment. Some of these things include:

- Whether or not you are having symptoms from the fibroids

- If you might want to become pregnant in the future

- The size of the fibroids

- The location of the fibroids

- Your age and how close to menopause you might be

If you have fibroids but do not have any symptoms, you may not need treatment. Your doctor will check during your regular exams to see if they have grown.

Medications

If you have fibroids and have mild symptoms, your doctor may suggest taking medication. Over-the-counter drugs such as ibuprofen or acetaminophen can be used for mild pain. If you have heavy bleeding during your period, taking an iron supplement can keep you from getting anemia or correct it if you already are anemic.

Several drugs commonly used for birth control can be prescribed to help control symptoms of fibroids. Low-dose birth control pills do not make fibroids grow and can help control heavy bleeding. The same is true of progesterone-like injections (e.g., Depo-Provera®). An IUD (intrauterine device) called Mirena® contains a small amount of progesterone-like medication, which can be used to control heavy bleeding as well as for birth control.

Other drugs used to treat fibroids are "gonadotropin releasing hormone agonists" (GnRHa). The one most commonly used is Lupron®. These drugs, given by injection, nasal spray, or implanted, can shrink your fibroids. Sometimes they are used before surgery to make fibroids easier to remove. Side effects of GnRHas can include hot flashes, depression, not being able to sleep, decreased sex drive, and joint pain. Most women tolerate GnRHas quite well. Most women do not get a period when taking GnRHas. This can be a big relief to women who have heavy bleeding. It also allows women with anemia to recover to a normal blood count. GnRHas can cause bone thinning, so their use is generally limited to six months or less. These drugs also are very expensive, and some insurance companies will cover only some or none of the cost. GnRHas offer temporary relief from the symptoms of fibroids; once you stop taking the drugs, the fibroids often grow back quickly.

Surgery

If you have fibroids with moderate or severe symptoms, surgery may be the best way to treat them. Here are the options:

- Myomectomy

- Hysterectomy

- Endometrial ablation

- uterine fibroid embolization (UFE), or uterine artery embolization (UAE)

New Treatments That Are Available for Uterine Fibroids

The following methods are not yet standard treatments, so your doctor may not offer them or health insurance may not cover them.

- **Radiofrequency ablation** uses heat to destroy the fibroid tissue without harming surrounding normal uterine tissue. The fibroids remain inside the uterus but shrink in size. Most women go home the same day and can return to normal activities within a few days.

- **Anti-hormonal drugs** may provide symptom relief without bone-thinning side effects.

415

Section 29.6

Vulvodynia

This section includes text excerpted from "Vulvodynia,"
Eunice Kennedy Shriver National Institute of Child Health and
Human Development (NICHD), January 26, 2017.

Vulvodynia is a term used to describe chronic pain (lasting at least 3 months) of the vulva that does not have a clear cause, such as an infection or cancer. The vulva refers to the external female genitalia, including the labia ("lips" or folds of skin at the opening of the vagina), the clitoris, and the vaginal opening. Vulvodynia is usually described as burning, stinging, irritation, or rawness.

Sometimes, vulvodynia is described with more specific terms.

- **Generalized vulvodynia** is pain or discomfort that can be felt in the entire vulvar area.

- **Localized vulvodynia** is felt in only one place on the vulva.

- **Provoked vulvodynia** is pain triggered by an activity or contact with the area, such as having sex, using a tampon, having a gynecological exam, or even wearing tight-fitting pants. Alternatively, **spontaneous vulvodynia** occurs when the pain is not initiated by any known trigger.

- **Provoked vestibulodynia** is vulvodynia with provoked pain that occurs in the vestibular region of the vulva, or the entry point to the vagina. This condition has formerly been called vulvar vestibulitis syndrome, focal vulvitis, vestibulodynia, or vulvar vestibulitis.

What Are the Symptoms of Vulvodynia?

The main symptom of vulvodynia is pain. The type of pain can be different for each woman.

Vulvodynia can cause burning, stinging, irritation, or rawness of the vulva. Some women may also have itching, aching, soreness, throbbing, or swelling. These symptoms may be caused by pressure on the vulvar area, such as during sex or when inserting a tampon. Symptoms may occur during exercise, after urinating, or even while sitting or resting.

Pain may move around or always be in the same place. It can be constant, or it can come and go.

How Many People Are Affected by or at Risk for Vulvodynia?

The exact number of women with vulvodynia is unknown. Researchers estimate that 9% to 18% of women between the ages of 18 and 64 may experience vulvar pain during their lifetimes.

The evidence suggests that many women either do not seek help at all or go from doctor to doctor seeking a diagnosis and treatment without receiving answers.

What Causes Vulvodynia?

Healthcare providers do not know what causes vulvodynia. It tends to be diagnosed when other causes of vulvar pain, such as infection or skin diseases, are ruled out.

Researchers think that one or more of the following may cause or contribute to vulvodynia:

- Injury to or irritation of the nerves that transmit pain and other sensations from the vulva

- Increased density of the nerve fibers in the vulvar vestibule

- Elevated levels of inflammatory substances in the vulvar tissue

- Abnormal response of vulvar cells to environmental factors

- Altered hormone receptor expression in the vulvar tissue

- Genetic factors such as susceptibility to chronic vestibular inflammation, susceptibility to chronic widespread pain, or inability to combat vulvovaginal infection

- Localized hypersensitivity to *Candida* or other vulvovaginal organisms

- Pelvic floor muscle weakness or spasm

How Do Healthcare Providers Diagnose Vulvodynia?

Vulvodynia tends to be diagnosed only when other causes of vulvar pain, such as infection or skin diseases, have been ruled out.

To diagnose vulvodynia, a healthcare provider will take a detailed medical history, including pain characteristics and any accompanying bowel, bladder, or sexual problems. The provider may recommend that a woman have blood drawn to assess levels of estrogen, progesterone, and testosterone. The provider may also perform a cotton swab test, applying gentle pressure to various vulvar sites and asking the patient to rate the severity of the pain. If any areas of skin appear suspicious, these areas may be further examined with a magnifying instrument or a tissue sample may be taken for biopsy.

Because vulvodynia is often a diagnosis of exclusion, it can be difficult and time-consuming to arrive at an actual diagnosis. The diagnostic process can be especially problematic for women who lack health insurance because they may not have the resources to continue seeking care to exclude the many possible causes of pain. Moreover, some women may be reluctant to discuss their pain or seek treatment.

What Are the Treatments for Vulvodynia?

There are several options to treat the symptoms of vulvodynia. These may include lifestyle changes and therapy, medical treatment, and surgical treatment.

A variety of treatment options may be presented to patients, including:

- Topical medications, such as lidocaine ointment (a local anesthetic) or hormonal creams

- Drug treatment, such as pain relievers, antidepressants, or anticonvulsants

- Biofeedback therapy, intended to help decrease pain sensation

- Physical therapy to strengthen pelvic floor muscles

- Injections of steroids or anesthetics

- Surgery to remove the affected skin and tissue in localized vulvodynia

- Changes in diet (for example, some physicians may suggest a diet low in oxalates, which can form crystals in the body if they aren't filtered out by the kidneys)

- Complementary or alternative therapies (including relaxation, massage, homeopathy, and acupuncture)

Chapter 30

Headaches

Chapter Contents

Section 30.1

Headaches: In Depth

This section includes text excerpted from "Headache:
Hope through Research," National Institute of Neurological
Disorders and Stroke (NINDS), April 2016.

You're sitting at your desk, working on a difficult task, when it suddenly feels as if a belt or vice is being tightened around the top of your head. Or you have periodic headaches that occur with nausea and increased sensitivity to light or sound. Maybe you are involved in a routine, non-stressful task when you're struck by head or neck pain.

Sound familiar? If so, you've suffered one of the many types of headache that can occur on its own or as part of another disease or health condition.

Anyone can experience a headache. Nearly 2 out of 3 children will have a headache by age 15. More than 9 in 10 adults will experience a headache sometime in their life. Headache is our most common form of pain and a major reason cited for days missed at work or school as well as visits to the doctor. Without proper treatment, headaches can be severe and interfere with daily activities.

Certain types of headache run in families. Episodes of headache may ease or even disappear for a time and recur later in life. It's possible to have more than one type of headache at the same time.

Primary headaches occur independently and are not caused by another medical condition. It's uncertain what sets the process of a primary headache in motion. A cascade of events that affect blood vessels and nerves inside and outside the head causes pain signals to be sent to the brain. Brain chemicals called neurotransmitters are involved in creating head pain, as are changes in nerve cell activity (called cortical spreading depression (CSD)). Migraine, cluster, and tension-type headache are the more familiar types of primary headache.

Secondary headaches are symptoms of another health disorder that causes pain-sensitive nerve endings to be pressed on or pulled or pushed out of place. They may result from underlying conditions including fever, infection, medication overuse, stress or emotional conflict, high blood pressure, psychiatric disorders, head injury or trauma, stroke, tumors, and nerve disorders (particularly trigeminal neuralgia, a chronic pain condition that typically affects a major nerve on one side of the jaw or cheek).

Headaches can range in frequency and severity of pain. Some individuals may experience headaches once or twice a year, while others may experience headaches more than 15 days a month. Some headaches may recur or last for weeks at a time. Pain can range from mild to disabling and may be accompanied by symptoms such as nausea or increased sensitivity to noise or light, depending on the type of headache.

Why Headaches Hurt

Information about touch, pain, temperature, and vibration in the head and neck is sent to the brain by the trigeminal nerve, one of 12 pairs of cranial nerves that start at the base of the brain.

The nerve has three branches that conduct sensations from the scalp, the blood vessels inside and outside of the skull, the lining around the brain (the *meninges*), and the face, mouth, neck, ears, eyes, and throat.

Brain tissue itself lacks pain-sensitive nerves and does not feel pain. Headaches occur when pain-sensitive nerve endings called nociceptors react to headache triggers (such as stress, certain foods or odors, or use of medicines) and send messages through the *trigeminal* nerve to the thalamus, the brain's "relay station" for pain sensation from all over the body. The thalamus controls the body's sensitivity to light and noise and sends messages to parts of the brain that manage awareness of pain and emotional response to it. Other parts of the brain may also be part of the process, causing nausea, vomiting, diarrhea, trouble concentrating, and other neurological symptoms.

When to See a Doctor

Not all headaches require a physician's attention. But headaches can signal a more serious disorder that requires prompt medical care. Immediately call or see a physician if you or someone you're with experience any of these symptoms:

- Sudden, severe headache that may be accompanied by a stiff neck.

- Severe headache accompanied by fever, nausea, or vomiting that is not related to another illness.

- "First" or "worst" headache, often accompanied by confusion, weakness, double vision, or loss of consciousness.

- Headache that worsens over days or weeks or has changed in pattern or behavior.

- Recurring headache in children.

- Headache following a head injury.

- Headache and a loss of sensation or weakness in any part of the body, which could be a sign of a stroke.

- Headache associated with convulsions.

- Headache associated with shortness of breath.

- Two or more headaches a week.

- Persistent headache in someone who has been previously headache-free, particularly in someone over age 50.

- New headaches in someone with a history of cancer or Human immunodeficiency virus infection and acquired immune deficiency syndrome (HIV/AIDS).

Diagnosing Your Headache

How and under what circumstances a person experiences a headache can be key to diagnosing its cause. Keeping a headache journal can help a physician better diagnose your type of headache and determine the best treatment. After each headache, note the time of day when it occurred; its intensity and duration; any sensitivity to light, odors, or sound; activity immediately prior to the headache; use of prescription and nonprescription medicines; amount of sleep the previous night; any stressful or emotional conditions; any influence from weather or daily activity; foods and fluids consumed in the past 24 hours; and any known health conditions at that time. Women should record the days of their menstrual cycles. Include notes about other family members who have a history of headache or other disorder. A pattern may emerge that can be helpful to reducing or preventing headaches.

Once your doctor has reviewed your medical and headache history and conducted a physical and neurological exam, lab screening and diagnostic tests may be ordered to either rule out or identify conditions that might be the cause of your headaches. Blood tests and urinalysis can help diagnose brain or spinal cord infections, blood vessel damage, and toxins that affect the nervous system. Testing a sample of the fluid that surrounds the brain and spinal cord can detect infections, bleeding in the brain (called a brain hemorrhage), and measure any buildup of pressure within the skull. Diagnostic imaging, such as with Computed Tomography (CT) and Magnetic Resonance Imaging (MRI), can detect irregularities in blood vessels and bones, certain brain tumors and cysts, brain damage from head injury, brain hemorrhage, inflammation, infection, and other disorders. Neuroimaging also gives doctors a way to see what's happening in the brain during headache attacks. An electroencephalogram (EEG) measures brain wave activity and can help diagnose brain tumors, seizures, head injury, and inflammation that may lead to headaches.

Headache Types and Their Treatment

The International Classification of Headache Disorders (ICHD), published by the International Headache Society (IHS), is used to classify more than 150 types of primary and secondary headache disorders.

Primary headache disorders are divided into four main groups: migraine, tension-type headache, trigeminal autonomic cephalgias (a group of short-lasting but severe headaches), and a miscellaneous group.

Migraine

If you suffer from migraine headaches, you're not alone. About 12 percent of the U.S. population experience migraines. Migraine headaches are characterized by throbbing and pulsating pain caused by the activation of nerve fibers that reside within the wall of brain blood vessels traveling within the meninges.

Migraines headaches are recurrent attacks of moderate to severe pain that is throbbing or pulsing and often strikes one side of the head. Untreated attacks last from 4 to 72 hours. Other common symptoms are increased sensitivity to light, noise, and odors; and nausea and vomiting. Routine physical activity, movement, or even coughing or sneezing can worsen the headache pain.

Tension-Type

Tension-type headache, previously called muscle contraction headache, is the most common type of headache. Its name indicates the role of stress and mental or emotional conflict in triggering the pain and contracting muscles in the neck, face, scalp, and jaw. Tension-type headaches may also be caused by jaw clenching, intense work, missed meals, depression, anxiety, or too little sleep. Sleep apnea may also cause tension-type headaches, especially in the morning. The pain is usually mild to moderate and feels as if constant pressure is being applied to the front of the face or to the head or neck. It also may feel as if a belt is being tightened around the head. Most often the pain is felt on both sides of the head. People who suffer tension-type headaches may also feel overly sensitive to light and sound but there is no pre-headache aura as with migraine. Typically, tension-type headaches usually disappear once the period of stress or related cause has ended.

Tension-type headaches affect women slightly more often than men. The headaches usually begin in adolescence and reach peak activity in the 30s. They have not been linked to hormones and do not have a strong hereditary connection.

There are two forms of tension-type headache: Episodic tension-type headaches occur between 10 and 15 days per month, with each attack lasting from 30 minutes to several days. Although the pain is not disabling, the severity of pain typically increases with the frequency of attacks. Chronic tension-type attacks usually occur more than 15 days per month over a 3-month period. The pain, which can be constant over a period of days or months, strikes both sides of the head and is more severe and disabling than episodic headache pain. Chronic tension headaches can cause sore scalps-even combing your hair can be painful. Most individuals will have had some form of episodic tension-type headache prior to onset of chronic tension-type headache.

Depression and anxiety can cause tension-type headaches. Headaches may appear in the early morning or evening, when conflicts in the office or at home are anticipated. Other causes include physical postures that strain head and neck muscles (such as holding your chin down while reading or holding a phone between your shoulder and ear), degenerative arthritis of the neck, and temporomandibular joint (TMJ) dysfunction (a disorder of the joints between the temporal bone located above the ear and the mandible, or lower jaw bone).

The first step in caring for a tension-type headache involves treating any specific disorder or disease that may be causing it. For example, arthritis of the neck is treated with anti-inflammatory medication and temporomandibular joint dysfunction may be helped by corrective devices for the mouth and jaw. A sleep study may be needed to detect sleep apnea and should be considered when there is a history of snoring, daytime sleepiness, or obesity.

A physician may suggest using analgesics, nonsteroidal anti-inflammatory drugs, or antidepressants to treat a tension-type headache that is not associated with a disease. Triptan drugs, barbiturates (drugs that have a relaxing or sedative effect), and ergot derivatives may provide relief to people who suffer from both migraine and tension-type headache.

Alternative therapies for chronic tension-type headaches include biofeedback, relaxation training, meditation, and cognitive-behavioral therapy to reduce stress. A hot shower or moist heat applied to the back of the neck may ease symptoms of infrequent tension headaches. Physical therapy, massage, and gentle exercise of the neck may also be helpful.

Trigeminal Autonomic Cephalgias

Some primary headaches are characterized by severe pain in or around the eye on one side of the face and autonomic (or involuntary) features on the same side, such as red and teary eye, drooping eyelid, and runny nose. These disorders, called trigeminal autonomic cephalgias (*cephalgia* meaning head pain), differ in attack duration and frequency, and have episodic and chronic forms. Episodic attacks occur on a daily or near-daily basis for weeks or months with pain-free remissions. Chronic attacks occur on a daily or near-daily basis for a year or more with only brief remissions.

Paroxysmal hemicrania is a rare form of primary headache that usually begins in adulthood. Pain and related symptoms may be similar to those felt in cluster headaches, but with shorter duration. Attacks typically occur 5 to 40 times per day, with each attack lasting 2 to 45 minutes. Severe throbbing, claw-like, or piercing pain is felt on one side of the face-in, around, or behind the eye and occasionally reaching to the back of the neck. Other symptoms may include red and watery eyes, a drooping or swollen eyelid on the affected side of the face, and nasal congestion. Individuals may also feel dull pain, soreness, or tenderness between attacks or increased sensitivity to light on the affected side of the face. Paroxysmal hemicrania has two forms: chronic, in which individuals experience attacks on a daily basis for a year or more, and episodic, in which the headaches may stop for months or years before recurring. Certain movements of the head or neck, external pressure to the neck, and alcohol use may trigger these headaches. Attacks occur more often in women than in men and have no familial pattern.

The nonsteroidal anti-inflammatory drug indomethacin can quickly halt the pain and related symptoms of paroxysmal hemicrania, but symptoms recur once the drug treatment is stopped. Non-prescription analgesics and calcium-channel blockers can ease discomfort, particularly if taken when symptoms first appear.

SUNCT (Short-lasting, Unilateral, Neuralgiform headache attacks with Conjunctival injection and Tearing) is a very rare type of headache with bursts of moderate to severe burning, piercing, or throbbing pain that is usually felt in the forehead, eye, or temple on one side of the head. The pain usually peaks within seconds of onset and may follow a pattern of increasing and decreasing intensity. Attacks typically occur during the day and last from 5 seconds to 4 minutes per episode. Individuals generally have five to six attacks per hour and are pain-free between attacks. This primary headache is slightly more common in men than in women, with onset usually after age 50. SUNCT may be episodic, occurring once or twice annually with headaches that remit and recur, or chronic, lasting more than 1 year.

Symptoms include reddish or bloodshot eyes (conjunctival injection), watery eyes, stuffy or runny nose, sweaty forehead, puffy eyelids, increased pressure within the eye on the affected side of the head, and increased blood pressure.

SUNCT is very difficult to treat. Anticonvulsants may relieve some of the symptoms, while anesthetics and corticosteroid drugs can treat some of the severe pain felt during these headaches. Surgery and glycerol injections to block nerve signaling along the trigeminal nerve have poor outcomes and provide only temporary relief in severe cases. Doctors are beginning to use deep brain stimulation (involving a surgically implanted battery-powered electrode that emits pulses of energy to surrounding brain tissue) to reduce the frequency of attacks in severely affected individuals.

Secondary Headache Disorders

Secondary headache disorders are caused by an underlying illness or condition that affects the brain. Secondary headaches are usually diagnosed based on other symptoms that occur concurrently and the characteristics of the headaches. Some of the more serious causes of secondary headache include:

- **Brain tumor.** A tumor that is growing in the brain can press against nerve tissue and pain-sensitive blood vessel walls, disrupting communication between the brain and the nerves or restricting the supply of blood to the brain. Headaches may develop, worsen, become more frequent, or come and go, often at irregular periods. Headache pain may worsen when coughing, changing posture, or straining, and may be severe upon waking. Treatment options include surgery, radiation therapy, and chemotherapy. However, the vast majority of individuals with headache do not have brain tumors.

- **Disorders of blood vessels in the brain, including stroke.** Several disorders associated with blood vessel formation and activity can cause headache. Most notable among these conditions is stroke. Headache itself can cause stroke or accompany a series of blood vessel disorders that can cause a stroke.

There are two forms of stroke. A hemorrhagic stroke occurs when an artery in the brain bursts, spilling blood into the surrounding tissue. An ischemic stroke occurs when an artery supplying the brain with blood becomes blocked, suddenly decreasing or stopping blood flow and causing brain cells to die.

Hemorrhagic Stroke

A hemorrhagic stroke is usually associated with disturbed brain function and an extremely painful headache that develops suddenly and may worsen with physical activity, coughing, or straining. Headache conditions associated with hemorrhagic stroke include:

- A **subarachnoid hemorrhage** is the rupture of a blood vessel located within the subarachnoid space-a fluid-filled space between layers of connective tissue (meninges) that surround the brain. The first sign of a subarachnoid hemorrhage is typically a severe headache with a split-second onset and no known cause. Neurologists call this a thunderclap headache. Pain may also be felt in the neck and lower back. This sudden flood of blood can contaminate the cerebrospinal fluid that flows within the spaces of the brain and cause extensive damage throughout the brain.

- **Intracerebral hemorrhage** is usually associated with severe headache. Several conditions can render blood vessels in the brain prone to rupture and hemorrhaging. Chronic hypertension can weaken the blood vessel wall. Poor blood clotting ability due to blood disorders or blood-thinning medications like warfarin further increase the risk of bleeding. And some venous strokes (caused by clots in the brain's veins) often cause bleeding into the brain. At risk are mothers in the postpartum period and persons with dehydration, cancer, or infections.

- An **aneurysm** is the abnormal ballooning of an artery that causes the artery wall to weaken. A ruptured cerebral aneurysm can cause hemorrhagic stroke and a sudden, incredibly painful headache that is generally different in severity and intensity from other headaches individuals may have experienced. Individuals usually describe the thunderclap-like headache as "the worst headache of my life." There may be loss of consciousness and other neurological features. "Sentinel" or sudden warning headaches sometimes occur from an aneurysm that leaks prior to rupture. Cerebral aneurysms that have leaked or ruptured are life-threatening and require emergency medical attention. Not all aneurysms burst, and people with very small aneurysms may be monitored to detect any growth or onset of symptoms. Treatment options include blocking the flow of blood to the aneurysm surgically (intra-arterial) and catheter techniques to fill the aneurysm with coils or balloons.

- **Arteriovenous malformation (AVM)**, an abnormal tangle of arteries and veins in the brain, causes headaches that vary in frequency, duration, and intensity as vascular malformations press on and displace normal tissue or leak blood into surrounding tissue. A headache consistently affecting one side of the head may be closely linked to the site of an AVM (although most one-sided headaches are caused by primary headache disorders). Symptoms may include seizures and hearing pulsating noises. Treatment options include decreasing blood flow to and from the malformation by injecting particles or glue, or through focused radiotherapy or surgery.

Ischemic Stroke

Headache that accompanies ischemic stroke can be caused by several problems with the brain's vascular system. Headache is prominent in individuals with clots in the brain's veins. Head pain occurs on the side of the brain in which the clot blocks blood flow and is often felt in the eyes or on the side of the head. Conditions of ischemic stroke that can cause headache include:

- Arterial dissection is a tear within an artery that supplies the brain with blood flow. The most common dissection occurs in the carotid artery in the neck, with head pain on the same side of the body where the tear occurs. Vertebral artery dissection causes pain in the rear upper part of the neck. Cervical artery dissection can lead to stroke or transient ischemic attacks (strokes that last only a few minutes but signal a subsequent, more severe stroke). They are usually caused by neck strain, i.e., trauma, chiropractic manipulation, sports injuries, or even pronounced bending of the head backwards over a sink for hair washing ("beauty parlor stroke"). Immediate medical attention can be lifesaving.

- Vascular inflammation can cause the buildup of plaque, which can lead to ischemic stroke. Cerebral vasculitis, an inflammation of the brain's blood vessel system, may cause headache, stroke, and/or progressive cognitive decline. Severe headache attributed to a chronic inflammatory disease of blood vessels on the outside of the head, called giant cell arteritis (previously known as temporal arteritis), usually affects people older than age 60. It also causes muscle pain and tenderness in the temple area. Individuals also may experience temporary, followed by permanent, loss of vision on one or both eyes, pain with chewing, a tender scalp, muscle aches, depression, and fatigue. Corticosteroids are typically used to treat vascular inflammation and can prevent blindness.

Children and Headache

Headaches are common in children. Headaches that begin early in life can develop into migraines as the child grows older. Migraines in children or adolescents can develop into tension-type headaches at any time. In contrast to adults with migraine, young children often feel migraine pain on both sides of the head and have headaches that usually last less than 2 hours. Children may look pale and appear restless or irritable before and during an attack. Other children may become nauseous, lose their appetite, or feel pain elsewhere in the body during the headache.

Headaches in children can be caused by a number of triggers, including emotional problems such as tension between family members, stress from school activities, weather changes, irregular eating and sleep, dehydration, and certain foods and drinks. Of special concern among children are headaches that occur after head injury or those accompanied by rash, fever, or sleepiness.

It may be difficult to identify the type of headache because children often have problems describing where it hurts, how often the headaches occur, and how long they last. Asking a child with a headache to draw a picture of where the pain is and how it feels can make it easier for the doctor to determine the proper treatment.

Migraine in particular is often misdiagnosed in children. Parents and caretakers sometimes have to be detectives to help determine that a child has migraine. Clues to watch for include sensitivity to light and noise, which may be suspected when a child refuses to watch television or use the computer, or when the child stops playing to lie down in a dark room. Observe whether or not a child is able to eat during a headache. Very young children may seem cranky or irritable and complain of abdominal pain (abdominal migraine).

Headache treatment in children and teens usually includes rest, fluids, and over-the-counter pain relief medicines. Always consult with a physician before giving headache medicines to a child. Most tension-type headaches in children can be treated with over-the-counter medicines that are marked for children with usage guidelines based on the child's age and weight. Headaches in some children may also be treated effectively using relaxation/behavioral therapy. Children with cluster headache may be treated with oxygen therapy early in the initial phase of the attacks.

Headache and Sleep Disorders

Headaches are often a secondary symptom of a sleep disorder. For example, tension-type headache is regularly seen in persons with insomnia or sleep-wake cycle disorders. Nearly three-fourths of individuals who suffer from narcolepsy complain of either migraine or cluster headache. Migraines and cluster headaches appear to be related to the number of and transition between rapid eye movement (REM) and other sleep periods an individual has during sleep. Hypnic headache awakens individuals mainly at night but may also interrupt daytime naps. Reduced oxygen levels in people with sleep apnea may trigger early morning headaches.

Getting the proper amount of sleep can ease headache pain. Generally, too little or too much sleep can worsen headaches, as can overuse of sleep medicines. Daytime naps often reduce deep sleep at night and can produce headaches in some adults. Some sleep disorders and secondary headache are treated using antidepressants. Check with a doctor before using over-the-counter medicines to ease sleep-associated headaches.

Coping with Headache

Headache treatment is a partnership between you and your doctor, and honest communication is essential. Finding a quick fix to your headache may not be possible. It may take some time for your doctor or specialist to determine the best course of treatment. Avoid using over-the-counter medicines more than twice a week, as they may actually worsen headache pain and the frequency of attacks. Visit a local headache support group meeting (if available) to learn how others with headache cope with their pain and discomfort. Relax whenever possible to ease stress and related symptoms, get enough sleep, regularly perform aerobic exercises, and eat a regularly scheduled and healthy diet that avoids food triggers. Gaining more control over your headache, stress, and emotions will make you feel better and let you embrace daily activities as much as possible.

Section 30.2

Hemicrania Continua

This section includes text excerpted from "Hemicrania Continua Information Page," National Institute of Neurological Disorders and Stroke (NINDS), February 11, 2012. Reviewed June 2017.

Hemicrania continua is a chronic and persistent form of headache marked by continuous pain that varies in severity, always occurs on the same side of the face and head, and is superimposed with additional debilitating symptoms on the continuous but fluctuating pain are occasional attacks of more severe pain. A small percentage of individuals with hemicrania continua have bilateral pain, or pain on both sides of the head. A headache is considered hemicrania continua if the person has had a one-sided daily or continuous headache of moderate intensity with occasional short, piercing head pain for more than 3 months without shifting sides or pain-free periods. The headache must also be completely responsive to treatment with the non-steroidal anti-inflammatory drug drug indomethacin. It must have at least one of the following symptoms: eye redness and/or tearing, nasal congestion and/or runny nose, ptosis (drooping eyelid) and miosis (contracture of the iris).

Occasionally, individuals will also have forehead sweating and migraine symptoms, such as throbbing pain, nausea and/or vomiting, or sensitivity to light and sound. The disorder has two forms: chronic, with daily headaches, and remitting, in which headaches may occur for a period as long as 6 months and are followed by a pain-free period of weeks to months until the pain returns. Most patients experience attacks of increased pain three to five times per 24-hour cycle. This disorder is more common in women than in men. Physical exertion and alcohol use may increase the severity of headache pain in some patients. The cause of this disorder is unknown.

Treatment of Hemicrania Continua

Indomethacin provides rapid relief from symptoms. Patients must take between 25 and 300 milligrams of indomethacin daily and indefinitely to decrease symptoms. Some individuals may need to take acid-suppression medicine due to a gastrointestinal side effect. For those who cannot tolerate the side effects, another Nonsteroidal Anti-inflammatory Drugs (NSAIDs), celecoxib, has been shown to have less complications and can be prescribed. Amitriptyline and other tricyclic antidepressants are also effective in some individuals with hemicrania continua as a preventative treatment.

Prognosis of Hemicrania Continua

Individuals may obtain complete to near-complete relief of symptoms with proper medical attention and daily medication. Some people may not be able to tolerate long-term use of indomethacin and may have to rely on less effective NSAIDs.

Section 30.3

Migraine

This section includes text excerpted from "Migraine Fact Sheet," Office on Women's Health (OWH), U.S. Department of Health and Human Services (HHS), July 16, 2012. Reviewed June 2017.

Migraine is a medical condition. A migraine headache is usually an intense, throbbing pain on one, or sometimes, both sides of the head. Migraine pain and symptoms affect 29.5 million Americans. About three out of four people who have migraines are women. Migraine is the most common form of disabling headache that sends patients to see their doctors.

What Is Migraine?

Most people who suffer from migraines get headaches that can be quite severe. A migraine headache is usually an intense, throbbing pain on one, or sometimes, both sides of the head. Most people with migraine headache feel the pain in the temples or behind one eye or ear, although any part of the head can be involved. Besides pain, migraine also can cause nausea and vomiting and sensitivity to light and sound. Some people also may see spots or flashing lights or have a temporary loss of vision.

Migraine can occur any time of the day, though it often starts in the morning. The pain can last a few hours or up to one or two days. Some people get migraines once or twice a week. Others, only once or twice a year. Most of the time, migraines are not a threat to your overall health. But migraine attacks can interfere with your day-to-day life.

Researchers don't know what causes migraine, but some things are more common in people who have them:

- Most often, migraine affects people between the ages of 15 and 55.

- Most people have a family history of migraine or of disabling headache.

- They are more common in women.

- Migraine often becomes less severe and less frequent with age.

How Common Are Migraines?

Migraine pain and symptoms affect 29.5 million Americans. Migraine is the most common form of disabling headache that sends patients to see their doctors.

What Causes Migraines?

The exact cause of migraine is not fully understood. Most researchers think that migraine is due to abnormal changes in levels of substances that are naturally produced in the brain. When the levels of these substances increase, they can cause inflammation. This inflammation then causes blood vessels in the brain to swell and press on nearby nerves, causing pain.

Genes also have been linked to migraine. People who get migraines may have abnormal genes that control the functions of certain brain cells.

Experts do know that people with migraines react to a variety of factors and events, called triggers. These triggers can vary from person to person and don't always lead to migraine. A combination of triggers—not a single thing or event—is more likely to set off an attack. A person's response to triggers also can vary from migraine to migraine. Many women with migraine tend to have attacks triggered by:

- Lack of or too much sleep
- Skipped meals
- Bright lights, loud noises, or strong odors
- Hormone changes during the menstrual cycle
- Stress and anxiety, or relaxation after stress
- Weather changes
- Alcohol (often red wine)
- Caffeine (too much or withdrawal)
- Foods that contain nitrates, such as hot dogs and lunch meats
- Foods that contain MSG (monosodium glutamate), a flavor enhancer found in fast foods, broths, seasonings, and spices
- Foods that contain tyramine, such as aged cheeses, soy products, fava beans, hard sausages, smoked fish, and Chianti wine
- Aspartame (NutraSweet® and Equal®)

To pinpoint your migraine triggers, keep a headache diary. Each day you have a migraine headache, put that in your diary. Also write down the:

- The time of day your headache started

- Where you were and what you were doing when the migraine started

- What you ate or drank 24 hours before the attack

- Each day you have your period, not just the first day (This can allow you and your doctor to see if your headaches occur at the same or similar time as your period.)

Talk with your doctor about what sets off your headaches to help find the right treatment for you.

Are There Different Kinds of Migraine?

Yes, there are many forms of migraine. The two forms seen most often are migraine with aura and migraine without aura.

Migraine with aura (previously called classical migraine). With a migraine with aura, a person might have these sensory symptoms (the so-called "aura") 10 to 30 minutes before an attack:

- Seeing flashing lights, zigzag lines, or blind spots

- Numbness or tingling in the face or hands

- Disturbed sense of smell, taste, or touch

- Feeling mentally "fuzzy"

Only one in five people who get migraine experience an aura. Women have this form of migraine less often than men.

Migraine without aura (previously called common migraine). With this form of migraine, a person does not have an aura but has all the other features of an attack.

How Can I Tell If I Have a Migraine or Just a Bad Tension-Type Headache?

Compared with migraine, tension-type headache is generally less severe and rarely disabling. Compare your symptoms with those in this chart to see what type of headache you might be having.

Table 30.1. Migraine versus Bad Tension-Type Headache

Symptom	Tension headache	Migraine headache
Intensity of pain: Mild-to-moderate	x	x
Intensity of pain: Moderate-to-severe		x
Quality of pain: Intense pounding or throbbing and/or debilitating		x
Quality of pain: Distracting, but not debilitating	x	
Quality of pain: Steady ache	x	x
Location of pain: One side of head		x
Location of pain: Both sides of head	x	x
Nausea, vomiting		x
Sensitivity to light and/or sounds	rare	x
Aura before onset of headache		x

Although fatigue and stress can bring on both tension and migraine headaches, migraines can be triggered by certain foods, changes in the body's hormone levels, and even changes in the weather.

There also are differences in how types of headaches respond to treatment with medicines. Although some over-the-counter drugs used to treat tension-type headaches sometimes help migraine headaches, the drugs used to treat migraine attacks do not work for tension-type headaches for most people.

You can't tell the difference between a migraine and a tension-type headache by how often they occur. Both can occur at irregular intervals. Also, in rare cases, both can occur daily or almost daily.

How Can I Tell If I Have a Migraine or a Sinus Headache?

Many people confuse a sinus headache with a migraine because pain and pressure in the sinuses, nasal congestion, and watery eyes often occur with migraine. To find out if your headache is sinus or migraine, ask yourself these questions:

In addition to my sinus symptoms, do I have:

1. Moderate-to-severe headache

2. Nausea

3. Sensitivity to light

If you answer "yes" to two or three of these questions, then most likely you have migraine with sinus symptoms. A true sinus headache is rare and usually occurs due to sinus infection. In a sinus infection, you would also likely have a fever and thick nasal secretions that are yellow, green, or blood-tinged. A sinus headache should go away with treatment of the sinus infection.

When Should I Seek Help for My Headaches?

Sometimes, headache can signal a more serious problem. You should talk to your doctor about your headaches if:

- You have several headaches per month and each lasts for several hours or days
- Your headaches disrupt your home, work, or school life
- You have nausea, vomiting, vision, or other sensory problems (such as numbness or tingling)
- You have pain around the eye or ear
- You have a severe headache with a stiff neck
- You have a headache with confusion or loss of alertness
- You have a headache with convulsions
- You have a headache after a blow to the head
- You used to be headache-free, but now have headaches a lot

What Tests Are Used to Find out If I Have Migraine?

If you think you get migraine headaches, talk with your doctor. Before your appointment, write down:

1. How often you have headaches
2. Where the pain is
3. How long the headaches last
4. When the headaches happen, such as during your period
5. Other symptoms, such as nausea or blind spots
6. Any family history of migraine
7. All the medicines that you are taking for all your medical problems, even the over-the-counter medicines (better still, bring the medicines in their containers to the doctor)

8. All the medicines you have taken in the past that you can recall and, if possible, the doses you took and any side effects you had

Your doctor may also do an exam and ask more questions about your health history. This could include past head injury and sinus or dental problems. Your doctor may be able to diagnose migraine just from the information you provide.

You may get a blood test or other tests, such as computerized tomography (CT) scan or MRI, if your doctor thinks that something else is causing your headaches. Work with your doctor to decide on the best tests for you.

Can Stress Cause Migraines?

Yes. Stress can trigger both migraine and tension-type headache. Events like getting married, moving to a new home, or having a baby can cause stress. But studies show that everyday stresses—not major life changes—cause most headaches. Juggling many roles, such as being a mother and wife, having a career, and financial pressures, can be daily stresses for women.

Making time for yourself and finding healthy ways to deal with stress are important. Some things you can do to help prevent or reduce stress include:

- Eating healthy foods

- Being active (at least 30 minutes most days of the week is best)

- Doing relaxation exercises

- Getting enough sleep

Try to figure out what causes you to feel stressed. You may be able to cut out some of these stressors. For example, if driving to work is stressful, try taking the bus or subway. You can take this time to read or listen to music, rather than deal with traffic. For stressors you can't avoid, keeping organized and doing as much as you can ahead of time will help you to feel in control.

How Are Migraines Treated?

Migraine has no cure. But your migraines can be managed with your doctor's help. Together, you will find ways to treat migraine symptoms when they happen, as well as ways to help make your migraines less frequent and severe. Your treatment plan may include some or all of these methods.

Medicine. There are two ways to approach the treatment of migraines with drugs: stopping a migraine in progress (called "abortive" or "acute" treatment) and prevention. Many people with migraine use both forms of treatment.

Acute treatment. Over-the-counter pain-relief drugs such as aspirin, acetaminophen, or NSAIDs (nonsteroidal anti-inflammatory drugs) like ibuprofen relieve mild migraine pain for some people. If these drugs don't work for you, your doctor might want you to try a prescription drug. Two classes of drugs that doctors often try first are:

- Triptans, which work by balancing the chemicals in the brain. Examples include sumatriptan (Imitrex®), rizatriptan (Maxalt®), zolmitriptan (Zomig®), almotriptan (Axert®), eletriptan (Relpax®), naratriptan (Amerge®), and frovatriptan (Frova®). Triptans can come as tablets that you swallow, tablets that dissolve on your tongue, nasal sprays, and as a shot. They should not be used if you have heart disease or high blood pressure.

- Ergot derivatives (ergotamine tartrate and dihydoergotamine), which work in the same way as triptans. They should not be used if you have heart disease or high blood pressure.

Most acute drugs for migraine work best when taken right away, when symptoms first begin. Always carry your migraine medicine with you in case of an attack. For people with extreme migraine pain, a powerful "rescue" drug might be prescribed, too. Because not everyone responds the same way to migraine drugs, you will need to work with your doctor to find the treatment that works best for you.

Prevention. Some medicines used daily can help prevent attacks. Many of these drugs were designed to treat other health conditions, such as epilepsy and depression. Some examples are:

- Antidepressants, such as amitriptyline (Elavil®) or venlafaxine (Effexor®)

- Anticonvulsants, such as divalproex sodium (Depakote®) or topiramate (Topamax®)

- Beta-blockers, such as propranolol (Inderal®) or timolol (Blocadren®)

- Calcium channel blockers, such as verapamil

These drugs may not prevent all migraines, but they can help a lot. Hormone therapy may help prevent attacks in women whose migraines seem to be linked to their menstrual cycle. Ask your doctor about prevention drugs if:

- Your migraines do not respond to drugs for symptom relief

- Your migraines are disabling or cause you to miss work, family activities, or social events

- You are using pain-relief drugs more than two times a week

Lifestyle changes. Practicing these habits can reduce the number of migraine attacks:

- Avoid or limit triggers.

- Get up and go to bed the same time every day.

- Eat healthy foods and do not skip meals.

- Engage in regular physical activity.

- Limit alcohol and caffeine intake.

- Learn ways to reduce and cope with stress.

Alternative methods. Biofeedback has been shown to help some people with migraine. It involves learning how to monitor and control your body's responses to stress, such as lowering heart rate and easing muscle tension. Other methods, such as acupuncture and relaxation, may help relieve stress. Counseling also can help if you think your migraines may be related to depression or anxiety. Talk with your doctor about these treatment methods.

What Are Rebound Migraines?

Women who use acute pain-relief medicine more than two or three times a week or more than 10 days out of the month can set off a cycle called rebound. As each dose of medicine wears off, the pain comes back, leading the patient to take even more. This overuse causes your medicine to stop helping your pain and actually start causing headaches. Rebound headaches can occur with both over-the-counter and prescription pain-relief medicines. They can also occur whether you take them for headache or for another type of pain. Talk to your doctor if you're caught in a rebound cycle.

What Are Some Ways I Can Prevent Migraine?

The best way to prevent migraine is to find out what triggers your attacks and avoid or limit these triggers. Since migraine headaches are more common during times of stress, finding healthy ways to cut down on and cope with stress might help. Talk with your doctor about starting a fitness program or taking a class to learn relaxation skills.

Talk with your doctor if you need to take your pain-relief medicine more than twice a week. Doing so can lead to rebound headaches. If your doctor has prescribed medicine for you to help prevent migraine, take them exactly as prescribed. Ask what you should do if you miss a dose and how long you should take the medicine. Talk with your doctor if the amount of medicine you are prescribed is not helping your headaches.

What Should I Do When a Migraine Begins?

Work with your doctor to come up with a plan for managing your migraines. Keeping a list of home treatment methods that have worked for you in the past also can help. When symptoms begin:

- If you take migraine medicine, take it right away.
- Drink fluids, if you don't have nausea during your migraine.
- Lie down and rest in a dark, quiet room, if that is practical.

Some people find the following useful:

- A cold cloth on your head
- Rubbing or applying pressure to the spot where you feel pain
- Massage or other relaxation exercises

Frequently Asked Questions

Are Migraine Headaches More Common in Women than Men?

Yes. About three out of four people who have migraines are women. Migraines are most common in women between the ages of 20 and 45. At this time of life women often have more job, family, and social duties. Women tend to report more painful and longer lasting headaches and more symptoms, such as nausea and vomiting. All these factors make it hard for a woman to fulfill her roles at work and at home when migraine strikes.

441

I Get Migraines Right before My Period. Could They Be Related to My Menstrual Cycle?

More than half of migraines in women occur right before, during, or after a woman has her period. This often is called "menstrual migraine." But, just a small fraction of women who have migraine around their period only have migraine at this time. Most have migraine headaches at other times of the month as well.

How the menstrual cycle and migraine are linked is still unclear. Researchers know that just before the cycle begins, levels of the female hormones, estrogen and progesterone, go down sharply. This drop in hormones may trigger a migraine, because estrogen controls chemicals in the brain that affect a woman's pain sensation.

Talk with your doctor if you think you have menstrual migraine. You may find that medicines, making lifestyle changes, and home treatment methods can prevent or reduce the pain.

Can Migraine Be Worse during Menopause?

If your migraine headaches are closely linked to your menstrual cycle, menopause may make them less severe. As you get older, the nausea and vomiting may decrease as well. About two-thirds of women with migraines report that their symptoms improve with menopause.

But for some women, menopause worsens migraine or triggers them to start. It is not clear why this happens. Menopausal hormone therapy, which is prescribed for some women during menopause, may be linked to migraines during this time. In general, though, the worsening of migraine symptoms goes away once menopause is complete.

Can Using Birth Control Pills Make My Migraines Worse?

In some women, birth control pills improve migraine. The pills may help reduce the number of attacks and their attacks may become less severe. But in other women, the pills may worsen their migraines. In still other women, taking birth control pills has no effect on their migraines.

The reason for these different responses is not well understood. For women whose migraines get worse when they take birth control pills, their attacks seem to occur during the last week of the cycle. This is because the last seven pills in most monthly pill packs don't have hormones; they are there to keep you in the habit of taking your birth control daily. Without the hormones, your body's estrogen levels drop sharply. This may trigger migraine in some women.

Talk with your doctor if you think birth control pills are making your migraines worse. Switching to a pill pack in which all the pills for the entire month contain hormones and using that for three months in a row can improve headaches. Lifestyle changes, such as getting on a regular sleep pattern and eating healthy foods, can help too.

I'm Pregnant. Can My Migraines Still Be Treated?

Some migraine medicines should not be used when you are pregnant because they can cause birth defects and other problems. This includes over-the-counter medicines, such as aspirin and ibuprofen. Talk with your doctor if migraine is a problem while you are pregnant or if you are planning to become pregnant. Your doctor might suggest a medicine that will help you and that is safe during pregnancy. Home treatment methods, such as doing relaxation exercises and using cold packs, also might help ease your pain. The good news is that for most women migraines improve or stop from about the third month of the pregnancy.

I Am Breastfeeding. Will Taking Medicine for Migraine Hurt My Baby?

Ask your doctor about what migraine medicines are safe to take while breastfeeding. Some medicines can be passed through breast milk and might be harmful to your baby.

Section 30.4

Cluster Headache

This section includes text excerpted from "Cluster Headache,"
Genetic and Rare Diseases Information Center (GARD), National
Center for Advancing Translational Sciences (NCATS), May 8, 2017.

Cluster headaches are a form of headache notable for their extreme pain and their pattern of occurring in "clusters," usually at the same time(s) of the day for several weeks. The headaches are accompanied by autonomic symptoms, and some people experience restlessness and agitation.

A cluster headache begins with severe pain strictly on one side of the head, often behind or around one eye. In some people, it may be preceded by a migraine-like "aura." The pain usually peaks over the next 5 to 10 minutes, and then continues at that intensity for up to three hours before going away. Typical attacks may strike up to eight times a day and are relatively short-lived. On average, a cluster period lasts 6 to 12 weeks. Autonomic symptoms may include: conjunctival injection (bloodshot eyes), swelling under or around the eye, excessive tearing of the eyes, drooping of the eyelid, runny nose and/or nasal congestion, and forehead and facial sweating. These symptoms generally occur only during the pain attack and are on the same side as the headache pain.

Cluster headaches usually begin between the ages of 20 and 50, although they can start at any age. Males are more commonly affected than females. Treatment can be divided into acute therapy aimed at stopping symptoms once they have started and preventive therapy aimed at preventing recurrent attacks during the cluster period.

Symptoms of Cluster Headache

People with cluster headaches describe the pain as piercing and unbearable. The headaches occur in "clusters" usually at the same time of the day and night for several weeks. The symptoms are usually experienced on one side of the head, often behind or around the eye. The nose and the eye on the affected side of the head may also get red, swollen, and runny. Some people will experience nausea; restlessness; changes in blood pressure and heart rate; and agitation, or sensitivities to light, sound, or smell. Most affected individuals have one to three cluster headaches a day and two cluster periods a year, separated by periods of freedom from symptoms.

A small group of people develop a chronic form of the disorder, characterized by bouts of cluster headaches that can go on for years with only brief periods (2 weeks or less) of remission.

Cause of Cluster Headache

Scientists aren't sure what causes cluster headaches, although there are currently several theories. The tendency of cluster headaches to occur during the same time(s) from day to day, and more often at night than during the daylight hours, suggests they could be caused by irregularities in the body's circadian rhythms, which are controlled by the brain and a family of hormones that regulate the sleep-wake cycle. The development of cluster headaches may additionally be related to the body's release of histamine (chemical released in the body during an allergic response) or serotonin (chemical made by nerve cells). It is also possible that a problem in a part of the brain called the hypothalamus may be involved.

Alcohol (especially red wine) provokes attacks in more than half of those with cluster headaches, but has no effect once the cluster period ends. Cluster headaches are also strongly associated with cigarette smoking. Glare, stress, or certain foods may also trigger an attack.

An increased familial risk of these headaches suggests that there may be a genetic cause, though more studies are needed to confirm this suspicion and identify specific genetic changes associated.

Treatment of Cluster Headache

Treatment does not cure cluster headaches. The goal of treatment is to relieve symptoms. Spontaneous remission may occur, or treatment may be required to prevent headaches.

There are medications available to lessen the pain of a cluster headache and suppress future attacks. Oxygen inhalation and triptan drugs (such as those used to treat migraine) administered as a tablet, nasal spray, or injection can provide quick relief from acute cluster headache pain. Lidocaine nasal spray, which numbs the nose and nostrils, may also be effective. Ergotamine and corticosteroids such as prednisone and dexamethasone may be prescribed to break the cluster cycle and then tapered off once headaches end. Verapamil may be used preventively to decrease the frequency and pain level of attacks. Lithium, valproic acid, and topiramate are sometimes also used preventively.

Chapter 31

Multiple Sclerosis Pain

Chapter Contents

Section 31.1

Multiple Sclerosis and Pain

This section contains text excerpted from the following sources:
Text in this section begins with excerpts from "Multiple Sclerosis,"
Genetics Home Reference (GHR), National Institutes of Health
(NIH), October 2015; Text beginning with the heading "What Are the
Signs and Symptoms of Multiple Sclerosis (MS)?" is excerpted from
"Multiple Sclerosis: Hope through Research," National Institute of
Neurological Disorders and Stroke (NINDS), March 10, 2017.

Multiple sclerosis (MS) is a condition characterized by areas of damage (lesions) on the brain and spinal cord. These lesions are associated with destruction of the covering that protects nerves and promotes the efficient transmission of nerve impulses (the myelin sheath) and damage to nerve cells. Multiple sclerosis is considered an autoimmune disorder; autoimmune disorders occur when the immune system malfunctions and attacks the body's own tissues and organs, in this case tissues of the nervous system.

Multiple sclerosis usually begins in early adulthood, between ages 20 and 40. The symptoms vary widely, and affected individuals can experience one or more effects of nervous system damage. Multiple sclerosis often causes sensory disturbances in the limbs, including a prickling or tingling sensation (paresthesia), numbness, pain, and itching. Some people experience Lhermitte sign, which is an electrical shock-like sensation that runs down the back and into the limbs. This sensation usually occurs when the head is bent forward. Problems with muscle control are common in people with multiple sclerosis. Affected individuals may have tremors, muscle stiffness (spasticity), exaggerated reflexes (hyperreflexia), weakness or partial paralysis of the muscles of the limbs, difficulty walking, or poor bladder control. Multiple sclerosis is also associated with vision problems, such as blurred or double vision or partial or complete vision loss. Infections that cause fever can make the symptoms worse.

There are several forms of multiple sclerosis: relapsing-remitting MS, secondary progressive MS, primary progressive MS, and progressive relapsing MS. The most common is the relapsing-remitting form, which affects approximately 80 percent of people with multiple sclerosis. Individuals with this form of the condition have periods during which they experience symptoms, called clinical attacks, followed by periods without any symptoms (remission). The triggers of clinical attacks and remissions are unknown. After about 10 years, relapsing-remitting MS usually develops into another form of the disorder called secondary progressive MS. In this form, there are no remissions, and symptoms of the condition continually worsen.

Primary progressive MS is the next most common form, affecting approximately 10 to 20 percent of people with multiple sclerosis. This form is characterized by constant symptoms that worsen over time, with no clinical attacks or remissions. Primary progressive MS typically begins later than the other forms, around age 40.

Progressive relapsing MS is a rare form of multiple sclerosis that initially appears like primary progressive MS, with constant symptoms. However, people with progressive relapsing MS also experience clinical attacks of more severe symptoms.

What Are the Signs and Symptoms of Multiple Sclerosis (MS)?

The symptoms of MS usually begin over one to several days, but in some forms, they may develop more slowly. They may be mild or severe and may go away quickly or last for months. Sometimes the initial symptoms of MS are overlooked because they disappear in a day or so and normal function returns. Because symptoms come and go in the majority of people with MS, the presence of symptoms is called an attack, or in medical terms, an exacerbation. Recovery from symptoms is referred to as remission, while a return of symptoms is called a relapse. This form of MS is therefore called relapsing-remitting MS, in contrast to a more slowly developing form called primary progressive MS. Progressive MS can also be a second stage of the illness that follows years of relapsing-remitting symptoms.

A diagnosis of MS is often delayed because MS shares symptoms with other neurological conditions and diseases.

The first symptoms of MS often include:

- vision problems such as blurred or double vision or optic neuritis, which causes pain in the eye and a rapid loss of vision.

- weak, stiff muscles, often with painful muscle spasms

- tingling or numbness in the arms, legs, trunk of the body, or face

- clumsiness, particularly difficulty staying balanced when walking

- bladder control problems, either inability to control the bladder or urgency

- dizziness that doesn't go away

MS may also cause later symptoms such as:

- mental or physical fatigue which accompanies the above symptoms during an attack

- mood changes such as depression or euphoria

- changes in the ability to concentrate or to multitask effectively

- difficulty making decisions, planning, or prioritizing at work or in private life

Some people with MS develop transverse myelitis, a condition caused by inflammation in the spinal cord. Transverse myelitis causes loss of spinal cord function over a period of time lasting from several hours to several weeks. It usually begins as a sudden onset of lower back pain, muscle weakness, or abnormal sensations in the toes and feet, and can rapidly progress to more severe symptoms, including paralysis. In most cases of transverse myelitis, people recover at least some function within the first 12 weeks after an attack begins. Transverse myelitis can also result from viral infections, arteriovenous malformations, or neuroinflammatory problems unrelated to MS. In such instances, there are no plaques in the brain that suggest previous MS attacks.

Neuromyelitis optica is a disorder associated with transverse myelitis as well as optic nerve inflammation. Patients with this disorder usually have antibodies against a particular protein in their spinal cord, called the aquaporin channel. These patients respond differently to treatment than most people with MS.

Most individuals with MS have muscle weakness, often in their hands and legs. Muscle stiffness and spasms can also be a problem. These symptoms may be severe enough to affect walking or standing. In some cases, MS leads to partial or complete paralysis. Many people with MS find that weakness and fatigue are worse when they have a fever or when they are exposed to heat. MS exacerbations may occur following common infections.

Tingling and burning sensations are common, as well as the opposite, numbness and loss of sensation. Moving the neck from side to side or flexing it back and forth may cause "Lhermitte sign," a characteristic sensation of MS that feels like a sharp spike of electricity coursing down the spine.

While it is rare for pain to be the first sign of MS, pain often occurs with optic neuritis and trigeminal neuralgia, a neurological disorder that affects one of the nerves that runs across the jaw, cheek, and face. Painful spasms of the limbs and sharp pain shooting down the legs or around the abdomen can also be symptoms of MS.

Most individuals with MS experience difficulties with coordination and balance at some time during the course of the disease. Some may have a continuous trembling of the head, limbs, and body, especially during movement, although such trembling is more common with other disorders such as Parkinson disease.

Fatigue is common, especially during exacerbations of MS. A person with MS may be tired all the time or may be easily fatigued from mental or physical exertion.

Urinary symptoms, including loss of bladder control and sudden attacks of urgency, are common as MS progresses. People with MS sometimes also develop constipation or sexual problems.

Depression is a common feature of MS. A small number of individuals with MS may develop more severe psychiatric disorders such as bipolar disorder and paranoia, or experience inappropriate episodes of high spirits, known as euphoria.

People with MS, especially those who have had the disease for a long time, can experience difficulty with thinking, learning, memory, and judgment. The first signs of what doctors call cognitive dysfunction may be subtle. The person may have problems finding the right word to say, or trouble remembering how to do routine tasks on the job or at home. Day-to-day decisions that once came easily may now be made more slowly and show poor judgment. Changes may be so small or happen so slowly that it takes a family member or friend to point them out.

What Causes MS?

The ultimate cause of MS is damage to myelin, nerve fibers, and neurons in the brain and spinal cord, which together make up the central nervous system (CNS). But how that happens, and why, are questions that challenge researchers. Evidence appears to show that MS is a disease caused by genetic vulnerabilities combined with environmental factors.

Although there is little doubt that the immune system contributes to the brain and spinal cord tissue destruction of MS, the exact target of the immune system attacks and which immune system cells cause the destruction isn't fully understood.

451

Researchers have several possible explanations for what might be going on. The immune system could be:

- fighting some kind of infectious agent (for example, a virus) that has components which mimic components of the brain (molecular mimicry)

- destroying brain cells because they are unhealthy

- mistakenly identifying normal brain cells as foreign

The last possibility has been the favored explanation for many years. Research now suggests that the first two activities might also play a role in the development of MS. There is a special barrier, called the blood-brain barrier, which separates the brain and spinal cord from the immune system. If there is a break in the barrier, it exposes the brain to the immune system for the first time. When this happens, the immune system may misinterpret the brain as "foreign."

Genetic Susceptibility

Susceptibility to MS may be inherited. Studies of families indicate that relatives of an individual with MS have an increased risk for developing the disease. Experts estimate that about 15 percent of individuals with MS have one or more family members or relatives who also have MS. But even identical twins, whose Deoxyribonucleic acid (DNA) is exactly the same, have only a 1 in 3 chance of both having the disease. This suggests that MS is not entirely controlled by genes. Other factors must come into play.

Current research suggests that dozens of genes and possibly hundreds of variations in the genetic code (called gene variants) combine to create vulnerability to MS. Some of these genes have been identified. Most of the genes identified so far are associated with functions of the immune system. Additionally, many of the known genes are similar to those that have been identified in people with other autoimmune diseases as type 1 diabetes, rheumatoid arthritis or lupus. Researchers continue to look for additional genes and to study how they interact with each other to make an individual vulnerable to developing MS.

Sunlight and Vitamin D

A number of studies have suggested that people who spend more time in the sun and those with relatively high levels of vitamin D are less likely to develop MS. Bright sunlight helps human skin produce vitamin D. Researchers believe that vitamin D may help regulate the immune system in ways that reduce the risk of MS. People from regions near the equator, where there is a great deal of bright sunlight, generally have a much lower risk of MS than people from temperate areas such as the United States and Canada. Other studies suggest that people with higher levels of vitamin D generally have less severe MS and fewer relapses.

Smoking

A number of studies have found that people who smoke are more likely to develop MS. People who smoke also tend to have more brain lesions and brain shrinkage than non-smokers. The reasons for this are currently unclear.

Infectious Factors and Viruses

A number of viruses have been found in people with MS, but the virus most consistently linked to the development of MS is Epstein-Barr virus (EBV), the virus that causes mononucleosis.

Only about 5 percent of the population has not been infected by EBV. These individuals are at a lower risk for developing MS than those who have been infected. People who were infected with EBV in adolescence or adulthood and who therefore develop an exaggerated immune response to EBV are at a significantly higher risk for developing MS than those who were infected in early childhood. This suggests that it may be the type of immune response to EBV that predisposes to MS, rather than EBV infection itself. However, there is still no proof that EBV causes MS.

Autoimmune and Inflammatory Processes

Tissue inflammation and antibodies in the blood that fight normal components of the body and tissue in people with MS are similar to those found in other autoimmune diseases. Along with overlapping evidence from genetic studies, these findings suggest that MS results from some kind of disturbed regulation of the immune system.

How Is MS Diagnosed?

There is no single test used to diagnose MS. Doctors use a number of tests to rule out or confirm the diagnosis. There are many other disorders that can mimic MS. Some of these other disorders can be cured, while others require different treatments than those used for MS. Therefore, it is very important to perform a thorough investigation before making a diagnosis.

In addition to a complete medical history, physical examination, and a detailed neurological examination, a doctor will order an MRI scan of the head and spine to look for the characteristic lesions of MS. MRI is used to generate images of the brain and/or spinal cord. Then a special dye or contrast agent is injected into a vein and the MRI is repeated. In regions with active inflammation in MS, there is disruption of the blood-brain barrier and the dye will leak into the active MS lesion.

Doctors may also order evoked potential tests, which use electrodes on the skin and painless electric signals to measure how quickly and accurately the nervous system responds to stimulation. In addition, they may request a lumbar puncture (sometimes called a "spinal tap") to obtain a sample of cerebrospinal fluid. This allows them to look for proteins and inflammatory cells associated with the disease and to rule out other diseases that may look similar to MS, including some infections and other illnesses. MS is confirmed when positive signs of the disease are found in different parts of the nervous system at more than one time interval and there is no alternative diagnosis.

Are There Treatments Available for MS?

There is still no cure for MS, but there are treatments for initial attacks, medications and therapies to improve symptoms, and drugs developed to slow the worsening of the disease. These drugs have been shown to reduce the number and severity of relapses and to delay the long-term progression of MS.

Treatments for Attacks

The usual treatment for an initial MS attack is to inject high doses of a steroid drug, such as methylprednisolone, intravenously (into a vein) over the course of 3 to 5 days. It may sometimes be followed by a tapered dose of oral steroids. Intravenous steroids quickly and potently suppress the immune system, and reduce inflammation. Clinical trials have shown that these drugs hasten recovery.

The drug mitoxantrone, which is administered intravenously four times a year, has been approved for especially severe forms of relapsing-remitting and secondary progressive MS. This drug has been associated with development of certain types of blood cancers in up to one percent of patients, as well as with heart damage. Therefore, this drug should be used as a last resort to treat patients with a form of MS that leads to rapid loss of function and for whom other treatments did not stop the disease.

Natalizumab works by preventing cells of the immune system from entering the brain and spinal cord. It is administered intravenously once a month. It is a very effective drug for many people, but it is associated with an increased risk of a potentially fatal viral infection of the brain called progressive multifocal encephalopathy (PML). People who take natalizumab must be carefully monitored for symptoms of PML, which include changes in vision, speech, and balance that do not remit like an MS attack. Therefore, natalizumab is generally recommended only for individuals who have not responded well to the other approved MS therapies or who are unable to tolerate them. Other side effects of natalizumab treatment include allergic and hypersensitivity reactions.

In March 2017, the FDA approved ocrelizumab (brand name Ocrevus) to treat adults with relapsing forms of MS and primary progressive multiple sclerosis.

Other FDA-approved drugs to treat relapsing forms of MS in adults include dimethyl fumarate and teriflunomide, both taken orally.

Table 31.1. Disease Modifying Drugs

Trade Name	Generic Name
Avonex	interferon beta-1a
Betaseron	interferon beta-1b
Rebif	interferon beta-1a
Copaxone	glatiramer acetate
Tysabri	natalizumab
Novantrone	mitoxantrone
Gilenya	fingolimod

Pain

People with MS may experience several types of pain during the course of the disease.

Trigeminal neuralgia is a sharp, stabbing, facial pain caused by MS affecting the trigeminal nerve as it exits the brainstem on its way to the jaw and cheek. It can be treated with anticonvulsant or antispasmodic drugs, alcohol injections, or surgery.

455

People with MS occasionally develop central pain, a syndrome caused by damage to the brain and/or spinal cord. Drugs such as gabapentin and nortriptyline sometimes help to reduce central pain.

Burning, tingling, and prickling (commonly called "pins and needles") are sensations that happen in the absence of any stimulation. The medical term for them is dysesthesias" They are often chronic and hard to treat.

Chronic back or other musculoskeletal pain may be caused by walking problems or by using assistive aids incorrectly. Treatments may include heat, massage, ultrasound treatments, and physical therapy to correct faulty posture and strengthen and stretch muscles.

Section 31.2

Multiple Sclerosis and CAM

This section includes text excerpted from "Multiple Sclerosis and Complementary Health Approaches," National Center for Complementary and Integrative Health (NCCIH), February 11, 2016.

Natural Products

Cannabinoids

Orally administered cannabinoids (cannabis extract, synthetic tetrahydrocannabinol (THC)), mucosally delivered cannabinoids (cannabis extract oral spray, nabiximols, and smoked cannabis have all been studied for therapeutic effects in MS. Based on available evidence, cannabinoids may relieve spasticity and/or pain in people with MS; however, no marijuana-derived medications are approved by the U.S. Food and Drug Administration (FDA) to treat MS. Sativex (nabiximols) is licensed in the UK for use as an add-on treatment for MS-related spasticity when people have shown inadequate response to other symptomatic treatments or found their side effects intolerable. There is insufficient data to determine if smoking marijuana ameliorates symptoms of MS. Additionally, the psychoactive properties and other potential adverse effects need to be considered.

Safety

- In the studies that were the basis for the 2014 American Academy of Neurology guidelines, cannabinoids were generally well tolerated, although some serious adverse effects were reported. Mild or moderate side effects including dizziness, somnolence, drowsiness, lightheadedness, memory disturbance, and difficulty concentrating were more common in participants receiving cannabinoids versus placebo. Less common effects included increased appetite, nausea, vomiting, constipation, and dry/sore mouth, myalgia, seizures, and others. The guidelines noted that because cannabinoids have known psychoactive properties, their potential for psychopathologic and neurocognitive adverse effects is a concern, especially in a patient population that may be vulnerable due to underlying disorders.

- The guidelines recommend that clinicians counsel patients about the potential for psychopathologic/cognitive and other adverse events associated with cannabinoids. Sativex oromucosal cannabinoid spray is not approved by FDA and is unavailable in the United States. Further, the guidelines suggest caution should be exercised with regard to extrapolation of results of trials of standardized oral cannabis extract (which are unavailable commercially) to other nonstandardized, non regulated cannabis extracts (which may be commercially available in states with medical marijuana laws).

Ginkgo Biloba

There is no evidence to support the use of ginkgo biloba as an effective treatment for cognitive function in people with MS.

Safety

- Side effects of ginkgo may include headache, nausea, gastrointestinal upset, diarrhea, dizziness, or allergic skin reactions. More severe allergic reactions have occasionally been reported.

- There are some data from animal models to suggest that ginkgo can have an effect on the pharmacokinetics of several drugs; however, current available clinical evidence suggests that low doses do not pose a risk for clinically relevant herb-drug interactions.

457

- Fresh ginkgo seeds contain large amounts of ginkgotoxin, which can cause serious adverse reactions, including seizures and death. Roasted seeds can also be toxic. Products made from standardized ginkgo leaf extracts contain little ginkgotoxin and appear to be safe when used orally and appropriately.

- National Toxicology Program (NTP) studies showed that rats and mice developed tumors after being given a specific ginkgo extract for up to 2 years. Further studies are needed to find out what substances in ginkgo caused the tumors and whether taking ginkgo as a dietary supplement affects the risk of cancer in people.

Omega-3 Fatty Acid Supplementation

There is insufficient data to assess any real beneficial effects of omega-3 fatty acid supplementation on MS. Evidence-based guidelines from the American Academy of Neurology concluded that a low-fat diet with fish oil supplementation is probably ineffective for reducing MS-related relapse, disability, or MRI lesions, or for improving fatigue or quality of life.

Safety

- Omega-3 fatty acid supplements generally do not have adverse effects. When adverse effects do occur, they typically consist of minor gastrointestinal symptoms.

- It is unclear whether people with fish or shellfish allergies can safely consume fish oil supplements.

- People who take anticoagulants or Nonsteroidal Antiinflammatory Drugs (NSAIDs) should use caution when taking omega-3 supplements, because they may extend bleeding time.

Vitamin D

There is insufficient evidence to support the use of vitamin D supplementation for MS. A 2010 Cochrane review suggests clinicians may want to consider relevant guidelines on vitamin D supplementation when advising patients with MS.

Safety

- Limited intervention studies in MS suggest that vitamin D supplements are generally well tolerated in MS.

- High doses may cause fatigue, abdominal cramps, nausea, vomiting, renal damage, and other adverse effects.

Bee Venom

Based on a few small studies, bee venom therapy seems to have no effect on either MS symptoms or disease progression. There are serious side effects associated with bee venom, including risk of anaphylactic reactions and death, which could limit any efficacy of bee venom therapy for the treatment of MS.

Safety

- There are serious side effects associated with bee venom, which could limit any efficacy of bee venom therapy in the treatment of MS.

Mind and Body Practices

Yoga

There is some limited evidence suggesting beneficial short-term effects of yoga on fatigue and mood in people with MS, but scientific studies overall had a high risk of bias and definitive conclusions could not be drawn.

Safety

- In the studies included in a 2014 systematic review and meta-analysis, yoga was not associated with serious adverse events.
- People with certain medical conditions, including MS, should modify or avoid some yoga poses.

Reflexology

There is insufficient evidence to support the use of reflexology for most symptoms of MS, including pain, health-related quality of life, disability, spasticity, fatigue, depression, and others. However, 2014 evidence-based guidelines from the American Academy of Neurology concluded that, based on four studies, reflexology is possibly effective for reducing MS-associated paresthesia over 11 weeks.

Safety

- Reflexology is generally considered safe for most people; however, vigorous pressure applied to the feet may cause discomfort for some people.

Magnet Therapy

There is some limited, low-level evidence that suggests that magnet therapy may have modest beneficial effects on spasticity outcomes in people with MS, but the studies have been of low methodological quality. There is also some evidence, based on two studies, suggesting that magnet therapy may be useful in reducing fatigue in people with relapsing-remitting MS.

Safety

- Magnets may interfere with the functioning of the medical device (e.g., pacemaker, insulin pump) and may not be safe for some people. Otherwise, magnets are generally considered safe when applied to the skin.

- Reports of side effects or complications have been rare.

Hyperbaric Oxygen Therapy

Although hyperbaric oxygen therapy is often heavily marketed to people with MS, there is no consistent evidence that supports the use of hyperbaric oxygen therapy for the treatment of MS.

Safety

- When safety guidelines are strictly adhered to, hyperbaric oxygen therapy appears to be generally safe. The predominant complication is pressure equalization problems within the middle ear. Serious complications are rare.

Chapter 32

Neuralgia and Neurological Pain

Chapter Contents

Section 32.1

Arachnoiditis

This section includes text excerpted from "Arachnoiditis," Genetic
and Rare Diseases Information Center (GARD), National Center for
Advancing Translational Sciences (NCATS), August 17, 2016.

Arachnoiditis is a pain disorder caused by inflammation of the
arachnoid, one of the membranes that surrounds and protects the
nerves of the spinal cord. The inflammation may occur due to irritation
from chemicals; infection; direct injury to the spine; chronic compression of spinal nerves; or complications from spinal surgery or other
spinal procedures. It may result in scar tissue and adhesions, which
cause the spinal nerves to "stick" together. If arachnoiditis affects the
function of nerves, it can cause symptoms such as numbness, tingling,
and a characteristic stinging and burning pain in the lower back or
legs. In some people. it may affect the bladder, bowel, and sexual
function. Very severe arachnoiditis can result in paralysis of the legs.
Treatment aims to relieve pain and improve symptoms that impair
function. Treatment may include pain medications, physical therapy,
and psychotherapy. Surgical treatment is controversial because it
offers only short-term relief and may increase formation of scar tissue.

Symptoms of Arachnoiditis

Arachnoiditis can cause a number of symptoms including numbness; tingling; loss of temperature sensation; and a characteristic stinging and burning pain in the lower back, limbs, and trunk. Pain is often
made worse by activity. Some people have debilitating muscle cramps
or spasms; loss of balance; tinnitus; problems with vision and hearing;
or bladder, bowel, or sexual dysfunction. In severe cases, arachnoiditis
may lead to paralysis of the legs.

Causes of Arachnoiditis

Arachnoiditis has many possible causes, including:

*   mechanical injury during spinal surgery, or complications from
    spinal surgery (about 60% of cases)

- trauma to the spinal cord
- one or more spinal taps
- steroid epidural injections or other injections
- spinal and epidural anesthesia
- myelography
- bacterial or viral spinal infections

The initial symptoms of arachnoiditis are caused by inflammation of the arachnoid, and the formation of scar tissue and adhesions later cause the more severe symptoms as the condition progresses.

Inheritance of Arachnoiditis

Arachnoiditis is generally not an inherited condition and typically results from inflammation due to prior spinal surgery, other procedures on the spine (such as injections), trauma, or infection. Familial cases of arachnoiditis have very rarely been reported. To researchers knowledge, only two families with multiple affected family members have been described, with possible autosomal dominant or multigenic inheritance (due to the interaction of multiple genes).

Treatment of Arachnoiditis

Arachnoiditis is difficult to treat. Management aims to relieve pain and improve symptoms that impair function. Treatment may involve pain management, physical therapy, and psychotherapy. Surgical intervention is controversial because it generally provides only short-term relief and may increase the formation of scar tissue, making the condition worse.

Can Two Back Surgeries, Multiple Spinal Injections and One Epidural Anesthetic Cause Arachnoiditis or Adhesive Arachnoiditis?

Arachnoiditis, which may progress to adhesive arachnoiditis, has been reported to occur due to spinal surgeries, steroid epidural injections, other types of injections into the spinal cord, and anesthetic spinal interventions. About 60 percent of cases are associated with spinal surgeries, and about 22 percent of cases may be due to spinal and epidural anesthesia. After a person has arachnoiditis, injections or any other invasions of the spine may worsen the disease significantly. However, researchers are unable to say whether specific interventions have caused arachnoiditis (or progression to adhesive arachnoiditis) in any one person. People with questions or concerns about arachnoiditis for themselves or family members are encouraged to speak with a spine specialist or other healthcare provider familiar with the condition.

How Does Arachnoiditis Progress to Adhesive Arachnoiditis?

Generally, arachnoiditis occurs as a progression of inflammatory changes. First it is characterized by inflammation of the arachnoid membrane (the "inflammatory phase"), which invades the space beneath the membrane. Over a period of time, the nerve roots may become inflamed and begin to adhere to each other and to the inner layer of the arachnoid membrane or the thecal sac. This is referred to as the "adhesive phase" or "proliferation stage" of arachnoiditis. The adhesions may then exert pressure on the nerve roots and may eventually result in scarring and fibrosis (thickening of tissue). Scarring and fibrosis may restrict blood flow to the affected area and eventually impede the free flow of cerebrospinal fluid (CSF).

Unfortunately, the disorder has no predictable pattern or severity of symptoms. Therefore, it is not possible to predict if or when arachnoiditis may progress. However, surgeries, injections or any other invasions of the spine may worsen the disease significantly.

What Is the Long-Term Outlook for People with Arachnoiditis?

Arachnoiditis causes chronic pain and neurological deficits. The disease does not improve significantly with treatment and does not have a predictable pattern of symptoms, severity, or progression. Some people with arachnoiditis may have milder symptoms which do not get much worse over time, although the aging process usually does add to the severity of the symptoms. Others may quickly progress to severe neurological symptoms that lead to paralysis. The majority of people with arachnoiditis appear to fall somewhere between these extremes.

Section 32.2

Central Pain Syndrome

This section includes text excerpted from "Central Pain Syndrome," Genetic and Rare Diseases Information Center (GARD), National Center for Advancing Translational Sciences (NCATS), April 10, 2017.

Central pain syndrome (CPS) is a rare neurological disorder caused by damage to or dysfunction of the pain-conducting pathways of the central nervous system (in the brain, brainstem, and spinal cord). Symptoms of CPS can vary greatly from one person to another, partly because the cause may differ. Primary symptoms are pain and loss of sensation, usually in the face, arms, and/or legs. Pain or discomfort may be felt after being touched, or even in the absence of a trigger. The pain may worsen by exposure to heat or cold and by emotional distress. CPS is usually associated with stroke, multiple sclerosis, tumors, epilepsy, brain or spinal cord trauma, or Parkinson disease. Treatment typically includes pain medications, but complete relief of pain may not be possible. Tricyclic antidepressants or anticonvulsants can sometimes be useful. Lowering stress levels appears to reduce pain.

Many different names have been used for this disorder, including Dejerine-Roussy syndrome, thalamic pain syndrome, central post-stroke syndrome, and others. The current name acknowledges that damage to various areas of the central nervous system can cause central pain, and that a stroke is not necessarily the cause. When CPS is due to a stroke, it may be referred to as the more specific term "central poststroke pain."

Symptoms of Central Pain Syndrome (CPS)

Central pain syndrome (CPS) often begins shortly after the injury or damage that caused it. However, it may be delayed by months or even years, especially if it is related to post-stroke pain. The characteristics of the pain associated with CPS differ widely, partly because of the variety of potential causes. It may affect a large portion of the body, or be restricted to specific areas such as the hands or feet.

465

The severity of pain is usually related to the cause of the central nervous system (CNS) injury or damage. Pain is typically constant, may be moderate to severe in intensity, and is often made worse by touch, movement, emotions, and temperature changes (usually cold temperatures).

People with CPS experience one or more types of pain sensations, the most prominent being burning. Mingled with the burning may be sensations of pins and needles, pressing, lacerating, aching, or brief, intolerable bursts of sharp pain. Some people also experience numbness. The burning and loss-of-touch sensations are usually most severe on the distal parts of the body, such as the feet or hands.

Diagnosis of CPS

A diagnosis of central pain syndrome (CPS) is based on the characteristic symptoms, a detailed patient history, a thorough clinical exam and a variety of specialized tests. CPS is suspected in people who complain of pain or other abnormal sensations following injury to the central nervous system. Other conditions that cause pain may need to be ruled out before a diagnosis of CPS is made. The clinical exam may include sensory testing to confirm and pinpoint the presence of sensory abnormalities, but also to rule out other causes of pain. Imaging tests such as a computerized tomography (CT) scan and magnetic resonance imaging (MRI) may be used to see tumors, infarcts, cerebral bleeding, and other lesions that may cause pain. MRI is the preferred technique when CPS is suspected.

Treatment of CPS

Treatment of central pain syndrome (CPS) is known to be challenging. The method of treatment may vary depending on the cause of the neurological damage. Pain medications (analgesics) often provide only some relief of pain.

In general, first-line management includes the use of tricyclic antidepressants such as nortriptyline, anticonvulsants such as gabapentin, or topical lidocaine. Second-line management involves the use of opioid analgesics such as tramadol, along with first-line medication. Third-line management may include other antidepressant or anticonvulsant medications.

Lowering stress levels appears to reduce pain. Other treatment alternatives have included the administration of a sympathetic blockade (a type of nerve block) and a guanethidine block, as well as psychological evaluation and treatment. Rarely, surgery is necessary. Stereotactic radiosurgery (SRS) of the pituitary has been used with some success. Other forms of potential treatments that have been discussed in the literature include transcutaneous electrical nerve stimulation (TENS); deep brain stimulation; and motor cortex stimulation.

Section 32.3

Glossopharyngeal Neuralgia

This section includes text excerpted from "Glossopharyngeal Neuralgia," Genetic and Rare Diseases Information Center (GARD), National Center for Advancing Translational Sciences (NCATS), January 28, 2013. Reviewed June 2017.

Glossopharyngeal neuralgia is a condition characterized by repeated episodes of severe pain in the tongue, throat, ear, and tonsils (areas connected to the ninth cranial nerve, or glossopharyngeal nerve). It typically occurs in individuals over age 40. Episodes of pain may last from a few seconds to a few minutes, and usually occur on one side. The pain may be triggered by swallowing, speaking, laughing, chewing or coughing. The condition is thought to be due to irritation of the nerve, although the source of irritation is unclear. The goal of treatment is to control pain, but over-the-counter pain medications are not very effective; the most effective drugs are anti-seizure medications. Some antidepressants help certain people. Surgery to cut or take pressure off of the glossopharyngeal nerve may be needed in severe cases.

What Are the Signs and Symptoms of Glossopharyngeal Neuralgia?

Glossopharyngeal neuralgia is characterized by repeated episodes of severe pain in areas connected to the ninth cranial nerve (glossopharyngeal nerve): the back of the nose and throat; back of the tongue; ear; tonsil area; and voice box. These episodes, or "attacks," may last for a few seconds or a few minutes. They may be triggered by actions such as coughing or sneezing, swallowing, talking, laughing, or chewing. Pain usually begins at the back of the tongue or throat, and it sometimes spreads to the ear or the back of the jaw. In rare cases the heartbeat may be affected, which can cause fainting.

What Causes Glossopharyngeal Neuralgia?

Glossopharyngeal neuralgia is believed to be caused by irritation of the glossopharyngeal nerve. In many cases, the source of the irritation is not found. Possible causes that have been proposed include various things pressing on the glossopharyngeal nerve such as an abnormally positioned artery, growths at the base of the skull, or tumors or infections of the throat and mouth. Rarely, the condition may be attributable to a tumor in the brain or neck, an abscess, an aneurysm in an artery in the neck, or multiple sclerosis.

Is Glossopharyngeal Neuralgia Inherited?

To researchers knowledge, there is no evidence that glossopharyngeal neuralgia is an inherited condition.

How Might Glossopharyngeal Neuralgia Be Treated?

The main goal of treatment for glossopharyngeal neuralgia is to control pain. Over-the-counter pain medications are generally not very effective in affected individuals. However, anti-seizure medications such as carbamazepine, gabapentin, pregabalin, and phenytoin have reportedly been effective. Some antidepressants may help some individuals. The application of local anesthetics to the affected region may also be beneficial. In severe cases, affected individuals may need surgery to cut or take pressure off of the glossopharyngeal nerve; these surgeries are generally considered effective. If an underlying cause for the condition is identified, treatment is generally aimed at the underlying problem.

Section 32.4

Pinched Nerve

This section includes text excerpted from "Pinched Nerve
Information Page," National Institute of Neurological
Disorders and Stroke (NINDS), January 21, 2017.

The term "pinched nerve" is a colloquial term and not a true medical
term. It is used to describe one type of damage or injury to a nerve or
set of nerves. The injury may result from compression, constriction, or
stretching. Symptoms include numbness, "pins and needles" or burning
sensations, and pain radiating outward from the injured area. One of
the most common examples of a single compressed nerve is the feeling
of having a foot or hand "fall asleep."

A "pinched nerve" frequently is associated with pain in the neck
or lower back. This type of pain can be caused by inflammation or
pressure on the nerve root as it exits the spine. If the pain is severe
or lasts a long time, you may need to have further evaluation from
your physician. Several problems can lead to similar symptoms
of numbness, pain, and tingling in the hands or feet but without
pain in the neck or back. These can include peripheral neuropathy,
carpal tunnel syndrome, and tennis elbow. The extent of such injuries
may vary from minor, temporary damage to a more permanent
condition. Early diagnosis is important to prevent further damage
or complications. Pinched nerve is a common cause of on-the-job
injury.

Treatment of Pinched Nerve

The most frequently recommended treatment for pinched nerve
is rest for the affected area. Nonsteroidal anti-inflammatory drugs
(NSAIDs) or corticosteroids may be recommended to help alleviate
pain. Physical therapy is often useful, and splints or collars may be
used to relieve symptoms. Depending on the cause and severity of the
pinched nerve, surgery may be needed.

Prognosis of Pinched Nerve

With treatment, most people recover from pinched nerve. However, in some cases, the damage is irreversible.

Section 32.5

Shingles and Postherpetic Neuralgia

This section includes text excerpted from "Shingles: Hope Through Research," National Institute of Neurological Disorders and Stroke (NINDS), March 2015.

Shingles is the reactivation of a viral infection in the nerves to the skin that causes pain, burning, or a tingling sensation, along with an itch and blisters in the skin supplied by the affected nerve. It is caused by the *varicella zoster virus,* or VZV—the same virus that causes chickenpox. When the itchy red spots of childhood chickenpox disappear, the virus remains in a dormant state in our nerve cells, ready to strike again in later life. This second eruption of the chickenpox virus is called shingles or herpes-zoster.

You cannot develop shingles unless you have had an earlier exposure to chickenpox. Shingles occurs when an unknown trigger causes the virus to become activated. Most adults who have the dormant virus in their body never get shingles.

What Are the Symptoms and Signs of Shingles?

The first symptom of shingles is often burning or tingling pain, or itch, generally in a band-like distribution on one side of the body, i.e., around the waist, chest, stomach, or back. Shingles pain can be mild or intense. Some people have mostly itching; some feel severe pain from the gentlest touch, such as the weight of bed linens or clothing. A few people may have general symptoms of a viral infection, like fatigue, fever, and headache.

After several days or up to two weeks after the first symptoms are felt, a rash of fluid-filled blisters (vesicles) appears. These are similar

470

to chickenpox but occur in a cluster rather than scattered over the body. The number of vesicles is variable. Some rashes merge and produce an area that looks like a burn. Other people may have just a few small scattered lesions. The clusters most often appear in a band called a dermatome, which contains nerves that branch out from the virus-affected nerve root exiting the spine. The second most common location is on one side of the face around the eye and on the forehead. However, shingles can involve any part of the body, including internal organs.

Recent studies have shown that subtle cases of shingles with only a few blisters, or none, are more common than previously thought. These cases may remain unrecognized.

What Is the Varicella-Zoster Virus and How Does It Cause Shingles?

The word "varicella" is derived from "variola," the Latin word for smallpox. "Zoster" is the Greek word for girdle; shingles often produces a girdle or belt of blisters or lesions around one side of the waist. This striking pattern also underlies the condition's common name: shingles comes from "cingulum," the Latin word for belt or girdle.

VZV belongs to a group of viruses called herpesviruses. This group includes the herpes simplex virus (HSV) that causes cold sores, fever blisters, and genital herpes. Like VZV, HSV can hide in the nervous system after an initial infection and then travel down nerve cell fibers to cause a renewed infection. Repeated episodes of cold sores on the lips are the most common example.

Most adults in the United States have had chickenpox, even if it was so mild as to pass unnoticed, and they are at risk for developing shingles later in life. In the original exposure to VZV (chickenpox), some of the virus particles settle into nerve cells (neurons) of sensory ganglia (a group of nerve cells that connect the sensory periphery and central nervous system), where they remain for many years in an inactive, hidden (latent) form. The neurons in the sensory ganglia have nerve fibers that supply the skin and relay information to the brain about what the body is sensing — heat, cold, touch, pain.

When the VZV reactivates, it spreads down the long nerve fibers (axons) that extend from the sensory cell bodies to the skin. As the virus multiplies, the telltale rash erupts. With shingles, the nervous system is more deeply involved than it was during the bout with chickenpox, and the symptoms are often more complex and severe.

How Are Chickenpox and Shingles Different?

When a person, usually a child, who has not received the chickenpox vaccine is exposed to VZV, he or she usually develops chickenpox, a highly contagious disease that can be spread by breathing as well as by contact with the rash. The infection begins in the upper respiratory tract where the virus incubates for 15 days or more. VZV then spreads to the bloodstream and migrates to the skin, giving rise to the familiar chickenpox rash.

In contrast, you can't catch shingles from someone else. You must already have been exposed to chickenpox and harbor the virus in your nervous system to develop shingles. When reactivated, the virus travels down nerves to the skin, causing the painful shingles rash. In shingles, the virus does not normally spread to the bloodstream or lungs, so the virus is not shed in air.

But a person with a shingles rash—which contains active virus particles—can pass the virus to someone who has never had chickenpox or who has not been vaccinated. In this case, the person will develop chickenpox, not shingles. A person must come into direct contact with the open sores of the shingles rash.

Merely being in the same room with someone who has shingles will not cause chickenpox. Children who develop chickenpox generally fully recover; however, adults who develop chickenpox can become seriously ill.

Likewise, a person with chickenpox cannot give shingles to someone else—but they can pass the virus to someone who has never had chickenpox.

Who Is at Risk for Shingles?

Anyone who had previously had chickenpox is at risk for shingles. About 25 percent of all adults, mostly otherwise healthy, will get shingles during their lifetime, usually after age 50. The incidence increases with age so that shingles is 10 times more likely to occur in adults over 60 than in children under 10. People with compromised immune systems, a natural consequence of aging or from use of immunosuppressive medications such as prednisone, are at increased risk of developing shingles. Immunosuppressive drugs are used to treat serious illnesses such as cancer or from chemotherapy or radiation treatment, or from infection with human immunodeficiency virus (HIV). Some individuals can also have re-eruptions and some, particularly those with impaired immunity from drugs and diseases, may have shingles that spread over the body significantly.

Youngsters whose mothers had chickenpox late in pregnancy—5 to 21 days before giving birth—or who had chickenpox in infancy have an increased risk of pediatric shingles. Sometimes these children are born with chickenpox or develop a typical case within a few days.

Most people who get shingles have it only once, but it is possible for the outbreak to appear again.

How Is Shingles Treated?

Currently, there is no cure for shingles, but attacks can be made less severe and shorter by using prescription antiviral drugs such as acyclovir, valacyclovir, or famciclovir as soon as possible after symptoms begin. Early treatment can reduce or prevent severe pain and help blisters dry faster. Antiviral drugs can reduce by about half the risk of being left with postherpetic neuralgia, which is chronic pain that can last for months or years after the shingles rash clears. Doctors recommend starting antiviral drugs at the first sign of the shingles rash, or if the telltale symptoms indicate that a rash is about to erupt. Other treatments to consider are anti-inflammatory corticosteroids such as prednisone. These are routinely used when the eye or other facial nerves are affected.

Most people with shingles can be treated at home.

People with shingles should also try to relax and reduce stress (stress can make pain worse and lead to depression); eat regular, well-balanced meals; and perform gentle exercises, such as walking or stretching to keep active and stop thinking about the pain (but check first with your physician). Placing a cool, damp washcloth on the blisters—but not when wearing a topical cream or patch—can help blisters dry faster and relieve pain. Keeping the area clean can help avoid a secondary bacterial infection.

Can Shingles Be Prevented?

Shingles Vaccine

In 2006, the U.S. Food and Drug Administration (FDA) approved a VZV vaccine (Zostavax) for use in people 60 and older who have had chickenpox. In March 2011, the FDA extended the approval to include adults ages 50–59.

The **Shingles Prevention Study**—a collaboration between the U.S. Department of Veterans Affairs (VA), the National Institute of Allergy and Infectious Diseases (NIAID), and Merck and Co., Inc.—involved more than 38,000 veterans aged 60 and older. The purpose was to find out how safe the vaccine is, and if it can prevent shingles. Half the study participants received the shingles vaccine, and half received a similar looking, inactive vaccine (placebo vaccine). Neither volunteers nor researchers knew if a particular subject had gotten active or placebo vaccine until after the end of the study (called a double-blind study). During more than 3 years of follow-up, the vaccine reduced shingles cases by 51 percent; 642 cases of shingles developed in the placebo group compared with only 315 in the vaccinated group. And in people who received the active vaccine and still got shingles, the severity and discomfort were reduced by 61 percent. The vaccine also reduced the number of cases of long-lasting nerve pain (postherpetic neuralgia) by two-thirds compared with the placebo.

The shingles vaccine is a preventive therapy and not a treatment for those who already have shingles or postherpetic neuralgia.

Chickenpox Vaccine

The chickenpox vaccine became available in the United States in 1995. Immunization with the varicella vaccine (or chickenpox vaccine)—now recommended in the United States for all children between 18 months and adolescence—can protect people from getting chickenpox. People who have been vaccinated against chickenpox are probably less likely to get shingles because the weak, "attenuated" strain of virus used in the chickenpox vaccine is less likely to survive in the body over decades.

What Is Postherpetic Neuralgia?

Sometimes, particularly in older people, shingles pain persists long after the rash has healed. This is postherpetic neuralgia, defined as pain lasting three months after onset of the rash. Pain can be mild or severe—the most severe cases can lead to insomnia, weight loss, depression, and disability. There may be other sensations, such as tingling, coldness, or loss of feeling. About 20 percent of people age 70 or greater who develop shingles may have long-lasting pain. Postherpetic neuralgia is not directly life-threatening and may get better over time.

About a dozen medications in four categories have been shown in clinical trials to provide some pain relief for postherpetic neuralgia. These include:

Tricyclic antidepressants (TCAs). TCAs are often the first type of drug given to people suffering from postherpetic neuralgia. The TCA amitriptyline was commonly prescribed in the past, but although effective, it has a high rate of side effects. Desipramine and nortriptyline have fewer side effects and are therefore better choices for older adults, the most likely group to have postherpetic neuralgia.

Common side effects of TCAs include dry eyes and mouth, constipation, and impaired memory. People with heart arrhythmias (irregular heartbeats), previous heart attacks, or narrow angle glaucoma should usually use a different class of drugs.

Anticonvulsants. Some drugs developed to reduce seizures can also treat postherpetic neuralgia because seizures and pain both involve abnormally increased firing of nerve cells. The antiseizure medication gabapentin is most often prescribed. Carbamazepine is effective for postherpetic neuralgia but has somewhat common side effects including drowsiness or confusion, dizziness, and sometimes ankle swelling. Some small studies have shown positive effects using divalproex sodium to treat postherpetic neuralgia.

Opioids. Opioids are strong pain medications used for all types of pain. They include oxycodone, morphine, tramadol, and methadone. Opioids can have side effects—including drowsiness, mental dulling, and constipation—and can be addictive, so their use must be monitored carefully in those with a history of addiction.

Topical local anesthetics. Local anesthetics are effective when applied directly to the skin of the painful area affected by postherpetic neuralgia. Lidocaine, the most commonly prescribed, is available in cream, gel, or spray form. It is also available in a patch that has been approved by the FDA for use specifically in postherpetic neuralgia. With topical local anesthetics, the drug stays in the skin and therefore does not cause problems such as drowsiness or constipation. Capsaicin cream may be somewhat effective and is available over the counter, but most people find that it causes severe burning pain during application. An alternative approach using a high concentration capsaicin patch has been reported to be effective.

Postherpetic Itch

The itch that sometimes occurs during or after shingles can be quite severe and painful. Clinical experience suggests that postherpetic itch is harder to treat than postherpetic neuralgia. Topical local anesthetics (which numb the skin) provide substantial relief to some individuals. Since postherpetic itch typically develops in skin that has severe sensory loss, it is particularly important to avoid scratching. Scratching numb skin too long or too hard can cause injury.

What Are Other Complications of Shingles?

Complications of zoster are more frequent in people with lesions in or around the eyes, forehead, and nose (ophthalmic shingles), or around the ear and on the face (herpes zoster oticus or Ramsay-Hunt syndrome). People with shingles in or near the eye should see an ophthalmologist immediately, as they can suffer painful eye infections and, in some cases, temporary or permanent vision loss. Symptoms can include redness and swelling involving just the white of the eye (sclera), the clear front of the eye (cornea), or internal parts of the eye. If the cornea is involved, treatment to avert permanent scarring is important to preventing lasting vision loss. The disease can cause damage to or death of the nerve cells that react to light (called acute retinal necrosis).

Shingles infections within or near the ear can cause hearing or balance problems as well as weakness of the muscles on the affected side of the face. These problems can be long-lasting or permanent.

In rare cases, shingles can spread into the brain or spinal cord and cause serious complications such as stroke or meningitis (an infection of the membranes outside the brain and spinal cord).

The varicella zoster virus also may involve blood vessels or provoke an immune reaction irritating the surface of blood vessels (vasculopathy). People with shingles have slightly increased risk of stroke, greatest in the first few weeks after vesicle eruption, but lasting for several months. The risk of stroke is highest in people with eye zoster, perhaps as much as five percent.

People with shingles need to seek immediate medical evaluation if they notice neurological symptoms outside the region of the primary shingles attack. People who are immunosuppressed, whether from diseases such as HIV or medications, have an increased risk of serious complications from shingles. They may develop shingles that spreads to involve more parts of the body, or shingles rashes that persist for long periods or return frequently. Many such individuals are helped by taking antiviral medications on a continuous basis. People taking immunosuppressive drugs, or with diseases such as HIV or leukemia, should see a doctor immediately for treatment to avoid possible serious complications.

Can Infection with VZV during Pregnancy Harm the Baby?

Some infections can be transmitted across the mother's bloodstream to the fetus or can be acquired by the baby during the birth process. Chickenpox during pregnancy poses some risk to the unborn child, depending upon the stage of pregnancy. During the first 30 weeks, maternal chickenpox may, in some cases, lead to congenital malformations (although such cases are rare). Most experts agree that shingles in a pregnant woman is even less likely to cause harm to the unborn child.

If a pregnant woman gets chickenpox between 21 to 5 days before giving birth, her newborn can have chickenpox at birth or develop it within a few days. But the time lapse between the start of the mother's illness and the birth of the baby generally allows the mother's immune system to react and produce antibodies to fight the virus. These antibodies can be transmitted to the unborn child and thus help fight the infection. Still, a small percent of the babies exposed to chickenpox in the 21 to 5 days before birth develop shingles in the first 5 years of life because the newborn's immune system is not yet fully functional and capable of keeping the virus latent.

If a mother contracts chickenpox at the time of birth, the newborn will have little ability to fight off the attack because its immune system is immature. If these babies develop chickenpox as a result, it can be fatal. They are given zoster immune globulin, a preparation made from the antibody-rich blood of adults who have recently recovered from chickenpox or shingles, to lessen the severity of their chickenpox.

Section 32.6

Tarlov Cysts

This section includes text excerpted from "Tarlov Cysts," Genetic
and Rare Diseases Information Center (GARD), National Center for
Advancing Translational Sciences (NCATS), May 25, 2016.

What Are Tarlov Cysts?

Tarlov cysts are fluid-filled sacs that most often affect nerve roots
in the sacrum, the group of bones at the base of the spine. These cysts
don't usually cause symptoms, but when compressing nerve roots,
they can cause lower back pain, sciatica (shock-like or burning pain
in the lower back, buttocks, and down one leg to below the knee),
urinary incontinence, headaches, sexual dysfunction, constipation,
and some loss of feeling or control of movement in the leg and/or foot.
Pressure on the nerves next to the cysts can also cause pain and deterioration of the surrounding bone. Asymptomatic tarlov cysts may
become symptomatic following shock, trauma, or exertion that causes
the buildup of cerebrospinal fluid. Current information indicates that
women are more commonly diagnosed with Tarlov cysts. The reason
for this is unknown. Treatment depends on the symptoms and size
of the cysts. Many methods have been described for treatment with
variable results.

Is There a Cure for Tarlov Cysts?

While there is no cure for Tarlov cysts, there are several treatment
options which have delivered mixed results in controlling the symptoms of the condition.

How Might Tarlov Cysts Be Treated?

While there is no standard accepted treatment for individuals with
symptomatic Tarlov cysts, many different therapies have been tried.
Tarlov cysts may be drained and shunted to relieve pressure and pain,
but relief is often only temporary and fluid build-up in the cysts will
recur. Corticosteroid injections may also temporarily relieve pain.

Nonsteroidal anti-inflammatory drugs (NSAIDs) may be prescribed to treat chronic pain and inflammation. Injecting the cysts with fibrin glue (a combination of naturally occurring substances based on the clotting factor in blood) may provide temporary relief of pain. Micro-surgical removal of the cyst wall may be an option in select individuals who do not respond to conservative treatments and who continue to experience pain or progressive neurological damage.

Transcutaneous electrical nerve stimulation (TENS) has been proven useful for some in pain management. TENS devices deliver electrical impulses through the skin to the nerves to control pain. Unlike medications and topical ointments, TENS does not have any known side effects, other than skin irritation from the electrodes in some patients.

A recent review analyzed the different surgical options, including the following:

- Sacral laminectomy with microsurgical cyst fenestration and cyst imbrication
- Sacral laminectomy with resection of the sacral cyst
- Microsurgical excision of the cyst along with duraplasty or plication of the cyst
- Release of the valve and imbrication of the sacral cysts with laminectomies
- Total or partial cyst wall removal, arranging the remaining nerve sheath, and repairing the local defect with muscle, gelfoam, and fibrin glue
- Removing of the cyst and closure of defect by fibrin glue
- Microscopic cyst resection and closure of defect by fibrin glue
- Microsurgical fenestration from the cyst to the thecal sac
- Fenestration of the cyst and closure of the opening by stitches and glue
- Cyst remodeling around the root using titanium clips
- Cyst excision and occlusion of its neck

Are There Surgical Options for Treatment of Tarlov Cysts?

There are a small number of physicians in the world who have surgical expertise in the treatment for Tarlov cysts. The short- and long-term outcome of surgery is improving but variable in individual patients at this time.

Who May Be Involved in the Management of a Patient with Tarlov Cysts?

Neurosurgeons and interventional neuroradiologists may treat individuals with Tarlov cysts. It is important that the treating physician is knowledgeable about the symptomatology of the cysts and the extended ramifications of untreated cysts that are present with no other spinal pathology. Pain management specialists are vital to the treatment of symptomatic Tarlov cysts. Family practice physicians (or other primary healthcare providers) play a key role in management of symptoms, including bowel and bladder dysfunction. A urologist might be consulted if the cysts are interfering with bladder function (urinary retention, increased frequency of urinary tract infections, or incontinence).

Chapter 33

Neuropathies

Chapter Contents

Section 33.1

Peripheral Neuropathy

This section includes text excerpted from "Peripheral Neuropathy Fact Sheet," National Institute of Neurological Disorders and Stroke (NINDS), December 2014.

An estimated 20 million people in the United States have some form of peripheral neuropathy, a condition that develops as a result of damage to the peripheral nervous system—the vast communications network that transmits information between the central nervous system (the brain and spinal cord) and every other part of the body. (Neuropathy means nerve disease or damage.) Symptoms can range from numbness or tingling, to pricking sensations (paresthesia), or muscle weakness. Areas of the body may become abnormally sensitive leading to an exaggeratedly intense or distorted experience of touch (allodynia). In such cases, pain may occur in response to a stimulus that does not normally provoke pain. Severe symptoms may include burning pain (especially at night), muscle wasting, paralysis, or organ or gland dysfunction. Damage to nerves that supply internal organs may impair digestion, sweating, sexual function, and urination. In the most extreme cases, breathing may become difficult, or organ failure may occur.

Peripheral nerves send sensory information back to the brain and spinal cord, such as a message that the feet are cold. Peripheral nerves also carry signals from the brain and spinal cord to the muscles to generate movement. Damage to the peripheral nervous system interferes with these vital connections. Like static on a telephone line, peripheral neuropathy distorts and sometimes interrupts messages between the brain and spinal cord and the rest of the body.

Peripheral neuropathies can present in a variety of forms and follow different patterns. Symptoms may be experienced over a period of days, weeks, or years. They can be acute or chronic. In acute neuropathies such as Guillain-Barré syndrome (in which the body's immune system attacks part of the peripheral nervous system and impairs sending and receiving nerve signals), symptoms appear suddenly, progress rapidly, and resolve slowly as damaged nerves heal. In chronic forms, symptoms begin subtly and progress slowly. Some people may have periods of relief followed by relapse. Others may reach a plateau stage where symptoms stay the same for many months or years. Many chronic neuropathies worsen over time. Although neuropathy may be painful and potentially debilitating, very few forms are fatal.

In diabetic neuropathy, one of the most common forms of peripheral neuropathy, nerve damage occurs in an ascending pattern. The first nerve fibers to malfunction are the ones that travel the furthest from the brain and the spinal cord. Pain and numbness often are felt symmetrically in both feet followed by a gradual progression up both legs. Later, the fingers, hands, and arms may become affected.

How Are the Peripheral Neuropathies Classified?

More than 100 types of peripheral neuropathy have been identified, each with its own symptoms and prognosis. In general, peripheral neuropathies are classified according to the type of damage to the nerves. Some forms of neuropathy involve damage to only one nerve and are called *mononeuropathies*. More frequently however, multiple nerves are affected, called *polyneuropathy*.

Some peripheral neuropathies are due to damage to the axons (the long, threadlike portion of the nerve cell), while others are due to damage to the myelin sheath, the fatty protein that coats and insulates the axon. Peripheral neuropathies may also be caused by a combination of both axonal damage and demyelination. Electrodiagnostic studies can help healthcare providers determine the type of damage involved.

What Are the Symptoms of Peripheral Nerve Damage?

Symptoms vary depending on whether motor, sensory, or autonomic nerves are damaged. Motor nerves control voluntary movement of muscles such as those used for walking, grasping things, or talking. Sensory nerves transmit information such as the feeling of a light touch or the pain from a cut. Autonomic nerves control organ activities that are regulated automatically such as breathing, digesting food, and heart and gland functions. Some neuropathies may affect all three types of nerves; others primarily affect one or two types. Doctors may use terms such as predominantly motor neuropathy, predominantly sensory neuropathy, sensory-motor neuropathy, or autonomic neuropathy to describe the types of nerves involved in an individual's condition.

Motor nerve damage is most commonly associated with muscle weakness. Other symptoms may include painful cramps and fasciculations (uncontrolled muscle twitching visible under the skin), muscle atrophy (severe shrinkage of muscle size), and decreased reflexes.

Sensory nerve damage causes a variety of symptoms because sensory nerves have a broad range of functions. Larger sensory fibers enclosed in myelin register vibration, light touch, and position sense. Damage to large sensory fibers impairs touch, resulting in a general decrease in sensation. Since this is felt most in the hands and feet, people may feel as if they are wearing gloves and stockings even when they are not. This damage to larger sensory fibers may contribute to the loss of reflexes. Loss of position sense often makes people unable to coordinate complex movements like walking or fastening buttons, or to maintain their balance when their eyes are shut.

Smaller sensory fibers without myelin sheaths transmit pain and temperature sensations. Damage to these fibers can interfere with the ability to feel pain or changes in temperature. People may fail to sense that they have been injured from a cut or that a wound is becoming infected. Others may not detect pain that warns of impending heart attack or other acute conditions. Loss of pain sensation is a particularly serious problem for people with diabetes, contributing to the high rate of lower limb amputations among this population.

Neuropathic pain is a common, often difficult to control symptom of sensory nerve damage and can seriously affect emotional well-being and overall quality of life. Often worse at night, neuropathic pain seriously disrupts sleep and adds to the emotional burden of sensory nerve damage. Neuropathic pain can often be associated with an over sensitization of pain receptors in the skin, so that people feel severe pain (allodynia) from stimuli that are normally painless. For example, some may experience pain from bed sheets draped lightly over the body. Over many years, sensory neuropathy may lead to changes in the skin, hair, as well as to joint and bone damage. Unrecognized injuries due to poor sensation contribute to these changes, so it is important for people with neuropathy to inspect numb areas for injury or damage.

Autonomic nerve damage symptoms are diverse since the parasympathetic and sympathetic nerves of the peripheral nervous system control nearly every organ in the body. Common symptoms of autonomic nerve damage include an inability to sweat normally, which may lead to heat intolerance; a loss of bladder control; and an inability to control muscles that expand or contract blood vessels to regulate blood pressure. A drop in blood pressure when a person moves suddenly from a seated to a standing position (a condition known as postural or orthostatic hypotension) may result in dizziness, lightheadedness, or fainting. Irregular heartbeats may also occur.

Gastrointestinal symptoms may accompany autonomic neuropathy. Malfunction of nerves controlling intestinal muscle contractions can lead to diarrhea, constipation, or incontinence. Many people also have problems eating or swallowing if autonomic nerves controlling these functions are affected.

What Causes Peripheral Neuropathy?

Peripheral neuropathy may be either inherited or acquired through disease processes or trauma. In many cases, however, a specific cause cannot be identified. Doctors usually refer to neuropathies with no known cause as idiopathic.

Causes of acquired peripheral neuropathy include:

Physical injury (trauma) is the most common cause of acquired nerve injury.

- Injury or sudden trauma

- Repetitive stress

Diseases or disorders and their related processes (such as inflammation) can be associated with peripheral neuropathy.

- Metabolic and endocrine disorders

- Small vessel disease

- Autoimmune diseases

- Kidney disorders

- Cancers

- Neuromas

- Infections

The human immunodeficiency virus (HIV) that causes Acquired immune deficiency syndrome (AIDS) is associated with several different forms of neuropathy, depending on the nerves affected and the specific stage of active immunodeficiency disease. A rapidly progressive, painful polyneuropathy affecting the feet and hands can be the first clinically apparent symptom of HIV infection. An estimated 30 percent of people who are HIV positive develop peripheral neuropathy; 20 percent develop distal neuropathic pain.

Exposure to toxins may damage nerves and cause peripheral neuropathy.

- Medication toxicity
- Environmental or industrial toxins
- Heavy alcohol consumption

Genetic mutations can either be inherited or arise de novo, meaning they are completely new mutations to an individual and are not passed along by either parent. Some genetic mutations lead to mild neuropathies with symptoms that begin in early adulthood and result in little, if any, significant impairment. More severe hereditary neuropathies often appear in infancy or childhood.

Advances in genetic testing in the last decade have led to significant strides in the ability to identify the genetic causes underlying peripheral neuropathies. For example, several genes have been found to play a role in different types of Charcot-Marie-Tooth, a group of disorders that are among the most common forms of inherited peripheral neuropathies. These neuropathies result from mutations in genes responsible for maintaining the health of the myelin sheath as well as the axons themselves. Key characteristics of Charcot- Marie-Tooth disorders include extreme weakening and wasting of muscles in the lower legs and feet, gait abnormalities, loss of tendon reflexes, and numbness in the lower limbs.

How Is Peripheral Neuropathy Diagnosed?

The symptoms of peripheral neuropathy are highly variable. A thorough neurological examination is required to sort out the cause of the symptoms and involves taking an extensive medical history (covering symptoms, work environment, social habits, exposure to toxins, alcohol use, risk of HIV or other infectious diseases, and family history of neurological diseases). In addition, tests are usually performed to identify the cause of the neuropathy as well as the extent and type of nerve damage.

A physical examination and various tests may reveal the presence of a systemic disease causing the nerve damage. Tests of muscle strength, as well as evidence of cramps or fasciculations, indicate motor fiber involvement. Evaluation of the person's ability to sense vibration, light touch, body position, temperature, and pain reveals any sensory nerve damage and may indicate whether small or large sensory nerve fibers are affected.

Blood tests can detect diabetes, vitamin deficiencies, liver or kidney dysfunction, other metabolic disorders, and signs of abnormal immune system activity. An examination of cerebrospinal fluid that surrounds the brain and spinal cord can reveal abnormal antibodies associated with some immune-mediated neuropathies. More specialized tests may reveal other blood or cardiovascular diseases, connective tissue disorders, or malignancies. Genetic tests are becoming available for a number of the inherited neuropathies.

Based on the results of the neurological exam, physical exam, patient history, and any previous screening or testing, the following additional tests may be ordered to help determine the nature and extent of the neuropathy:

- Nerve conduction velocity (NCV)

- Electromyography (EMG)

- Nerve biopsy

- Skin biopsy

What Treatments Are Available?

Address Underlying Conditions

The first step in treating peripheral neuropathy is to address any contributing causes such as infection, toxin exposure, medication-related toxicity, vitamin deficiencies, hormonal deficiencies, autoimmune disorders, or compression that can lead to neuropathy. Peripheral nerves have the ability to regenerate axons, as long as the nerve cell itself has not died, which may lead to functional recovery over time. Correcting an underlying condition often can result in the neuropathy resolving on its own as the nerves recover or regenerate.

The adoption of healthy lifestyle habits such as maintaining optimal weight, avoiding exposure to toxins, exercising, eating a balanced diet, correcting vitamin deficiencies, and limiting or avoiding alcohol consumption can reduce the effects of peripheral neuropathy. Exercise can reduce cramps, improve muscle strength, and prevent muscle wasting. Various dietary strategies can improve gastrointestinal symptoms. Timely treatment of injuries can help prevent permanent damage. Smoking cessation is particularly important because smoking constricts the blood vessels that supply nutrients to the peripheral nerves and can worsen neuropathic symptoms. Self-care skills such as meticulous foot care and careful wound treatment in people with diabetes and others who have an impaired ability to feel pain can alleviate symptoms and improve quality of life. Such changes often create conditions that encourage nerve regeneration.

Systemic diseases frequently require more complex treatments. Strict control of blood glucose levels has been shown to reduce neuropathic symptoms and help people with diabetic neuropathy avoid further nerve damage.

Inflammatory and autoimmune conditions leading to neuropathy can be controlled in several ways. Immunosuppressive drugs such as prednisone, cyclosporine, or azathioprine may be beneficial. Plasmapheresis—a procedure in which blood is removed, cleansed of immune system cells and antibodies, and then returned to the body—can help reduce inflammation or suppress immune system activity. Large intravenously administered doses of immunoglobulins (antibodies that alter the immune system, and agents such as rituximab that target specific inflammatory cells) also can suppress abnormal immune system activity.

Symptom Management

Neuropathic pain, or pain caused by the injury to a nerve or nerves, is often difficult to control. Mild pain may sometimes be alleviated by over-the-counter analgesics such as nonsteroidal anti-inflammatory drugs (NSAIDs). More chronic and discomforting pain may need to be addressed through the care of a physician. Medications that are used for chronic neuropathic pain fall under several classes of drugs: antidepressants, anticonvulsant medications, antiarrhythmic medications, and narcotic agents. The antidepressant and anticonvulsant medications modulate pain through their mechanism of action on the peripheral nerves, spinal cord, or brain and tend to be the most effective types of medications to control neuropathic pain. Antidepressant medications include tricyclic antidepressants such as amitriptyline or newer serotonin-norepinephrine reuptake inhibitors such as duloxetine hydrochloride or venlafaxine. Anticonvulsant medications that are frequently used include gabapentin, pregabalin, topiramate, and carbamazepine, although other medications used for treating epilepsy may also be useful. Mexiletine is an antiarrhythmic medication that may be used for treatment of chronic painful neuropathies.

For pain that does not respond to the previously described medications, the addition of narcotic agents may be considered. Because the use of prescription obtained pain relievers that contain opioids can lead to dependence and addiction, their use is recommended only after other means of controlling the pain have failed. One of the newest narcotic medications approved for the treatment of diabetic neuropathy is tapentadol, a drug with both opioid activity and norepinephrine-reuptake inhibition activity of an antidepressant.

Topically administered medications are another option for neuropathic pain. Two agents are topical lidocaine, an anesthetic agent, and capsaicin, a substance found in hot peppers that modifies peripheral pain receptors. Topical agents are generally most appropriate for localized chronic pain such as herpes zoster neuralgia (shingles) pain. Their usefulness for treating diffuse chronic diabetic neuropathy is more limited.

Transcutaneous electrical nerve stimulation (TENS) is a non-invasive intervention used for pain relief in a range of conditions, and a number of studies have described its use for neuropathic pain. The therapy involves attaching electrodes to the skin at the site of pain or near associated nerves and then administering a gentle electrical current. Although data from controlled clinical trials are not available to broadly establish its efficacy for peripheral neuropathies, TENS has been shown in some studies to improve peripheral neuropathy symptoms associated with diabetes.

Other complementary approaches may provide additional support and pain relief. For example, mechanical aids such as hand or foot braces can help reduce pain and physical disability by compensating for muscle weakness or alleviating nerve compression. Orthopedic shoes can improve gait disturbances and help prevent foot injuries in people with a loss of pain sensation. Acupuncture, massage, and herbal medications also are considered in the treatment of neuropathic pain.

Surgical intervention can be considered for some types of neuropathies. Injuries to a single nerve caused by focal compression such as at the carpal tunnel of the wrist, or other entrapment neuropathies, may respond well to surgery that releases the nerve from the tissues compressing it. Some surgical procedures reduce pain by destroying the nerve; this approach is appropriate only for pain caused by a single nerve and when other forms of treatment have failed to provide relief. Peripheral neuropathies that involve more diffuse nerve damage, such as diabetic neuropathy, are not amenable to surgical intervention.

Section 33.2

Diabetic Neuropathies

This section includes text excerpted from "Nerve Damage (Diabetic Neuropathies)," National Institute of Diabetes and Digestive and Kidney Diseases (NIDDK), November 2013. Reviewed June 2017.

Diabetic neuropathies are a family of nerve disorders caused by diabetes. People with diabetes can, over time, develop nerve damage throughout the body. Some people with nerve damage have no symptoms. Others may have symptoms such as pain, tingling, or numbness—loss of feeling—in the hands, arms, feet, and legs. Nerve problems can occur in every organ system, including the digestive tract, heart, and sex organs.

About 60 to 70 percent of people with diabetes have some form of neuropathy. People with diabetes can develop nerve problems at any time, but risk rises with age and longer duration of diabetes. The highest rates of neuropathy are among people who have had diabetes for at least 25 years. Diabetic neuropathies also appear to be more common in people who have problems controlling their blood glucose, also called blood sugar, as well as those with high levels of blood fat and blood pressure and those who are overweight.

What Causes Diabetic Neuropathies?

The causes are probably different for different types of diabetic neuropathy. Researchers are studying how prolonged exposure to high blood glucose causes nerve damage. Nerve damage is likely due to a combination of factors:

- Metabolic factors, such as high blood glucose, long duration of diabetes, abnormal blood fat levels, and possibly low levels of insulin

- Neurovascular factors, leading to damage to the blood vessels that carry oxygen and nutrients to nerves

- Autoimmune factors that cause inflammation in nerves

- Mechanical injury to nerves, such as carpal tunnel syndrome
- Inherited traits that increase susceptibility to nerve disease
- Lifestyle factors, such as smoking or alcohol use

What Are the Symptoms of Diabetic Neuropathies?

Symptoms depend on the type of neuropathy and which nerves are affected. Some people with nerve damage have no symptoms at all. For others, the first symptom is often numbness, tingling, or pain in the feet. Symptoms are often minor at first, and because most nerve damage occurs over several years, mild cases may go unnoticed for a long time. Symptoms can involve the sensory, motor, and autonomic— or involuntary—nervous systems. In some people, mainly those with focal neuropathy, the onset of pain may be sudden and severe.

Symptoms of nerve damage may include:

- Numbness, tingling, or pain in the toes, feet, legs, hands, arms, and fingers
- Wasting of the muscles of the feet or hands
- Indigestion, nausea, or vomiting
- Diarrhea or constipation
- Dizziness or faintness due to a drop in blood pressure after standing or sitting up
- Problems with urination
- Erectile dysfunction in men or vaginal dryness in women
- Weakness

Symptoms that are not due to neuropathy, but often accompany it, include weight loss and depression.

What Are the Types of Diabetic Neuropathy?

Diabetic neuropathy can be classified as peripheral, autonomic, proximal, or focal. Each affects different parts of the body in various ways.

- **Peripheral neuropathy**, the most common type of diabetic neuropathy, causes pain or loss of feeling in the toes, feet, legs, hands, and arms.

- **Autonomic neuropathy** causes changes in digestion, bowel and bladder function, sexual response, and perspiration. It can also affect the nerves that serve the heart and control blood pressure, as well as nerves in the lungs and eyes. Autonomic neuropathy can also cause hypoglycemia unawareness, a condition in which people no longer experience the warning symptoms of low blood glucose levels.

- **Proximal neuropathy** causes pain in the thighs, hips, or buttocks and leads to weakness in the legs.

- **Focal neuropathy** results in the sudden weakness of one nerve or a group of nerves, causing muscle weakness or pain. Any nerve in the body can be affected.

Neuropathy Affects Nerves throughout the Body

Peripheral neuropathy affects:

- toes
- feet
- legs
- hands
- arms

Autonomic neuropathy affects:

- heart and blood vessels
- digestive system
- urinary tract
- sex organs
- sweat glands
- eyes
- lungs

Proximal neuropathy affects:

- thighs
- hips
- buttocks
- legs

Focal neuropathy affects:

- eyes
- facial muscles
- ears
- pelvis and lower back
- chest
- abdomen
- thighs
- legs
- feet

What Is Peripheral Neuropathy?

Peripheral neuropathy, also called distal symmetric neuropathy or sensorimotor neuropathy, is nerve damage in the arms and legs. Feet and legs are likely to be affected before hands and arms. Many people with diabetes have signs of neuropathy that a doctor could notice but could not feel symptoms themselves. Symptoms of peripheral neuropathy may include:

- numbness or insensitivity to pain or temperature
- a tingling, burning, or prickling sensation
- sharp pains or cramps
- extreme sensitivity to touch, even light touch
- loss of balance and coordination

These symptoms are often worse at night.

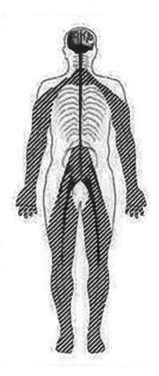

Figure 33.1. *Impact of Peripheral Neuropathy across the Body*

Peripheral neuropathy affects the nerves in your toes, feet, legs, hands, and arms.

Peripheral neuropathy may also cause muscle weakness and loss of reflexes, especially at the ankle, leading to changes in the way a person walks. Foot deformities, such as hammertoes and the collapse of the midfoot, may occur. Blisters and sores may appear on numb areas of the foot because pressure or injury goes unnoticed. If an infection occurs and is not treated promptly, the infection may spread to the bone, and the foot may then have to be amputated. Many amputations are preventable if minor problems are caught and treated in time.

What Is Autonomic Neuropathy?

Autonomic neuropathy affects the nerves that control the heart, regulate blood pressure, and control blood glucose levels. Autonomic neuropathy also affects other internal organs, causing problems with digestion, respiratory function, urination, sexual response, and vision. In addition, the system that restores blood glucose levels to normal after a hypoglycemic episode may be affected, resulting in loss of the warning symptoms of hypoglycemia.

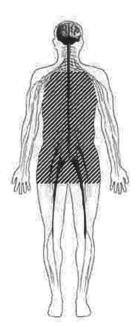

Figure 33.2. *Impact of Autonomic neuropathy across the Body*

Autonomic neuropathy affects the nerves in your heart, stomach, intestines, bladder, sex organs, sweat glands, eyes, and lungs.

What Is Proximal Neuropathy?

Proximal neuropathy, sometimes called lumbosacral plexus neuropathy, femoral neuropathy, or diabetic amyotrophy, starts with pain in the thighs, hips, buttocks, or legs, usually on one side of the body. This type of neuropathy is more common in those with type 2 diabetes and in older adults with diabetes. Proximal neuropathy causes weakness in the legs and the inability to go from a sitting to a standing position without help. Treatment for weakness or pain is usually needed. The length of the recovery period varies, depending on the type of nerve damage.

What Is Focal Neuropathy?

Focal neuropathy appears suddenly and affects specific nerves, most often in the head, torso, or leg. Focal neuropathy may cause:

- inability to focus the eye
- double vision
- aching behind one eye
- paralysis on one side of the face, called Bell palsy
- severe pain in the lower back or pelvis
- pain in the front of a thigh
- pain in the chest, stomach, or side
- pain on the outside of the shin or inside of the foot
- chest or abdominal pain that is sometimes mistaken for heart disease, a heart attack, or appendicitis

Focal neuropathy is painful and unpredictable and occurs most often in older adults with diabetes. However, it tends to improve by itself over weeks or months and does not cause long-term damage.

People with diabetes also tend to develop nerve compressions, also called entrapment syndromes. One of the most common is carpal tunnel syndrome, which causes numbness and tingling of the hand and sometimes muscle weakness or pain. Other nerves susceptible to entrapment may cause pain on the outside of the shin or the inside of the foot.

Can Diabetic Neuropathies Be Prevented?

The best way to prevent neuropathy is to keep blood glucose levels as close to the normal range as possible. Maintaining safe blood glucose levels protects nerves throughout the body.

How Are Diabetic Neuropathies Diagnosed?

Doctors diagnose neuropathy on the basis of symptoms and a physical exam. During the exam, the doctor may check blood pressure, heart rate, muscle strength, reflexes, and sensitivity to position changes, vibration, temperature, or light touch.

Foot Exam

Experts recommend that people with diabetes have a comprehensive foot exam each year to check for peripheral neuropathy. People diagnosed with peripheral neuropathy need more frequent foot exams. A comprehensive foot exam assesses the skin, muscles, bones, circulation, and sensation of the feet. The doctor may assess protective sensation or feeling in the feet by touching them with a nylon monofilament—similar to a bristle on a hairbrush—attached to a wand or by pricking them with a pin. People who cannot sense pressure from a pinprick or monofilament have lost protective sensation and are at risk for developing foot sores that may not heal properly. The doctor may also check temperature perception or use a tuning fork, which is more sensitive than touch pressure, to assess vibration perception.

Other Tests

The doctor may perform other tests as part of the diagnosis.

- Nerve conduction studies or electromyography
- A check of heart rate variability
- Ultrasound

How Are Diabetic Neuropathies Treated?

The first treatment step is to bring blood glucose levels within the normal range to help prevent further nerve damage. Blood glucose monitoring, meal planning, physical activity, and diabetes medicines or insulin will help control blood glucose levels. Symptoms may get worse when blood glucose is first brought under control, but over time, maintaining lower blood glucose levels helps lessen symptoms. Good blood glucose control may also help prevent or delay the onset of further problems. As scientists learn more about the underlying causes of neuropathy, new treatments may become available to help slow, prevent, or even reverse nerve damage.

As described below additional treatment depends on the type of nerve problem and symptom.

Pain Relief

Doctors usually treat painful diabetic neuropathy with oral medications, although other types of treatments may help some people. People with severe nerve pain may benefit from a combination of medications or treatments and should consider talking with a healthcare provider about treatment options.

Medications used to help relieve diabetic nerve pain include:

- tricyclic antidepressants, such as amitriptyline, imipramine, and desipramine (Norpramin, Pertofrane)

- other types of antidepressants, such as duloxetine (Cymbalta), venlafaxine, bupropion (Wellbutrin), paroxetine (Paxil), and citalopram (Celexa)

- anticonvulsants, such as pregabalin (Lyrica), gabapentin (Gabarone, Neurontin), carbamazepine, and lamotrigine (Lamictal)

- opioids and opioid like drugs, such as controlled-release oxycodone, an opioid; and tramadol (Ultram), an opioid that also acts as an antidepressant

Duloxetine and pregabalin are approved by the U.S. Food and Drug Administration (FDA) specifically for treating painful diabetic peripheral neuropathy.

People do not have to be depressed for an antidepressant to help relieve their nerve pain. All medications have side effects, and some are not recommended for use in older adults or those with heart disease. Because over-the-counter pain medicines such as acetaminophen and ibuprofen may not work well for treating most nerve pain and can have serious side effects, some experts recommend avoiding these medications.

Treatments that are applied to the skin—typically to the feet— include capsaicin cream and lidocaine patches (Lidoderm, Lidopain). Studies suggest that nitrate sprays or patches for the feet may relieve pain. Studies of alpha-lipoic acid, an antioxidant, and evening primrose oil suggest they may help relieve symptoms and improve nerve function in some patients.

A device called a bed cradle can keep sheets and blankets from touching sensitive feet and legs. Acupuncture, biofeedback, or physical therapy may help relieve pain in some people. Treatments that involve electrical nerve stimulation, magnetic therapy, and laser or light therapy may be helpful but need further study. Researchers are also studying several new therapies in clinical trials.

Foot Care

People with neuropathy need to take special care of their feet. The nerves to the feet are the longest in the body and are the ones most often affected by neuropathy. Loss of sensation in the feet means that sores or injuries may not be noticed and may become ulcerated or infected. Circulation problems also increase the risk of foot ulcers. Smoking increases the risk of foot problems and amputation. A healthcare provider may be able to provide help with quitting smoking.

More than 60 percent of all nontraumatic lower-limb amputations in the United States occur in people with diabetes. Nontraumatic amputations are those not caused by trauma such as severe injuries from an accident. Comprehensive foot care programs can reduce amputation rates by 45 to 85 percent.

Careful foot care involves:

- cleaning the feet daily using warm—not hot—water and a mild soap. Soaking the feet should be avoided. A soft towel can be used to dry the feet and between the toes.

- inspecting the feet and toes every day for cuts, blisters, redness, swelling, calluses, or other problems. Using a mirror—handheld or placed on the floor—may be helpful in checking the bottoms of the feet, or another person can help check the feet. A healthcare provider should be notified of any problems.

- using lotion to moisturize the feet. Getting lotion between the toes should be avoided.

- filing corns and calluses gently with a pumice stone after a bath or shower.

- cutting toenails to the shape of the toes and filing the edges with an emery board each week or when needed.

- always wearing shoes or slippers to protect feet from injuries. Wearing thick, soft, seamless socks can prevent skin irritation.

- wearing shoes that fit well and allow the toes to move. New shoes can be broken in gradually by first wearing them for only an hour at a time.

- looking shoes over carefully before putting them on and feeling the insides to make sure the shoes are free of tears, sharp edges, or objects that might injure the feet.

People who need help taking care of their feet should consider making an appointment to see a foot doctor, also called a podiatrist.

Chapter 34

Phantom Pain

About Phantom Pain

When a limb is traumatically severed, pain perceived in the part of the body that no longer exists often develops. This is called "phantom limb" pain, and is different from "stump" pain, which is pain within the part of the limb that remains intact. Unfortunately, phantom pain resolves in only 16 percent of people, with the rest experiencing this pain for the remainder of the lives. There is currently no reliable treatment for phantom limb pain.

Causes and Treatment

The exact reason that phantom limb pain occurs is unclear, but when a nerve is cut—as happens with a traumatic amputation— changes occur in the brain and spinal cord that actually worsen with increasing phantom pain. These abnormal changes may often be corrected by putting local anesthetic—termed a "peripheral nerve block"—on the injured nerve, keeping any "bad signals" from reaching

This chapter contains text excerpted from the following sources: Text in this chapter begins with excerpts from "Treating Phantom Limb Pain Using Continuous Peripheral Nerve Blocks: A Department of Defense Funded Multicenter Study (DoD-PLP-Tx)," ClinicalTrials.gov, National Institutes of Health (NIH), October 27, 2016; Text under the heading "Recent Findings" is excerpted from "Pain: Hope through Research," National Institute of Neurological Disorders and Stroke (NINDS), January 2014.

501

the brain, with resolution of the phantom limb pain. However, when the nerve block ends after a few hours, the phantom pain returns. But, this demonstrates that the brain abnormalities—and phantom pain—that occur with an amputation may be dependent upon the "bad" signals being sent from the injured nerve(s), suggesting that a very long peripheral nerve block—lasting many days rather than hours—may permanently reverse the abnormal changes in the brain, and provide lasting relief from phantom pain.

Until recently, extending a peripheral nerve block beyond 16 hours was unrealistic. However, a treatment option called a "continuous peripheral nerve block" is now available. This technique involves the placement of a tiny tube—smaller than a piece of spaghetti—through the skin and next to the nerves supplying the amputated limb. The tiny tube may be placed with minimal discomfort in about 15 minutes. Numbing medicine called local anesthetic is then infused through the tube, blocking any signals that the injured nerve sends to the spinal cord and brain. Using a small, portable infusion pump, this prolonged nerve block may be provided in individuals' own homes.

Recent Findings

Researchers understanding of phantom pain has improved tremendously in recent years. Investigators previously believed that brain cells affected by amputation simply died off. They attributed sensations of pain at the site of the amputation to irritation of nerves located near the limb stump. Now, using imaging techniques such as positron emission tomography (PET) and magnetic resonance imaging (MRI), scientists can actually visualize increased activity in the brain's cortex when an individual feels phantom pain. When study participants move the stump of an amputated limb, neurons in the brain remain dynamic and excitable. Surprisingly, the brain's cells can be stimulated by other body parts, often those located closest to the missing limb.

Treatments for phantom pain may include analgesics, anticonvulsants, and other types of drugs; nerve blocks; electrical stimulation; psychological counseling, biofeedback, hypnosis, and acupuncture; and, in rare instances, surgery.

Chapter 35

Sickle Cell Pain

What Is Sickle Cell Disease?

The term sickle cell disease (SCD) describes a group of inherited red blood cell disorders. People with SCD have abnormal hemoglobin, called hemoglobin S or sickle hemoglobin, in their red blood cells.

Hemoglobin is a protein in red blood cells that carries oxygen throughout the body.

"Inherited" means that the disease is passed by genes from parents to their children. SCD is not contagious. A person cannot catch it, like a cold or infection, from someone else.

People who have SCD inherit two abnormal hemoglobin genes, one from each parent. In all forms of SCD, at least one of the two abnormal genes causes a person's body to make hemoglobin S. When a person has two hemoglobin S genes, Hemoglobin SS, the disease is called sickle cell anemia. This is the most common and often most severe kind of SCD.

Hemoglobin SC disease and hemoglobin Sβ thalassemia are two other common forms of SCD.

Some forms of sickle cell disease includes:

- Hemoglobin SS

- Hemoglobin SC

This chapter includes text excerpted from "Sickle Cell Disease," National Heart, Lung, and Blood Institute (NHLBI), August 2, 2016.

- Hemoglobin Sβ0 thalassemia
- Hemoglobin Sβ+ thalassemia
- Hemoglobin SD
- Hemoglobin SE

What Causes Sickle Cell Disease?

Abnormal hemoglobin, called hemoglobin S, causes sickle cell disease (SCD).

The problem in hemoglobin S is caused by a small defect in the gene that directs the production of the beta globin part of hemoglobin. This small defect in the beta globin gene causes a problem in the beta globin part of hemoglobin, changing the way that hemoglobin works.

Inheritance

When the hemoglobin S gene is inherited from only one parent and a normal hemoglobin gene is inherited from the other, a person will have sickle cell trait. People with sickle cell trait are generally healthy.

Only rarely do people with sickle cell trait have complications similar to those seen in people with SCD. But people with sickle cell trait are carriers of a defective hemoglobin S gene. So, they can pass it on when they have a child.

If the child's other parent also has sickle cell trait or another abnormal hemoglobin gene (like thalassemia, hemoglobin C, hemoglobin D, hemoglobin E), that child has a chance of having SCD.

It is important to keep in mind that each time this couple has a child, the chances of that child having sickle cell disease remain the same. In other words, if the first-born child has sickle cell disease, there is still a 25 percent chance that the second child will also have the disease. Both boys and girls can inherit sickle cell trait, sickle cell disease, or normal hemoglobin.

If a person wants to know if he or she carries a sickle hemoglobin gene, a doctor can order a blood test to find out.

Who Is at Risk for Sickle Cell Disease?

In the United States, most people with sickle cell disease (SCD) are of African ancestry or identify themselves as black.

- About 1 in 13 African American babies is born with sickle cell trait.

- About 1 in every 365 black children is born with sickle cell disease.

There are also many people with this disease who come from Hispanic, southern European, Middle Eastern, or Asian Indian backgrounds.

Approximately 100,000 Americans have SCD.

What Are the Signs and Symptoms of Sickle Cell Disease?

Early Signs and Symptoms

If a person has sickle cell disease (SCD), it is present at birth. But most infants do not have any problems from the disease until they are about 5 or 6 months of age. Every state in the United States, the District of Columbia, and the U.S. territories requires that all newborn babies receive screening for SCD. When a child has SCD, parents are notified before the child has symptoms.

Some children with SCD will start to have problems early on, and some later. Early symptoms of SCD may include:

- Painful swelling of the hands and feet, known as dactylitis

- Fatigue or fussiness from anemia

- A yellowish color of the skin, known as jaundice, or whites of the eyes, known as icterus, that occurs when a large number of red cells hemolyze

The signs and symptoms of SCD will vary from person to person and can change over time. Most of the signs and symptoms of SCD are related to complications of the disease.

Major Complications of Sickle Cell Disease

Acute Pain (Sickle Cell or Vaso-occlusive) Crisis

Pain episodes (crises) can occur without warning when sickle cells block blood flow and decrease oxygen delivery. People describe this pain as sharp, intense, stabbing, or throbbing. Severe crises can be even more uncomfortable than postsurgical pain or childbirth.

Pain can strike almost anywhere in the body and in more than one spot at a time. But the pain often occurs in the:

- Lower back

505

- Legs
- Arms
- Abdomen
- Chest

A crisis can be brought on by:

- Illness
- Temperature changes
- Stress
- Dehydration (not drinking enough)
- Being at high altitudes

Chronic Pain

Many adolescents and adults with SCD suffer from chronic pain. This kind of pain has been hard for people to describe, but it is usually different from crisis pain or the pain that results from organ damage.

Chronic pain can be severe and can make life difficult. Its cause is not well understood.

Severe Anemia

People with SCD usually have mild to moderate anemia. At times, however, they can have severe anemia. Severe anemia can be life threatening. Severe anemia in an infant or child with SCD may be caused by:

- **Splenic sequestration crisis.** The spleen is an organ that is located in the upper left side of the belly. The spleen filters germs in the blood, breaks up blood cells, and makes a kind of white blood cell. A splenic sequestration crisis occurs when red blood cells get stuck in the spleen, making it enlarge quickly. Since the red blood cells are trapped in the spleen, there are fewer cells to circulate in the blood. This causes severe anemia. A big spleen may also cause pain in the left side of the belly. A parent can usually palpate or feel the enlarged spleen in the belly of his or her child.

- **Aplastic crisis.** This crisis is usually caused by a parvovirus B19 infection, also called fifth disease or slapped cheek syndrome. Parvovirus B19 is a very common infection, but in SCD it can cause the bone marrow to stop producing new red cells for a while, leading to severe anemia.

Splenic sequestration crisis and aplastic crisis most commonly occur in infants and children with SCD. Adults with SCD may also experience episodes of severe anemia, but these usually have other causes.

No matter the cause, severe anemia may lead to symptoms that include:

- Shortness of breath

- Being very tired

- Feeling dizzy

- Having pale skin

Babies and infants with severe anemia may feed poorly and seem very sluggish.

Infections

The spleen is important for protection against certain kinds of germs. Sickle cells can damage the spleen and weaken or destroy its function early in life.

People with SCD who have damaged spleens are at risk for serious bacterial infections that can be life-threatening. Some of these bacteria include:

- Pneumococcus

- Hemophilus influenza type B

- Meningococcus

- Salmonella

- Staphylococcus

- Chlamydia

- *Mycoplasma pneumoniae*

Bacteria can cause:

- Blood infection (septicemia)

- Lung infection (pneumonia)

- Infection of the covering of the brain and spinal cord (meningitis)

- Bone infection (osteomyelitis)

Acute Chest Syndrome

Sickling in blood vessels of the lungs can deprive a person's lungs of oxygen. When this happens, areas of lung tissue are damaged and cannot exchange oxygen properly. This condition is known as acute chest syndrome. In acute chest syndrome, at least one segment of the lung is damaged.

This condition is very serious and should be treated right away at a hospital.

Acute chest syndrome often starts a few days after a painful crisis begins. A lung infection may accompany acute chest syndrome.

Symptoms may include:

- Chest pain

- Fever

- Shortness of breath

- Rapid breathing

- Cough

Brain Complications

Clinical stroke. A stroke occurs when blood flow is blocked to a part of the brain. When this happens, brain cells can be damaged or can die. In SCD, a clinical stroke means that a person shows outward signs that something is wrong. The symptoms depend upon what part of the brain is affected. Symptoms of stroke may include:

- Weakness of an arm or leg on one side of the body

- Trouble speaking, walking, or understanding

- Loss of balance

- Severe headache

As many as 24 percent of people with hemoglobin SS and 10 percent of people with hemoglobin SC may suffer a clinical stroke by age 45.

In children, clinical stroke occurs most commonly between the ages of 2 and 9, but recent prevention strategies have lowered the risk.

Silent stroke and thinking problems. Brain imaging and tests of thinking (cognitive studies) have shown that children and adults with hemoglobin SS and hemoglobin Sβ0 thalassemia often have signs of silent brain injury, also called silent stroke. Silent brain injury is damage to the brain without showing outward signs of stroke.

This injury is common. Silent brain injury can lead to learning problems or trouble making decisions or holding down a job.

Eye Problems

Sickle cell disease can injure blood vessels in the eye.

The most common site of damage is the retina, where blood vessels can overgrow, get blocked, or bleed. The retina is the light-sensitive layer of tissue that lines the inside of the eye and sends visual messages through the optic nerve to the brain.

Detachment of the retina can occur. When the retina detaches, it is lifted or pulled from its normal position. These problems can cause visual impairment or loss.

Heart Disease

People with SCD can have problems with blood vessels in the heart and with heart function. The heart can become enlarged. People can also develop pulmonary hypertension.

People with SCD who have received frequent blood transfusions may also have heart damage from iron overload.

Pulmonary Hypertension

In adolescents and adults, injury to blood vessels in the lungs can make it hard for the heart to pump blood through them. This causes the pressure in lung blood vessels to rise. High pressure in these blood vessels is called pulmonary hypertension. Symptoms may include shortness of breath and fatigue.

When this condition is severe, it has been associated with a higher risk of death.

Kidney Problems

The kidneys are sensitive to the effects of red blood cell sickling.

SCD causes the kidneys to have trouble making the urine as concentrated as it should be. This may lead to a need to urinate often and to have bedwetting or uncontrolled urination during the night (nocturnal enuresis). This often starts in childhood. Other problems may include:

- Blood in the urine
- Decreased kidney function
- Kidney disease
- Protein loss in the urine

Priapism

Males with SCD can have unwanted, sometimes prolonged, painful erections. This condition is called priapism.

Priapism happens when blood flow out of the erect penis is blocked by sickled cells. If it goes on for a long period of time, priapism can cause permanent damage to the penis and lead to impotence.

If priapism lasts for more than 4 hours, emergency medical care should be sought to avoid complications.

Gallstones

When red cells hemolyze, they release hemoglobin. Hemoglobin gets broken down into a substance called bilirubin. Bilirubin can form stones that get stuck in the gallbladder. The gallbladder is a small, sac-shaped organ beneath the liver that helps with digestion. Gallstones are a common problem in SCD.

Gallstones may be formed early on but may not produce symptoms for years. When symptoms develop, they may include:

- Right-sided upper belly pain
- Nausea
- Vomiting

If problems continue or recur, a person may need surgery to remove the gallbladder.

Liver Complications

There are a number of ways in which the liver may be injured in SCD.

Sickle cell intrahepatic cholestasis is an uncommon, but severe, form of liver damage that occurs when sickled red cells block blood vessels in the liver. This blockage prevents enough oxygen from reaching liver tissue.

These episodes are usually sudden and may recur. Children often recover, but some adults may have chronic problems that lead to liver failure.

People with SCD who have received frequent blood transfusions may develop liver damage from iron overload.

Leg Ulcers

Sickle cell ulcers are sores that usually start small and then get larger and larger.

The number of ulcers can vary from one to many. Some ulcers will heal quickly, but others may not heal and may last for long periods of time. Some ulcers come back after healing.

People with SCD usually don't get ulcers until after the age of 10.

Joint Complications

Sickling in the bones of the hip and, less commonly, the shoulder joints, knees, and ankles, can decrease oxygen flow and result in severe damage. This damage is a condition called avascular or aseptic necrosis. This disease is usually found in adolescents and adults.

Symptoms include pain and problems with walking and joint movement. A person may need pain medicines, surgery, or joint replacement if symptoms persist.

Delayed Growth and Puberty

Children with SCD may grow and develop more slowly than their peers because of anemia. They will reach full sexual maturity, but this may be delayed.

Pregnancy

Pregnancies in women with SCD can be risky for both the mother and the baby.

Mothers may have medical complications including:

- Infections
- Blood clots
- High blood pressure
- Increased pain episodes

They are also at higher risk for:

- Miscarriages

- Premature births

- "Small-for-dates babies" or underweight babies

Mental Health

As in other chronic diseases, people with SCD may feel sad and frustrated at times. The limitations that SCD can impose on a person's daily activities may cause them to feel isolated from others. Sometimes they become depressed.

People with SCD may also have trouble coping with pain and fatigue, as well as with frequent medical visits and hospitalizations.

How Is Sickle Cell Disease Diagnosed?

Screening Tests

People who do not know whether they make sickle hemoglobin (hemoglobin S) or other abnormal hemoglobin (such as C, β thalassemia, E) can find out by having their blood tested. This way, they can learn whether they carry a gene (i.e., have the trait) for an abnormal hemoglobin that they could pass on to a child.

When each parent has this information, he or she can be better informed about the chances of having a child with some type of sickle cell disease (SCD), such as hemoglobin SS, SC, Sβ thalassemia, or others.

Newborn Screening

When a child has SCD, it is very important to diagnose it early to better prevent complications.

Every state in the United States, the District of Columbia, and the U.S. territories require that every baby is tested for SCD as part of a newborn screening program.

In newborn screening programs, blood from a heel prick is collected in "spots" on a special paper. The hemoglobin from this blood is then analyzed in special labs.

Newborn screening results are sent to the doctor who ordered the test and to the child's primary doctor.

If a baby is found to have SCD, health providers from a special follow-up newborn screening group contact the family directly to make sure that the parents know the results. The child is always retested to be sure that the diagnosis is correct.

Newborn screening programs also find out whether the baby has an abnormal hemoglobin trait. If so, parents are informed, and counseling is offered.

Remember that when a child has sickle cell trait or SCD, a future sibling, or the child's own future child, may be at risk. These possibilities should be discussed with the primary care doctor, a blood specialist called a hematologist, and/or a genetics counselor.

Prenatal Screening

Doctors can also diagnose SCD before a baby is born. This is done using a sample of amniotic fluid, the liquid in the sac surrounding a growing embryo, or tissue taken from the placenta, the organ that attaches the umbilical cord to the mother's womb.

Testing before birth can be done as early as 8–10 weeks into the pregnancy. This testing looks for the sickle hemoglobin gene rather than the abnormal hemoglobin.

How Is Sickle Cell Disease Treated?

Hydroxyurea

What Is Hydroxyurea?

Hydroxyurea is an oral medicine that has been shown to reduce or prevent several SCD complications.

This medicine was studied in patients with SCD because it was known to increase the amount of fetal hemoglobin (hemoglobin F) in the blood. Increased hemoglobin F provides some protection against the effects of hemoglobin S.

Hydroxyurea was later found to have several other benefits for a person with SCD, such as decreasing inflammation.

- **Use in adults.** Many studies of adults with hemoglobin SS or hemoglobin Sβ thalassemia showed that hydroxyurea reduced the number of episodes of pain crises and acute chest syndrome. It also improved anemia and decreased the need for transfusions and hospital admissions.

- **Use in children.** Studies in children with severe hemoglobin SS or Sβ thalassemia showed that hydroxyurea reduced the number of vaso-occlusive crises and hospitalizations. A study of very young children (between the ages of 9 and 18 months) with hemoglobin SS or hemoglobin Sβ thalassemia also showed that hydroxyurea decreased the number of episodes of pain and dactylitis.

Who Should Use Hydroxyurea?

Since hydroxyurea can decrease several complications of SCD, most experts recommend that children and adults with hemoglobin SS or Sβ0 thalassemia who have frequent painful episodes, recurrent chest crises, or severe anemia take hydroxyurea daily.

Some experts offer hydroxyurea to all infants over 9 months of age and young children with hemoglobin SS or Sβ0 thalassemia, even if they do not have severe clinical problems, to prevent or reduce the chance of complications. There is no information about how safe or effective hydroxyurea is in children under 9 months of age.

Some experts will prescribe hydroxyurea to people with other types of SCD who have severe, recurrent pain. There is little information available about how effective hydroxyurea is for these types of SCD.

In all situations, people with SCD should discuss with their doctors whether or not hydroxyurea is an appropriate medication for them.

Pregnant women should not use hydroxyurea.

How Is Hydroxyurea Taken?

To work properly, hydroxyurea should be taken by mouth daily at the prescribed dose. When a person does not take it regularly, it will not work as well, or it won't work at all.

A person with SCD who is taking hydroxyurea needs careful monitoring. This is particularly true in the early weeks of taking the medicine. Monitoring includes regular blood testing and dose adjustments.

What Are the Risks of Hydroxyurea?

Hydroxyurea can cause the bloods' white cell count or platelet count to drop. In rare cases, it can worsen anemia. These side effects usually go away quickly if a person stops taking the medication. When a person restarts it, a doctor usually prescribes a lower dose.

Other short-term side effects are less common.

It is still unclear whether hydroxyurea can cause problems later in life in people with SCD who take it for many years. Studies so far suggest that it does not put people at a higher risk of cancer and does not affect growth in children. But further studies are needed.

Red Blood Cell Transfusions

Doctors may use acute and chronic red blood cell transfusions to treat and prevent certain SCD complications. The red blood cells in a transfusion have normal hemoglobin in them.

A transfusion helps to raise the number of red blood cells and provides normal red blood cells that are more flexible than red blood cells with sickle hemoglobin. These cells live longer in the circulation. Red blood cell transfusions decrease vaso-occlusion (blockage in the blood vessel) and improve oxygen delivery to the tissues and organs.

Acute Transfusion in SCD

Doctors use blood transfusions in SCD for complications that cause severe anemia. They may also use them when a person has an acute stroke, in many cases of acute chest crises, and in multi-organ failure.

A person with SCD usually receives blood transfusions before surgery to prevent SCD-related complications afterwards.

Chronic Transfusion

Doctors recommend regular or ongoing blood transfusions for people who have had an acute stroke, since transfusions decrease the chances of having another stroke.

Doctors also recommend chronic blood transfusions for children who have abnormal TCD ultrasound results because transfusions can reduce the chance of having a first stroke.

Some doctors use this approach to treat complications that do not improve with hydroxyurea. They may also use transfusions in people who have too many side effects from hydroxyurea.

What Are the Risks of Transfusion Therapy?

Possible complications include:

- Hemolysis
- Iron overload, particularly in people receiving chronic transfusions (can severely impair heart and lung function)
- Infection
- Alloimmunization (can make it hard to find a matching unit of blood for a future transfusion)

All blood banks and hospital personnel have adopted practices to reduce the risk of transfusion problems.

People with SCD who receive transfusions should be monitored for and immunized against hepatitis. They should also receive regular screenings for iron overload. If a person has iron overload, the doctor will give chelation therapy, a medicine to reduce the amount of iron in the body and the problems that iron overload causes.

Hematopoietic Stem Cell Transplantation

At the present time, hematopoietic stem cell transplantation (HSCT) is the only cure for SCD. People with SCD and their families should ask their doctor about this procedure.

What Are Stem Cells?

Stem cells are special cells that can divide over and over again. After they divide, these cells can go on to become blood red cells, white cells, or platelets.

A person with SCD has stem cells that make red blood cells that can sickle. People without SCD have stem cells that make red cells that usually won't sickle.

What Stem Cells Are Used in HSCT?

In HSCT, stem cells are taken from the bone marrow or blood of a person who does not have sickle cell disease (the donor). The donor, however, may have sickle cell trait.

The donor is often the person's sister or brother. This is because the safest and most successful transplants use stem cells that are matched for special proteins called HLA antigens. Since these antigens are inherited from parents, a sister or brother is the most likely person to have the same antigens as the person with SCD.

What Are the Risks?

HSCT is successful in about 85 percent of children when the donor is related and HLA matched. Even with this high success rate, HSCT still has risks.

Complications can include severe infections, seizures, and other clinical problems. About 5 percent of people have died. Sometimes transplanted cells attack the recipient's organs (graft versus host disease).

Medicines are given to prevent many of the complications, but they still can happen.

How Can Sickle Cell Disease Be Prevented?

People who do not know whether they carry an abnormal hemoglobin gene can ask their doctor to have their blood tested.

Couples who are planning to have children and know that they are at risk of having a child with sickle cell disease (SCD) may want to meet with a genetics counselor. A genetics counselor can answer questions about the risk and explain the choices that are available.

Living with Sickle Cell Disease

If you or your child has sickle cell disease (SCD), you should learn as much as you can about the disease. Your healthcare providers are there to help you, and you should feel comfortable asking questions.

Prevent and Control Complications

Avoid situations that may set off a crisis. Extreme heat or cold, as well as abrupt changes in temperature, are often triggers. When swimming, ease into the pool rather than jumping right in.

Avoid overexertion and dehydration. Take time out to rest and drink plenty of fluids.

Do not travel in an aircraft cabin that is unpressurized.

Take your medicines as your doctor prescribes. Get any medical and lab tests or immunizations that your doctor orders.

See a doctor right away if you have any of the following danger signs:

- Fever
- Stroke symptoms
- Problems breathing
- Symptoms of splenic enlargement
- Sudden loss of vision
- Symptoms of severe anemia

If your child attends daycare, preschool, or school, speak to his or her teacher about the disease. Teachers need to know what to watch for and how to accommodate your child.

Get Ongoing Care

Make and keep regular appointments with your SCD doctor or medical team. These visits will help to reduce the number of acute problems that need immediate care. Avoid seeing your doctor only when you or your child has an urgent problem that needs care right away.

Your SCD medical team can help prevent complications and improve your quality of life.

Coping with Pain

Every person experiences pain differently. Work with your doctor to develop a pain management plan that works for you. This often includes over-the-counter medicines, as well as stronger medicines that you get with a prescription.

You may find other methods that help your pain, such as:

- A heating pad
- A warm bath
- A massage
- Physical therapy
- Acupuncture
- Distracting and relaxing activities, such as listening to music, talking on the phone, or watching TV

Chapter 36

Sinus Pain

What Is Sinusitis?

Sinusitis means your sinuses are inflamed. The cause can be an infection or another problem. Your sinuses are hollow air spaces within the bones surrounding the nose. They produce mucus, which drains into the nose. If your nose is swollen, this can block the sinuses and cause pain. There are several types of sinusitis, including:

- Acute, which lasts up to 4 weeks

- Subacute, which lasts 4 to 12 weeks

- Chronic, which lasts more than 12 weeks and can continue for months or even years

- Recurrent, with several attacks within a year

Acute sinusitis often starts as a cold, which then turns into a bacterial infection. Allergies, nasal problems, and certain diseases can also cause acute and chronic sinusitis.

This chapter contains text excerpted from the following sources: Text under the heading "What Is Sinusitis?" is excerpted from "Sinusitis," U.S. National Library of Medicine (NLM), National Institutes of Health (NIH), January 26, 2017; Text beginning with the heading "Causes" is excerpted from "Sinus Infection (Sinusitis)," Centers for Disease Control and Prevention (CDC), April 17, 2015; Text under the heading "Alternative Approach To Chronic Sinusitis" is excerpted from "Is Rinsing Your Sinuses with Neti Pots Safe?" Centers for Disease Control and Prevention (CDC), January 24, 2017.

Causes

Sinus infections occur when fluid is trapped or blocked in the sinuses, allowing germs to grow. Sinus infections are usually (9 out of 10 cases in adults; 5-7 out of 10 cases in children) caused by a virus. They are less commonly (1 out of 10 cases in adults; 3-5 out of 10 cases in children) caused by bacteria.

Other conditions can cause symptoms similar to a sinus infection, including:

- Allergies
- Pollutants (airborne chemicals or irritants)
- Fungal infections

Risk Factors

Several conditions can increase your risk of getting a sinus infection:

- A previous respiratory tract infection, such as the common cold
- Structural problems within the sinuses
- A weak immune system or taking drugs that weaken the immune system
- Nasal polyps
- Allergies

In children, the following are also risk factors for a sinus infection:

- Going to daycare
- Using a pacifier
- Drinking a bottle while laying down
- Being exposed to secondhand smoke

Signs and Symptoms

Common signs and symptoms of a sinus infection include:

- Headache
- Stuffy or runny nose
- Loss of the sense of smell
- Facial pain or pressure

- Postnasal drip (mucus drips down the throat from the nose)
- Sore throat
- Fever
- Coughing
- Fatigue (being tired)
- Bad breath

When to Seek Medical Care

See a healthcare professional if you or your child has any of the following:

- Temperature higher than 100.4 °F
- Symptoms that are getting worse or lasting more than 10 days
- Multiple sinus infections in the past year
- Symptoms that are not relieved with over-the-counter medicines
- You may have chronic sinusitis if your sinus infection lasts more than 8 weeks or if you have more than 4 sinus infections each year. If you are diagnosed with chronic sinusitis, or believe you may have chronic sinusitis, you should visit your healthcare professional for evaluation. Chronic sinusitis can be caused by nasal growths, allergies, or respiratory tract infections (viral, bacterial, or fungal).

Diagnosis and Treatment

Your healthcare professional will determine if you or your child has a sinus infection by asking about symptoms and doing a physical examination. Sometimes they will also swab the inside of your nose.

Antibiotics may be needed if the sinus infection is likely to be caused by bacteria. Antibiotics will not help a sinus infection caused by a virus or an irritation in the air (like secondhand smoke). These infections will almost always get better on their own. Antibiotic treatment in these cases may even cause harm in both children and adults.

If symptoms continue for more than 10 days, schedule a follow-up appointment with your healthcare professional for re-evaluation.

Symptom Relief

Rest, over-the-counter medicines and other self-care methods may help you or your child feel better. For more information about symptomatic relief, talk to your healthcare professional, including your pharmacist. Always use over-the-counter products as directed since many over-the-counter products are not recommended for children of certain ages.

Prevention

There are several steps you can take to help prevent a sinus infection, including:

- Practice good hand hygiene

- Keep you and your child up to date with recommended immunizations

- Avoid close contact with people who have colds or other upper respiratory infections

- Avoid smoking and exposure to secondhand smoke

- Use a clean humidifier to moisten the air at home

Alternative Approach to Chronic Sinusitis

Little teapots with long spouts have become a fixture in many homes to flush out clogged nasal passages and help people breathe easier. Along with other nasal irrigation systems, these devices—commonly called neti pots—use a saline, or saltwater, solution to treat congested sinuses, colds and allergies. They're also used to moisten nasal passages exposed to dry indoor air. But be careful. According to the U.S. Food and Drug Administration (FDA), improper use of these neti pots and other nasal rinsing devices can increase your risk of infection. These nasal rinse devices—which include bulb syringes, squeeze bottles, and battery-operated pulsed water devices—are usually safe and effective products when used and cleaned properly, says Eric A. Mann, MD, PhD, a doctor at FDA.

Sinus rinsing can remove dust, pollen and other debris, as well as help to loosen thick mucus. It can also help relieve nasal symptoms of sinus infections, allergies, colds and flu. Plain water can irritate your nose. The saline allows the water to pass through delicate nasal membranes with little or no burning or irritation.

Tap water isn't safe for use as a nasal rinse because it's not adequately filtered or treated. Some tap water contains low levels of organisms—such as bacteria and protozoa, including amoebas—that may be safe to swallow because stomach acid kills them. But in your nose, these organisms can stay alive in nasal passages and cause potentially serious infections. They can even be fatal in some rare cases, according to the Centers for Disease Control and Prevention (CDC).

What Types of Water Are Safe to Use?

- Distilled or sterile water, which you can buy in stores. The label will state "distilled" or "sterile."

- Boiled and cooled tap water—boiled for 3 to 5 minutes, then cooled until it is lukewarm. Previously boiled water can be stored in a clean, closed container for use within 24 hours.

- Water passed through a filter designed to trap potentially infectious organisms.

Chapter 37

Somatoform Pain Disorder

A somatoform disorder is a physical disorder in which medical professionals can identify no physiological causes and psychological factors are instead thought to be involved. Patients experience physical symptoms but not as a consequence of a medical condition or due to the effect of a substance or drug. Somatoform pain disorder is one among many somatoform disorders described in the *Diagnostic and Statistical Manual for Mental Disorders, Fourth Edition, Text Revision* (DSM-IV-TR). The pain in somatoform pain disorders is very real and not feigned by patients. Psychological causes play a very import role in the onset, severity, worsening, or maintenance of pain.

How Is Somatoform Pain Disorder Diagnosed?

Somatoform pain disorder is diagnosed after a thorough physical examination and testing have ruled out any physical cause of pain that is severe enough to disrupt daily life and relationships of the patient.

What Are the Common Symptoms Exhibited?

Somatoform pain disorder affects people of all ages. The major symptom of somatoform pain disorder is chronic pain that lasts for months leading to inability in carrying on everyday life in terms of work, mundane tasks, and relationships. Other symptoms include:

- Pain that requires medical intervention

"Somatoform Pain Disorder," © 2017 Omnigraphics. Reviewed June 2017.

- Worry and stress because of pain

- Insomnia, fatigue, and related problems

- Depression and anxiety

- Negative feelings such as helplessness and hopelessness

- Compromised relationships at home, work, and school

- Long periods of inactivity

What Are the Causes of Somatoform Pain Disorder?

The actual cause of somatoform pain disorders remains unknown but researchers believe psychological distress is a major contributing factor. Patients may also have an anxiety disorder. Victims of physical and sexual abuse are more likely to be diagnosed with somatoform pain disorders; though not all individuals with somatoform pain disorder have such a history. Researchers have also begun to study links between emotional well-being and how the brain perceives pain.

What Are the Medical Tests That Are Prescribed during Diagnosis?

Diagnostic scans such as magnetic resonance imaging (MRI), computed tomography (CT), Ultrasound, X-rays are prescribed to rule out physical and anatomical causes that may be causing pain. An array of lab tests may also be ordered for the same reason.

What Is the Treatment for Somatoform Pain Disorder?

Medical professionals generally treat somatoform pain disorder with a combination of antidepressants and talk therapy. Pain medication is not prescribed since it has little to no effect and can potentially become habit forming. Before treatment can begin, patients must also accept the diagnosis, and in some cases he or she may resist the idea that pain being experienced is caused by psychological and not physical causes. Cognitive behavior therapy (CBT) is a type of talk therapy that helps patients deal with pain following a process of identifying what kind of thoughts lead to the experience of physical pain how to handle them effectively. Classes of psychiatric medication such as selective serotonin reuptake inhibitors (SSRIs), serotonin–norepinephrine reuptake inhibitors (SNRIs), and tricyclic antidepressants are used in conjunction with talk therapy to help ease the pain.

Additional treatment options include the following:

- Acupuncture
- Exercise
- Hypnotherapy
- Massage therapy
- Medication
- Music therapy
- Yoga

What Is the Prognosis for Somatoform Pain Disorder?

In the case of acute pain, the prognosis for remission is good but as promising for chronic pain. The chances for remission are good if the patient is employed and continues to work and follows a treatment regimen of cognitive behavior therapy and antidepressants.

References

1. "Somatoform Pain Disorder," University of Maryland Medical Center (UMMC), 2017.

2. "Pain Disorder," Advameg, Inc., 2017.

3. "Pain Disorder," Internet Brands, Inc., 2017.

4. Protagoras-Lianos, Dolores. "Pain Somatoform Disorder," Medscape, Oct 4, 2013.

Chapter 38

Stroke and Pain

Pain is common after a stroke. Pain means that the body is hurt or something is wrong. Every stroke survivor's pain is different. The pain may be mild or severe. It may last for a short time or be constant.

What Do You Need to Know?

Pain after a stroke is caused by many things. Your loved one can have one or more types of pain. The key is to find the cause of the pain so it can be treated.

Local Pain

Local pain results from physical problems. After a part of the body is paralyzed (unable to move) or weakened, the muscles may become tight and stiff. These changes in the muscles can cause pain. This pain is often felt in the joints, most often in the shoulders. Your loved one may also have sore muscles from learning new ways to walk or move. Pain may be caused by lying or sitting in one place too long. Other common causes are pressure sores or painful leg cramps at night.

Central Pain

Central pain is a direct result of damage to the brain from the stroke. Sensations like light touch are felt as pain when they should not be painful. This pain is described as burning or aching. The pain is usually on the side of the body affected by the stroke. It is often

---

This chapter includes text excerpted from "Pain after Stroke," U.S. Department of Veterans Affairs (VA), May 10, 2011. Reviewed June 2017.

constant and may get worse over time. Changes in cold and hot temperatures may increase the pain. Movement or touching may increase the pain.

Why Is It Important to Get Help?

Talk to the healthcare team about your loved one's pain. Pain often leads to other problems. For instance, pain can cause depression and loss of sleep. Your loved one may stop moving a painful part of the body. Over time, the joint of this body part may "lock up" and your loved one will lose movement.

What Treatments Should You Discuss with Your Healthcare Team?

Pain usually lessens with treatment. There are many treatments to ask about.

Pain Medicines

Pain medicines are one of the most important treatments. Use pain medicines that your healthcare team suggests. Follow the directions on the label of the medicine. Give pain medicines on a regular basis. Do not wait until the pain gets bad to give pain medicines. Do not stop using medicines for fear of addiction. When pain medicines are used correctly, they do not cause addiction.

Over-the-counter (OTC) pain medicines, like Tylenol®** or Advil®** relieve mild pain. These OTC medicines may interact with other medicines your loved one takes. Check with your healthcare team before taking any OTC medicines. For more severe pain, stronger prescription pain medicines like narcotics are often needed.

Medicines used to treat depression, spasticity (tightness and stiffness of muscles) or seizures may relieve central pain. Shots or injections of cortisone (steroids) into joints like the shoulder may help.

Exercises

Exercises to strengthen muscles can help your loved one move better. For example, stretching exercises decrease the tightness and soreness of the muscles. Talk with a physical therapist about the best exercise plan.

Heat Therapy

Heat therapy like heating pads and warm baths may soothe sore muscles and stiff joints.

Electrical Nerve Stimulation

Electrical nerve stimulation (often called TENS or TNS) improves the strength of the muscles and often reduces pain. Patches or electrodes are placed on the skin. A mild electrical current runs through these patches. This is not painful.

Complementary or Alternative Therapies

Complementary or alternative therapies like acupuncture, massage therapy, and yoga often relieve pain.

What if the Pain Continues?

Everyone has the right to good pain control. Ask your healthcare team to try different treatments to relieve the pain. If the pain continues, ask about other types of care.

- Pain clinics are helpful for people whose pain is difficult to treat. Ask about pain clinics in your area.

- Psychologists help stroke survivors find ways to live with pain that cannot be completely relieved. Psychologists also help survivors who are sad or depressed due to living with pain.

How Can You Help Your Loved One Describe the Pain?

Your healthcare team needs to know how your loved one feels. Ask your loved one to rate the pain. Use a pain scale of "0-10," with "0" being no pain and "10" being the worst pain your loved one has ever felt. If your loved one can't speak, use a pain scale.

Take note of where your loved one hurts. What things bring on the pain? What makes it worse? When does the pain occur? How does it feel? Report these symptoms to your healthcare team.

Remember that some stroke survivors have trouble speaking. Watch for signs of pain such as moaning or changes in behaviors. Some stroke survivors may not feel pain. They may not know when they are cut or burned by hot water. Watch for sores and other injuries.

Talk with Your Loved One About the Pain

- Pain almost always is a real problem. Believe your loved one's complaints.

- Allow time for your loved one to talk about the pain.

- Talk about feelings of sadness related to the pain. Watch for signs of depression. Report problems to your healthcare team. Learn more about depression after stroke.

Helpful Tips

- Help your loved one remain active to keep muscles strong and reduce pain.

- Talk with your healthcare team about correct ways to exercise. Also ask about how best to position paralyzed or weak arms and legs. Splints or other devices may be helpful.

- Support a weak or paralyzed arm to reduce pain in the shoulder. Ask your healthcare team about using an arm sling. Provide support for the arm on a lapboard or raised armrest. Use pillows while lying in bed.

- Have your loved one wear loose, comfortable clothing.

- Help your loved one relax. Find an activity that your loved one enjoys such as playing with the dog or watching television. Suggest activities like listening to music, reading a book, prayer or meditation.

- Use warm baths, showers, warm washcloths or heating pads. Be sure to check the temperature so as not to cause burns. Cool cloths and ice may also help. Talk with your healthcare team about the best plan.

Remember

- Pain is almost always a real problem. Believe your loved one. Get help for any signs or problems of pain.

- Pain can cause other problems like depression and loss of sleep.

- Treatment is based on what is causing the pain. Ask about the pain. Help your loved one describe the pain to the healthcare team.

- Everyone has the right to good pain control. Ask for different treatments if the pain is not relieved.

Chapter 39

Surgical Pain

Chapter Contents

Section 39.1

What You Need to Know about Pain Control during and after Surgery

This section contains text excerpted from the following
sources: Text in this section begins with excerpts from "Managing
Pain from a Broken Hip: A Guide for Adults and Their Caregivers,"
Agency for Healthcare Research and Quality (AHRQ), U.S.
Department of Health and Human Services (HHS), May 17, 2011.
Reviewed June 2017; Text beginning with the heading "What
to Expect after Surgery" is excerpted from "Tips for Decreasing
Pain Medications after Surgery," U.S. Department of Veterans
Affairs (VA), July 3, 2016.

The amount of pain and type of pain can change during your treatment. For example, the pain can be different before and after an operation, during rehabilitation, and after you come home from the hospital.

Uncontrolled pain can also interfere with treatments for your other medical conditions. Pain can also slow down your physical therapy and recovery. Your doctor, nurse, or physical therapist will ask you about your pain. They may ask you to rate your pain so that they can see if treatment is helping. It is important to let them know if you are still in pain.

If you are caring for someone who has difficulty thinking or expressing thoughts (called "dementia"), he or she may not be able to tell you about the pain. It is still important that the pain is managed.

Understanding Your Choices

Usual Care for Pain

Your doctor may give you medicines to treat the pain before or after an operation. Some of these include:

- **Acetaminophen.** This non-aspirin pain medicine is often used for many types of pain, such as body aches and headaches. It usually is not strong enough by itself to relieve the pain.

- **Opioid analgesics.** Some common names for these drugs are morphine, codeine, and oxycodone. You may get these medicines as a pill, a shot, or through a tube in your arm (called an "IV").

Common side effects of opioid analgesics include:

- Nausea, vomiting, and constipation.
- Sleepiness and confusion.
- Itchiness.

Nonsteroidal anti-inflammatory drugs or NSAIDs. Some common names for these drugs are ibuprofen and naproxen. These medicines come as a pill or a liquid.
Some of the common side effects of NSAIDs include:

- Dizziness.
- Nausea.
- Diarrhea.
- Excess gas.
- Irritation and bleeding of the stomach and intestines.

Be sure to tell your doctor if you experience any of these side effects. Your doctor may give you medicines to help.

Additional Ways to Reduce Pain

Researchers have studied other ways to manage pain. These other treatments include:

- Nerve blocks.
- Acupressure.
- Muscle-relaxation therapy.
- Neurostimulation.

Nerve blocks

What is a nerve block?
A nerve block uses a medicine called an "anesthetic" to numb the nerves so that you do not feel pain for a little while. Anesthetics are

the same kind of medicine dentists use to numb teeth and gums. The nerve block will make a part of your body numb for a little while.

Your doctor might use a nerve block to help ease your pain if you cannot take medicines like NSAIDs or opioids. Nerve blocks may be used before, during, or after an operation.

There are many types of nerve blocks. They are named for the part of the body where the doctor injects the anesthetic. Your doctor (or anesthesiologist or nurse anesthetist) may inject these medicines into more than one place in your body to give you the most pain relief. For a broken hip, injections are often given around the hip and groin area.

What are the benefits of using a nerve block?

Some research shows that nerve blocks used before, during, or after an operation may ease short-term pain more than the usual treatment of opioid or NSAID pain medication. Nerve blocks may help you avoid "delirium," or confusion and cloudy thinking, which can be caused by pain or by opioid pain medicines.

Are there any side effects from using a nerve block?

Researchers cannot say if nerve blocks cause more or less side effects than other treatments for the pain from a broken hip.

Traction

Traction is a treatment where a part of the body is pulled into a certain position. Traction is usually used before an operation.

There have been only a few studies on traction. They show that traction before an operation does not help relieve pain more than using pain medicines alone, but there is not enough research to know for sure.

Traction may be needed for reasons other than pain.

It is not known if using both traction and medicines for pain increases your risks of serious side effects compared to taking only medicines.

Acupressure, Muscle-Relaxation Therapy, and Neurostimulation (TENS)

Although some studies show that these methods might help, there is not enough research to say if these options can lessen pain. These therapies can be used before or after an operation.

What is acupressure?

"Acupressure" is when a trained therapist presses on specific parts of the body to relieve pain in other body parts.

What is muscle-relaxation therapy?

"Muscle-relaxation therapy" involves breathing and relaxation routines to reduce muscle tension.

What is neurostimulation?

"Neurostimulation," also known as "TENS," involves giving small amounts of electricity to excite the nerves around the painful area.

Will acupressure, muscle-relaxation therapy, or TENS help relieve my pain?

Doctors do not know if the pain will be improved or relieved by acupressure, relaxation therapy, or TENS more than by medicines like opioid and NSAID medicines.

What are the risks of acupressure, muscle-relaxation therapy, and TENS?

There is not enough research to say if these options have any risks or can cause any side effects for people.

Making a Decision

Ask your doctor:

- Which options do you think are best to manage my pain?
- How quickly can I expect relief from my pain?
- How long do you think I will need to manage my pain?
- Are you concerned about side effects from any of these options?

What to Expect after Surgery

You may be taking a prescription medication for your pain. The medication is often also called a narcotic or opioid and is different from pain medications like Tylenol© or Advil©. As your body heals, pain will decrease. Decrease (wean) the amount of pain pills you take until you're not taking any. This guideline instructs how to decrease your medication given to you after your surgery.

If you were taking medication before surgery, continue taking that as prescribed by your provider.

Important Tips

- Opioids can lead to addiction if you don't manage them carefully. It's important to gradually stop taking them over several weeks or days.

- You may have to accept some amount of pain in order to wean off the meds.

- DO NOT stop taking the pain medication all at once.

- DO slowly decrease the amount you take until you're not taking any.

How do I Control the Pain?

As you slowly decrease your opioid pain meds, you can control your pain other ways:

- Tylenol © Acetaminophen)

- Advil © (Ibuprofen)

- Ice and/or heat

Ask your doctor before taking any medications!

To Wean off Medication Given for Surgery

There are 2 parts:

1. **Increase the Amount of Time between Doses**

    For example, if you are taking a pain med every 4 hours, stretch the time between doses:

    - Take same dose every 5–6 hours for 5–7 days.

    - Then, take same dose every 7–8 hours for 5–7 days.

2. **Decrease the Dose**

    - For example, if you are taking 2 pills at a time, start taking 1 pill each time for 5–7 days.

    - If taking 1 pill each time, cut pill in half and only take a half each dose for 5–7 days.

    - Then, try to stop taking the medication completely.

What Happens If I Stop Suddenly?

If you stop taking opioid pain meds suddenly, you may have symptoms of withdrawal 6–24 hours later, which can include:

- Shaking
- Fever/sweating for no reason
- Nausea (wanting to throw up)
- Vomiting (throwing up)
- Diarrhea
- More pain
- Feeling worried
- Feeling irritable
- Trouble sleeping or very tired

Symptoms often resolve in 1–2 days. However, call your healthcare provider if you are concerned!

Section 39.2

Codeine and Tramadol Can Cause Breathing Problems for Children

This section includes text excerpted from "Codeine and Tramadol Can Cause Breathing Problems for Children," U.S. Food and Drug Administration (FDA), April 20, 2017.

Codeine and tramadol are opioid medicines that may be used to treat pain. Codeine is also in some cough and cold remedies.

These medicines can cause life-threatening breathing problems in children. Some children and adults break down codeine and tramadol into their active forms faster than other people. That can cause the level of opioids in these people to rise too high and too quickly.

Nursing mothers who are taking codeine or tramadol can pass unsafe levels of opioids to their babies through breast milk. Those infants can become too sleepy, have difficulty breastfeeding, or have serious breathing problems.

That's why the U.S. Food and Drug Administration (FDA) is strengthening drug labels for codeine and tramadol to protect children and nursing babies.

Beware of Giving Kids Codeine or Tramadol

The FDA is warning that children younger than 12 shouldn't take codeine products to treat pain or cough or tramadol to treat pain.

The FDA hasn't approved tramadol for use in children. Kids younger than 18 shouldn't take tramadol to treat pain after surgery to remove the tonsils (tonsillectomy) or adenoids (adenoidectomy). (Codeine labeling already warns that children should not be treated for post-surgery pain with codeine in these cases.)

Youths ages 12 through 18 who are obese or have obstructive sleep apnea (blocked airflow during sleep) or a weakened respiratory system shouldn't take codeine or tramadol. These risk factors can increase their chances of serious breathing problems.

Tramadol is available only for adults and by prescription to treat pain. Codeine products are available by prescription and, in some states, over-the-counter (OTC). Codeine is often combined with acetaminophen in prescription pain medicines and with other cold medicines for treatment of cough.

Alternatives to Codeine and Tramadol

There are several alternatives for pain management in children, which you should discuss with your healthcare professional or pharmacist.

There are also alternative OTC and prescription medications available for cough. The FDA doesn't recommend OTC cold and cough medicines for children younger than 2. Even in older children who have colds, coughs are generally mild and go away in a few days, so they may not need to take any medicine.

How to Know If Your Child's Medicine Has Codeine or Tramadol

Read the label to make sure the medicine doesn't have codeine or tramadol. Also, ask your healthcare provider or pharmacist if your medicine has codeine or tramadol.

Chapter 40

Urological Pain

Chapter Contents

Section 40.1

Interstitial Cystitis
(Painful Bladder Syndrome)

This section includes text excerpted from "Interstitial Cystitis
(Painful Bladder Syndrome)," National Institute of Diabetes and
Digestive and Kidney Diseases (NIDDK), January 2017.

Definition and Facts

What Is Interstitial Cystitis (IC)?

Interstitial cystitis (IC), also called bladder pain syndrome, is a
chronic, or long-lasting, condition that causes painful urinary symptoms. Symptoms of IC may be different from person to person. For
example, some people feel mild discomfort, pressure, or tenderness in
the pelvic area. Other people may have intense pain in the bladder
or struggle with urinary urgency, the sudden need to urinate, or frequency, the need to urinate more often.

Healthcare professionals diagnose IC by ruling out other conditions
with similar symptoms.

Researchers don't know the exact cause of IC. Some researchers
believe IC may result from conditions that cause inflammation in
various organs and parts of the body.

Severe IC symptoms can affect your quality of life. You may feel
like you can't exercise or leave your home because you have to use the
bathroom too often, or perhaps your relationship is suffering because
sex is painful.

Working with healthcare professionals, including a urologist or
urogynecologist, along with a pain specialist, may help improve your
IC symptoms.

How Common Is IC?

IC is common. The condition may affect between 3 million and 8
million women and between 1 million and 4 million men in the United
States.

Who Is More Likely to Develop IC?

IC can occur at any age, including during childhood, but is most common in adult women and men. About twice as many women are affected as men. However, more men may struggle with IC than researchers originally thought.

Some research suggests that women are more likely to develop IC if they have a history of being sexually abused or physically traumatized.

What Other Health Problems Do People with IC Have?

Many women with IC are more likely to have other conditions such as irritable bowel syndrome, fibromyalgia, and chronic fatigue syndrome. Allergies and some autoimmune diseases are also associated with IC.

Vulvodynia, which is chronic pain in the vulva that often causes a burning or stinging feeling, or rawness, is commonly associated with IC. Vulvodynia has symptoms that overlap with IC.

What Are the Complications of IC?

The symptoms of IC—such as urgency, frequency, and pain—may lead you to decrease your physical and social activity and negatively affect your quality of life.

Women with pelvic pain or vulvodynia often have pain during sexual intercourse, which can damage your relationships and self-image. Men also can experience pelvic pain that causes uncomfortable or painful sex. Sometimes sex can increase bladder pain attacks, also called symptom flares.

Sexual complications may cause people to avoid further intimacy, possibly leading to depression and guilt. Like many people who deal with chronic pain, people with IC are more likely to struggle with sleep loss due to the frequent need to urinate, and with anxiety and depression.

Medical tests such as pelvic exams and Pap tests often are painful for women with IC symptoms, especially those who may have pelvic floor muscle spasm. Don't avoid these tests. Talk with a healthcare professional about how to make pelvic exams and Pap tests more comfortable and how often you should have them.

Symptoms and Causes

What Are the Symptoms of IC?

People with interstitial cystitis (IC) have repeat discomfort, pressure, tenderness or pain in the bladder, lower abdomen, and pelvic area. Symptoms vary from person to person, may be mild or severe, and can even change in each person as time goes on.

Symptoms may include a combination of these symptoms:

Urgency

Urgency is the feeling that you need to urinate right now. A strong urge is normal if you haven't urinated for a few hours or if you have been drinking a lot of liquids. With IC, you may feel pain or burning along with an urgent need to urinate before your bladder has had time to fill.

Frequency

Frequency is urinating more often than you think you should need to, given the amount of liquid you are drinking. Most people urinate between four and seven times a day. Drinking large amounts of liquid can cause more frequent urinating. Taking blood pressure medicines called diuretics, or water pills, can also cause more frequent urinating. Some people with IC feel a strong, painful urge to urinate many times a day.

Pain

As your bladder starts to fill, you may feel pain—rather than just discomfort—that gets worse until you urinate. The pain usually improves for a while once you empty your bladder. People with IC rarely have constant bladder pain. The pain may go away for weeks or months and then return. People with IC sometimes refer to an attack of bladder pain as a symptom flare.

Some people may have pain without urgency or frequency. This pain may come from a spasm in the pelvic floor muscles, the group of muscles that is attached to your pelvic bones and supports your bladder, bowel, and uterus or prostate. Pain from pelvic floor muscle spasm may get worse during sex.

What Causes IC?

Researchers don't know the exact cause of IC. Researchers are working to understand the causes of IC and to find effective treatments.

Diagnosis

How Do Healthcare Professionals Diagnose IC?

Healthcare professionals will use your medical history, a physical exam, and lab tests to diagnose IC.

A healthcare professional will ask if you have a history of health problems related to IC. He or she will ask questions about your symptoms and other questions to help find the cause of your bladder problems.

If you are a woman who has IC symptoms, a healthcare professional may also perform a pelvic exam. During the pelvic exam, the healthcare professional will check your pelvic floor muscles to see if any of your painful symptoms are related to spasm in your pelvic floor muscles.

For men, a healthcare professional may perform a digital rectal exam to check for prostate problems and to check your pelvic floor muscles.

Doctors diagnose IC based on:

- pain in or near the bladder, usually with urinary frequency and urgency

- the absence of other diseases and conditions that could cause similar symptoms, such as urinary tract infections (UTIs), bladder cancer, endometriosis in women, or prostatitis—infection or inflammation of the prostate—in men.

What Tests Do Doctors Use to Diagnose IC?

A healthcare professional may use the following tests to look inside your urethra and bladder, and may even take a tissue sample from inside your bladder. The healthcare professional will use tests to rule out certain diseases and conditions, such as UTI and bladder cancer. If the test results are normal and all other diseases and conditions are ruled out, your doctor may diagnose IC.

- Urinalysis and Urine Culture

- Cystoscopy

Treatment

How Do Doctors Treat IC?

Researchers have not found one treatment for interstitial cystitis (IC) that works for everyone. Doctors aim current treatments at relieving symptoms in each person on an individual basis.

A healthcare professional will work with you to find a treatment plan that meets your needs. Your plan may include:

- lifestyle changes
  - Change your eating habits

- Quit smoking
- Reduce stress
- Be physically active
- Get support
- bladder training
- physical therapy
- medicines
  - acetaminophen (Tylenol)
  - aspirin (Bayer)
  - ibuprofen (Advil, Motrin)
  - pentosan polysulfate (Elmiron)
  - tricyclic antidepressants or antihistamines
  - botulinum toxin A (Botox) injections into your detrusor muscle
  - cyclosporine
- bladder procedures
  - Bladder instillation
  - Bladder stretching
- Surgery
  - Bladder augmentation
  - Bladder removal
  - Urinary diversion

Some treatments may work better for you than others. You also may need to use a combination of these treatments to relieve your symptoms.

A healthcare professional may ask you to fill out a form, called a symptom scale, with questions about how you feel. The symptom scale may allow a healthcare professional to better understand how you are responding to treatment.

You may have to try several different treatments before you find one that works for you. Your symptoms may disappear with treatment, a change in what you eat, or without a clear reason. Even when your symptoms go away, they may return after days, weeks, months, or even years. Researchers do not know why. With time, you and your doctor should be able to find a treatment that gives you some relief and helps you cope with IC.

Eating, Diet, and Nutrition

Can What I Eat or Drink Relieve or Prevent IC?

No research consistently links certain foods or drinks to IC. However, some research strongly suggests a relationship between diet and symptoms. Healthy eating and staying hydrated are important for your overall health, including bladder health.

Some people with IC find that certain foods or drinks trigger or worsen their symptoms, such as alcohol, tomatoes, spices, chocolate, caffeinated and citrus beverages, and high-acid foods. Some people also note that their symptoms get worse after eating or drinking products with artificial sweeteners, or sweeteners that are not found naturally in foods and beverages.

Learning which foods trigger or worsen symptoms may take some effort. Keep a food diary and note the times you have bladder pain. For example, the diary might reveal that your symptom flares always happen after you eat tomatoes or oranges.

Stopping certain foods and drinks—and then adding them back to what you normally eat and drink one at a time—may help you figure out which foods or drinks, if any, affect your symptoms. Talk with your healthcare professional about how much liquid you should drink to prevent dehydration based on your health, how active you are, and where you live. Water is the best liquid for bladder health.

Some doctors recommend taking an antacid with meals. This medicine reduces the amount of acid that gets into the urine.

Section 40.2

Kidney Stones

This section includes text excerpted from "Kidney Stones,"
National Institute of Diabetes and Digestive and Kidney
Diseases (NIDDK), September 2016.

Definition and Facts

What Are Kidney Stones?

Kidney stones are hard, pebble-like pieces of material that form in one or both of your kidneys when high levels of certain minerals are in your urine. Kidney stones rarely cause permanent damage if treated by a healthcare professional.

Kidney stones vary in size and shape. They may be as small as a grain of sand or as large as a pea. Rarely, some kidney stones are as big as golf balls. Kidney stones may be smooth or jagged and are usually yellow or brown.

A small kidney stone may pass through your urinary tract on its own, causing little or no pain. A larger kidney stone may get stuck along the way. A kidney stone that gets stuck can block your flow of urine, causing severe pain or bleeding.

If you have symptoms of kidney stones, including severe pain or bleeding, seek care right away. A doctor, such as a urologist, can treat any pain and prevent further problems, such as a urinary tract infection (UTI).

Do Kidney Stones Have Another Name?

The scientific name for a kidney stone is renal calculus or nephrolith. You may hear healthcare professionals call this condition nephrolithiasis or urolithiasis.

What Type of Kidney Stones Do I Have?

You probably have one of four main types of kidney stones. Treatment for kidney stones usually depends on their size, location, and what they are made of.

Calcium Stones

Calcium stones, including calcium oxalate stones and calcium phosphate stones, are the most common types of kidney stones. Calcium oxalate stones are more common than calcium phosphate stones.

Calcium from food does not increase your chance of having calcium oxalate stones. Normally, extra calcium that isn't used by your bones and muscles goes to your kidneys and is flushed out with urine. When this doesn't happen, the calcium stays in the kidneys and joins with other waste products to form a kidney stone.

Uric Acid Stones

A uric acid stone may form when your urine contains too much acid. Eating a lot of fish, shellfish, and meat—especially organ meat—may increase uric acid in urine.

Struvite Stones

Struvite stones may form after you have a UTI. They can develop suddenly and become large quickly.

Cystine Stones

Cystine stones result from a disorder called cystinuria that is passed down through families. Cystinuria causes the amino acid cystine to leak through your kidneys and into the urine.

How Common Are Kidney Stones?

Kidney stones are common and are on the rise. About 11 percent of men and 6 percent of women in the United States have kidney stones at least once during their lifetime.

Who Is More Likely to Develop Kidney Stones?

Men are more likely to develop kidney stones than women. If you have a family history of kidney stones, you are more likely to develop them. You are also more likely to develop kidney stones again if you've had them once.

You may also be more likely to develop a kidney stone if you don't drink enough liquids.

People with Certain Conditions

You are more likely to develop kidney stones if you have certain conditions, including:

- a blockage of the urinary tract

- chronic, or long-lasting, inflammation of the bowel

- cystic kidney diseases, which are disorders that cause fluid-filled sacs to form on the kidneys

- cystinuria

- digestive problems or a history of gastrointestinal tract surgery

- gout, a disorder that causes painful swelling of the joints

- hypercalciuria, a condition that runs in families in which urine contains unusually large amounts of calcium; this is the most common condition found in people who form calcium stones

- hyperoxaluria, a condition in which urine contains unusually large amounts of oxalate

- hyperparathyroidism, a condition in which the parathyroid glands release too much parathyroid hormone, causing extra calcium in the blood

- hyperuricosuria, a disorder in which too much uric acid is in the urine

- obesity

- repeated, or recurrent, UTIs

- renal tubular acidosis, a disease that occurs when the kidneys fail to remove acids into the urine, which causes a person's blood to remain too acidic

People Who Take Certain Medicines

You are more likely to develop kidney stones if you are taking one or more of the following medicines over a long period of time:

- diuretics, often called water pills, which help rid your body of water

- calcium-based antacids

- indinavir, a protease inhibitor used to treat human immunodeficiency virus (HIV) infection

- topiramate, an antiseizure medication

What Are the Complications of Kidney Stones?

Complications of kidney stones are rare if you seek treatment from a healthcare professional before problems occur.

If kidney stones are not treated, they can cause:

- hematuria, or blood in the urine

- severe pain

- UTIs, including kidney infections

- loss of kidney function

Symptoms and Causes

What Are the Symptoms of Kidney Stones?

Symptoms of kidney stones include:

- sharp pains in your back, side, lower abdomen, or groin

- pink, red, or brown blood in your urine, also called hematuria

- a constant need to urinate

- pain while urinating

- inability to urinate or can only urinate a small amount

- cloudy or bad-smelling urine

See a healthcare professional right away if you have any of these symptoms. These symptoms may mean you have a kidney stone or a more serious condition.

Your pain may last for a short or long time or may come and go in waves. Along with pain, you may have:

- nausea

- vomiting

Other symptoms include:

- fever

- chills

What Causes Kidney Stones?

Kidney stones are caused by high levels of calcium, oxalate, and phosphorus in the urine. These minerals are normally found in urine and do not cause problems at low levels.

Certain foods may increase the chances of having a kidney stone in people who are more likely to develop them.

What Causes Kidney Stones?

Diagnosis

How Do Healthcare Professionals Diagnose Kidney Stones?

Healthcare professionals use your medical history, a physical exam, and lab and imaging tests to diagnose kidney stones.

A healthcare professional will ask if you have a history of health conditions that make you more likely to develop kidney stones. The healthcare professional also may ask if you have a family history of kidney stones and about what you typically eat. During a physical exam, the healthcare professional usually examines your body. The healthcare professional will ask you about your symptoms.

What Tests Do healthcare Professionals Use to Diagnose Kidney Stones?

Healthcare professionals may use lab or imaging tests to diagnose kidney stones.

- Lab Tests
  - Urinalysis
  - Blood tests
- Imaging Tests
  - Abdominal X-ray
  - Computed tomography (CT) scans

Treatment

How Do Healthcare Professionals Treat Kidney Stones?

Healthcare professionals usually treat kidney stones based on their size, location, and what type they are.

Small kidney stones may pass through your urinary tract without treatment. If you're able to pass a kidney stone, a healthcare professional may ask you to catch the kidney stone in a special container. A healthcare professional will send the kidney stone to a lab to find out what type it is. A healthcare professional may advise you to drink plenty of liquids if you are able to help move a kidney stone along. The healthcare professional also may prescribe pain medicine.

Larger kidney stones or kidney stones that block your urinary tract or cause great pain may need urgent treatment. If you are vomiting and dehydrated, you may need to go to the hospital and get fluids through an IV.

Kidney Stone Removal

A urologist can remove the kidney stone or break it into small pieces with the following treatments:

- Shock wave lithotripsy
- Cystoscopy and ureteroscopy
- Percutaneous nephrolithotomy

After these procedures, sometimes the urologist may leave a thin flexible tube, called a ureteral stent, in your urinary tract to help urine flow or a stone to pass. Once the kidney stone is removed, your doctor sends the kidney stone or its pieces to a lab to find out what type it is.

The healthcare professional also may ask you to collect your urine for 24 hours after the kidney stone has passed or been removed. The healthcare professional can then measure how much urine you produce in a day, along with mineral levels in your urine. You are more likely to form stones if you don't make enough urine each day or have a problem with high mineral levels.

How Can I Prevent Kidney Stones?

To help prevent future kidney stones, you also need to know what caused your previous kidney stones. Once you know what type of kidney stone you had, a healthcare professional can help you make changes to your eating, diet, and nutrition to prevent future kidney stones.

Drinking Liquids

In most cases, drinking enough liquids each day is the best way to help prevent most types of kidney stones. Drinking enough liquids keeps your urine diluted and helps flush away minerals that might form stones.

Though water is best, other liquids such as citrus drinks may also help prevent kidney stones. Some studies show that citrus drinks, such as lemonade and orange juice, protect against kidney stones because they contain citrate, which stops crystals from turning into stones.

Unless you have kidney failure, you should drink six to eight, 8-ounce glasses a day. If you previously had cystine stones, you may need to drink even more. Talk with a healthcare professional if you can't drink the recommended amount due to other health problems, such as urinary incontinence, urinary frequency, or kidney failure.

The amount of liquid you need to drink depends on the weather and your activity level. If you live, work, or exercise in hot weather, you may need more liquid to replace the fluid you lose through sweat. A healthcare professional may ask you to collect your urine for 24 hours to determine the amount of urine you produce a day. If the amount of urine is too low, the healthcare professional may advise you to increase your liquid intake.

Medicines

If you have had a kidney stone, a healthcare professional also may prescribe medicines to prevent future kidney stones. Depending on the type of kidney stone you had and what type of medicine the healthcare professional prescribes, you may have to take the medicine for a few weeks, several months, or longer.

For example, if you had struvite stones, you may have to take an oral antibiotic for 1 to 6 weeks, or possibly longer.

If you had another type of stone, you may have to take a potassium citrate tablet 1 to 3 times daily. You may have to take potassium citrate for months or even longer until a healthcare professional says you are no longer at risk for kidney stones.

Table 40.1. Medicines

Type of kidney stone	Possible medicines prescribed by your doctor
Calcium Stones	• potassium citrate, which is used to raise the citrate and pH levels in urine • diuretics, often called water pills, help rid your body of water
Uric Acid Stones	• allopurinol, which is used to treat high levels of uric acid in the body • potassium citrate

Table 40.1. Continued

Type of kidney stone	Possible medicines prescribed by your doctor
Struvite Stones	• antibiotics, which are bacteria-fighting medications • acetohydroxamic acid, a strong antibiotic, used with another long-term antibiotic medication to prevent infection
Cystine Stones	• mercaptopropionyl glycine, an antioxidant used for heart problems • potassium citrate

Talk with a healthcare professional about your health history prior to taking kidney stone medicines. Some kidney stone medicines have minor to serious side effects. Side effects are more likely to occur the longer you take the medicine and the higher the dose. Tell the healthcare professional about any side effects that occur when you take kidney stone medicine.

Hyperparathyroidism Surgery

People with hyperparathyroidism, a condition that results in too much calcium in the blood, sometimes develop calcium stones. Treatment for hyperparathyroidism may include surgery to remove the abnormal parathyroid gland. Removing the parathyroid gland cures hyperparathyroidism and can prevent kidney stones. Surgery sometimes causes complications, including infection.

Eating, Diet, and Nutrition

Can I Help Prevent Kidney Stones by Changing What I Eat or Drink?

Drinking enough liquid, mainly water, is the most important thing you can do to prevent kidney stones. Unless you have kidney failure, many healthcare professionals recommend that you drink six to eight, 8-ounce glasses a day. Talk with a healthcare professional about how much liquid you should drink.

Studies have shown that the Dietary Approaches to Stop Hypertension (DASH) diet can reduce the risk of kidney stones.

Studies have shown that being overweight increases your risk of kidney stones. A dietitian can help you plan meals to help you lose weight.

Does the Type of Kidney Stone I Had Affect Food Choices I Should Make?

Yes. If you have already had kidney stones, ask your healthcare professional which type of kidney stone you had. Based on the type of kidney stone you had, you may be able to prevent kidney stones by making changes in how much sodium, animal protein, calcium, or oxalate is in the food you eat.

You may need to change what you eat and drink for these types of kidney stones:

- Calcium Oxalate Stones

- Calcium Phosphate Stones

- Uric Acid Stones

- Cystine Stones

A dietitian who specializes in kidney stone prevention can help you plan meals to prevent kidney stones. Find a dietitian who can help you.

Section 40.3

Loin Pain Hematuria Syndrome

This section includes text excerpted from "Loin Pain Hematuria Syndrome," Genetic and Rare Diseases Information Center (GARD), National Center for Advancing Translational Sciences (NCATS), April 1, 2015.

Loin pain hematuria syndrome (LPHS) is a condition that is characterized by persistent or recurrent loin pain and hematuria (blood in the urine). Other signs and symptoms include nausea and vomiting; a low-grade fever (up to 101°F); and/or dysuria during episodes of pain. The exact underlying cause of LPHS is currently unknown; however, scientists suspect that it may be due to abnormalities of the glomerular basement membranes (the tissues in the kidney that filter blood); bleeding disorders; or crystal and/or stone formation in the kidneys. Treatment is symptomatic and usually consists of pain management.

Symptoms

As the name of the condition suggests, loin pain hematuria syndrome (LPHS) is characterized primarily by recurrent or persistent loin pain and/or hematuria (blood in the urine). The loin pain is sometimes described as burning or throbbing and may worsen with exercise or when lying in a supine (face upward) position. Although some may only experience pain on one side initially, most people with LPHS will eventually develop bilateral (on both sides) loin pain. During episodes of pain, affected people may also experience nausea and vomiting; a low-grade fever (up to 101°F); and/or dysuria.

Cause

The exact underlying cause of loin pain hematuria syndrome (LPHS) is currently unknown. However, scientists have proposed several theories. For example, some cases of LPHS may be due to abnormal glomerular basement membranes, which are the tissues in the kidney that filter blood. If these tissues are abnormal, red blood cells may be allowed to enter the urinary space, leading to both loin pain and hematuria (blood in the urine). Other factors that may lead to the signs and symptoms of LPHS include:

- Blood disorders, called coagulopathies, which impair the blood's ability to clot

- Spasms in the kidney's blood vessels which may restrict blood flow to certain tissues and lead to tissue death

Up to 50 percent of people affected by LPHS also experience kidney stones. Some scientists, therefore, suspect that the formation of crystals and/or stones in the kidney may also contribute to the condition as they may block or injure the renal tubules (the long narrow tubes in the kidney that concentrate and transport urine).

Diagnosis

A diagnosis of loin pain hematuria syndrome is suspected based on the presence of characteristic signs and symptoms, after other conditions that cause similar features have been excluded. Severe hematuria (blood in urine) may be obvious; however, a urinalysis can be performed to detect microscopic levels of hematuria. In some cases, a kidney biopsy may also be recommended to evaluate the structure and function of the kidney.

Treatment

Treatment of loin pain hematuria syndrome (LPHS) typically consists of pain management. Narcotics or oral opioids may be prescribed to help control pain. Patients with severe pain may need high-dose opioids daily and may occasionally require hospitalization for intravenous pain relievers and control of nausea.

Limited evidence suggests that drugs that inhibit angiotensin may reduce the frequency and severity of episodes of loin pain and severe hematuria. People with debilitating pain who do not respond to other therapies may be offered surgery (i.e., a nerve block, nephrectomy, kidney auto-transplantation); however, surgical treatment of LPHS is controversial as studies suggest that it has limited value for treating recurrent pain.

Prognosis

The long-term outlook (prognosis) for people with loin pain hematuria syndrome (LPHS) is poorly understood. However, it generally does not lead to kidney failure or a shortened lifespan. Unfortunately, the pain associated with LPHS is often severe and may interfere with quality of life. In many cases, pain can only be managed through high doses of pain relievers and/or hospitalization.

Part Four

Medical
Management of Pain

Chapter 41

Pain Treatment

Chapter Contents

Section 41.1

Treatments for Pain

This section includes text excerpted from "Pain: You
Can Get Help," National Institute on Aging (NIA),
National Institutes of Health (NIH), May 2015.

Everyone reacts to pain differently. Many older people have been
told not to talk about their aches and pains. Some people feel they
should be brave and not complain when they hurt. Other people are
quick to report pain and ask for help.

Worrying about pain is a common problem. This worry can make
you afraid to stay active, and it can separate you from your friends
and family. Working with your doctor, you can find ways to continue
to take part in physical and social activities despite being in pain.

Some people put off going to the doctor because they think pain is
just part of aging and nothing can help. This is not true! It is important
to see a doctor if you have a new pain. Finding a way to manage your
pain is often easier if it is addressed early.

Describing Pain

Many people have a hard time describing pain. Think about these
questions when you explain how the pain feels:

- Where does it hurt?

- When did it start? Does the pain come and go?

- What does it feel like? Is the pain sharp, dull, or burning? Would
  you use some other word to describe it?

- Do you have other symptoms?

- When do you feel the pain? In the morning? In the evening?
  After eating?

- Is there anything you do that makes the pain feel better or
  worse? For example, does using a heating pad or ice pack help?
  Does changing your position from lying down to sitting up make
  it better? Have you tried any over-the-counter medications for it?

Your doctor or nurse may ask you to rate your pain on a scale of 0 to 10, with 0 being no pain and 10 being the worst pain you can imagine. Or, your doctor may ask if the pain is mild, moderate, or severe. Some doctors or nurses have pictures of faces that show different expressions of pain. You point to the face that shows how you feel.

Treating Pain

Treating, or managing, chronic pain is important. The good news is that there are ways to care for pain. Some treatments involve medications, and some do not. Your doctor may make a treatment plan that is specific for your needs.

Most treatment plans do not just focus on reducing pain. They also include ways to support daily function while living with pain.

Pain doesn't always go away overnight. Talk with your doctor about how long it may take before you feel better. Often, you have to stick with a treatment plan before you get relief. It's important to stay on a schedule. Sometimes this is called "staying ahead" or "keeping on top" of your pain. As your pain lessens, you can likely become more active and will see your mood lift and sleep improve.

Medicines to Treat Pain

Your doctor may prescribe one or more of the following pain medications:

- **Acetaminophen** may help all types of pain, especially mild to moderate pain. Acetaminophen is found in over-the-counter and prescription medicines. People who drink a lot of alcohol or who have liver disease should not take acetaminophen. Be sure to talk with your doctor about whether it is safe for you to take and what would be the right dose.

- **Nonsteroidal anti-inflammatory drugs (NSAIDs)** include medications like aspirin, naproxen, and ibuprofen. Some types of NSAIDs can cause side effects, like internal bleeding, which make them unsafe for many older adults. For instance, you may not be able to take ibuprofen if you have high blood pressure or had a stroke. Talk to your doctor before taking NSAIDs to see if they are safe for you.

- **Narcotics** (also called opioids) are used for severe pain and require a doctor's prescription. They may be habit-forming. Examples of narcotics are codeine, morphine, and oxycodone.

563

- **Other medications** are sometimes used to treat pain. These include antidepressants, anticonvulsive medicines, local painkillers like nerve blocks or patches, and ointments and creams.

As people age, they are at risk for developing more serious side effects from medication. It's important to take exactly the amount of pain medicine your doctor prescribes.

Mixing any pain medication with alcohol or other drugs, such as tranquilizers, can be dangerous. Make sure your doctor knows all the medicines you take, including over-the-counter drugs and herbal supplements, as well as the amount of alcohol you drink.

What Other Treatments Help with Pain?

In addition to drugs, there are a variety of complementary and alternative approaches that may provide relief. Talk to your doctor about these treatments. It may take both medicine and other treatments to feel better.

- **Acupuncture** uses hair-thin needles to stimulate specific points on the body to relieve pain.

- **Biofeedback** helps you learn to control your heart rate, blood pressure, and muscle tension. This may help reduce your pain and stress level.

- **Cognitive behavioral therapy (CBT)** is a form of short-term counseling that may help reduce your reaction to pain.

- **Distraction** can help you cope with pain by learning new skills that may take your mind off your discomfort.

- **Electrical nerve stimulation** uses electrical impulses in order to relieve pain.

- **Guided imagery** uses directed thoughts to create mental pictures that may help you relax, manage anxiety, sleep better, and have less pain.

- **Hypnosis** uses focused attention to help manage pain.

- **Massage therapy** can release tension in tight muscles.

- **Physical therapy** uses a variety of techniques to help manage everyday activities with less pain and teaches you ways to improve flexibility and strength.

Helping Yourself

There are things you can do yourself that might help you feel better. Try to:

- **Keep a healthy weight**. Putting on extra pounds can slow healing and make some pain worse. Keeping a healthy weight might help with knee pain, or pain in the back, hips, or feet.

- **Be active**. Try to keep moving. Pain might make you inactive, which can lead to a cycle of more pain and loss of function. Mild activity can help.

- **Get enough sleep**. It will improve healing and your mood.

- **Avoid tobacco, caffeine, and alcohol**. They can get in the way of your treatment and increase your pain.

- **Join a pain support group**. Sometimes, it can help to talk to other people about how they deal with pain. You can share your ideas and thoughts while learning from others.

- **Participate in activities you enjoy**. Taking part in activities that you find relaxing, like listening to music or doing art, might help take your mind off of some of the pain.

Section 41.2

Models of Pain Treatment

This section includes text excerpted from "Chronic Pain Primer,"
U.S. Department of Veterans Affairs (VA), June 17, 2015.

There are four primary models of chronic pain service delivery, which are based on the results of the International Association for the Study of Pain (IASP) Task Force on Guidelines for Desirable Characteristics for Pain Treatment Facilities.

Single service clinics or modality-oriented clinics are outpatient clinics that provide a specific type of treatment for pain but do not provide comprehensive assessment or management. Most often

565

they are staffed by individuals from a single discipline with some expertise in a range of pain interventions falling within their areas of specialty training. Examples include a nerve block clinic, a transcutaneous nerve stimulation (TENS) clinic, or a biofeedback clinic. In general, these approaches are best suited for individuals with chronic pain, but without a chronic pain syndrome. The goal of treatment is pain reduction.

The next level of intervention occurs within a **pain clinic.** These outpatient clinics specifically focus on the diagnosis and management of individuals with chronic pain. They are staffed by individuals from one or more disciplines with specialized training in chronic pain. They may focus only on selected pain problems (e.g., a "headache clinic" or a "back pain clinic"), or on more general pain conditions. They may refer to outside consultants or staff for services not available within the clinic. They are most appropriate for individuals with more severe pain but without a chronic pain syndrome. However, those with mild chronic pain syndromes also may be appropriate.

As healthcare professionals increase in treatment intensity and complexity, they next come to the **multidisciplinary (or interdisciplinary) pain clinic.** This level of intervention includes a specific outpatient or inpatient program of treatment which typically includes at a minimum physical restoration, medical, educational, and psychological services delivered by an identifiable team of individuals from a range of disciplines with extensive training and experience in chronic pain interventions. These pain programs are most suited for those with mild to moderate chronic pain syndromes who require more global and intensive treatment of their pain and their related areas of dysfunction. Goals include improvement in pain, activity level, flexibility, strength, endurance, and psychosocial functioning.

The final type of treatment delivery is provided through a **multidisciplinary (or interdisciplinary) pain center.** The pain center is the largest and most complex type of pain treatment model, and typically is associated with a medical school or teaching hospital. Such centers offer treatment of both acute and chronic pain using a dedicated, interdisciplinary staff working in a team setting. Staff specialize in pain treatment. Unlike the multidisciplinary pain clinic, pain centers also must engage in active pain-related research and staff education. Pain centers are most appropriate for individuals with moderate to severe chronic pain syndromes, and for those with less severe pain syndromes but very complex and refractory pain problems. They also are most appropriate for individuals with chronic pain whose rehabilitation is complicated by concurrent medical or emotional problems that require closer monitoring and the immediate availability of emergent and supportive services.

Examples of Popular Pain Treatment Modalities

- Pain medications (e.g., narcotic analgesics, Non-Steroidal Anti-Inflammatory Drugs (NSAIDs), Tricyclic antidepressants, anticonvulsant medications, "muscle relaxants," etc.)

- Bed rest/braces for pain reduction

- Surgery

- Nerve blocks/steroid injections

- Trigger point injections

- Acupuncture

- Patient controlled analgesia pump

- Dorsal column stimulator implant

- Physical Therapy-passive modalities (e.g., ultrasound, infrared, massage)

- Electrical Stimulation Therapy

- Physical Therapy-active treatments (e.g., exercise, TENS, gait training)

- Manipulation

- Biofeedback

- Relaxation

- Group therapy

- Individual therapy

- Behavior therapy

- Cognitive behavioral therapy (CBT)

- Hypnosis

- Education

- Multidisciplinary pain management programs

Unfortunately, popularity of a treatment does not guarantee its effectiveness. It is up to the individual practitioners to determine whether a given treatment is potentially effective for the condition, and to ascertain if professional or state guidelines or standards of care governing the treatment of certain pain conditions exist.

Chapter 42

Diagnosing and Evaluating Pain

Chapter Contents

Section 42.1

Chronic Pain Assessment

This section contains text excerpted from the following
sources: Text in this section begins with excerpts from "Chronic
Pain Primer," U.S. Department of Veterans Affairs (VA), June
2015; Text under the heading "Pain Numeric Rating Scale" is
excerpted from "Numeric Pain Rating Scale," U.S. Department of
Veterans Affairs (VA), May 27, 2007. Reviewed June 2017.

The presence of chronic pain does not always mean that the individual with pain is in distress. Surprisingly, pain may be experienced, but may not be perceived as unpleasant. Therefore, when measuring chronic pain, one needs both quantitative, qualitative, and distress measures.

Assessment

Quantitative measures are used to judge the "amount" of pain. The best quantitative measure is a scaled self-report of pain. Many of these scales exist. They include verbal descriptive scales, nonverbal scales, scales for children, and number scales. The easiest and perhaps best-validated quantitative measure is the pain Visual Analog Scale (VAS), using either a 0–100 or 0–10 reference line. A typical 10-point VAS, and the version healthcare professionals use, follows:

NAME _____

DATE _____

TIME _____

TIME _____

Place a vertical mark across the line at a point which shows what your current pain level is.

| _____ |

NO PAIN UNBEARABLE PAIN

The line length is 10 cm. Scoring the response simply involves measuring the distance between the "no pain" endpoint and the individual's response, in centimeters (e.g., a score of 5.2).

Measures of tissue damage, autonomic levels, and reports of others have not been found to be very reliable or accurate quantitative measures. In fact, correlations between medical staff estimates of an individual's pain level and the person's own rating generally are quite low. Behavioral measures of pain (e.g., facial expressions, postural changes, etc.) are accurate but usually require much more time to score.

Qualitative measures are used to differentiate between possible etiologies. Suggestions for gathering some qualitative pain information follow:

- Have the person describe the pain in their own terms. If they have difficulty, provide a verbal list of possible descriptors as examples (e.g., "Is the pain throbbing, aching, pulsating, cutting, burning, shooting, stabbing, pounding, or burning?").

- Determine if it is constant or intermittent. If it is intermittent, ask how often it is present, and what, if anything, seems to trigger it.

- Ask what makes the pain better, and what makes it worse.

Distress measures provide us with information as to how much the pain interferes with the person's life. The more it interferes, the more unpleasant it is perceived. Distress measures include assessment of emotional distress, marital/family dysfunction due to pain, financial pressures due to pain, and a variety of other indicators.

In order to effectively diagnose and treat chronic pain healthcare professionals typically need to incorporate measures from all three of these pain domains (i.e., quantitative, qualitative, and distress) at a minimum. At present there are no universally accepted means of measuring these pain domains.

Pain Numeric Rating Scale

1. On a scale of 0 to 10, with 0 being no pain at all and 10 being the worst pain imaginable, how would you rate your pain RIGHT NOW.

0	1	2	3	4	5	6	7	8	9
No Pain									Worst Pain Imaginable

2. On the same scale, how would you rate your USUAL level of pain during the last week.

0	1	2	3	4	5	6	7	8	9
No Pain									Worst Pain Imaginable

3. On the same scale, how would you rate your BEST level of pain during the last week.

0	1	2	3	4	5	6	7	8	9
No Pain									Worst Pain Imaginable

4. On the same scale, how would you rate your WORST level of pain during the last week.

0	1	2	3	4	5	6	7	8	9
No Pain									Worst Pain Imaginable

Section 42.2

X-Rays

This section includes text excerpted from "Medical X-Ray Imaging,"
U.S. Food and Drug Administration (FDA), June 3, 2017.

Medical imaging has led to improvements in the diagnosis and treatment of numerous medical conditions in children and adults.

There are many type—or modalities—of medical imaging procedures, each of which uses different technologies and techniques. Computed tomography (CT), fluoroscopy, and radiography ("conventional X-ray" including mammography) all use ionizing radiation to generate images of the body. Ionizing radiation is a form of radiation that has enough energy to potentially cause damage to DNA and may elevate a person's lifetime risk of developing cancer.

CT, radiography, and fluoroscopy all work on the same basic principle: an X-ray beam is passed through the body where a portion of the X-rays are either absorbed or scattered by the internal structures, and the remaining X-ray pattern is transmitted to a detector (e.g., film or a computer screen) for recording or further processing by a computer. These exams differ in their purpose:

- Radiography—a single image is recorded for later evaluation. Mammography is a special type of radiography to image the internal structures of breasts.

- Fluoroscopy—a continuous X-ray image is displayed on a monitor, allowing for real-time monitoring of a procedure or passage of a contrast agent ("dye") through the body. Fluoroscopy can result in relatively high radiation doses, especially for complex interventional procedures (such as placing stents or other devices inside the body) which require fluoroscopy be administered for a long period of time.

- CT—many X-ray images are recorded as the detector moves around the patient's body. A computer reconstructs all the individual images into cross-sectional images or "slices" of internal organs and tissues. A CT exam involves a higher radiation dose than conventional radiography because the CT image is reconstructed from many individual X-ray projections.

Benefits/Risks

Benefits

The discovery of X-rays and the invention of CT represented major advances in medicine. X-ray imaging exams are recognized as a valuable medical tool for a wide variety of examinations and procedures. They are used to:

- noninvasively and painlessly help to diagnosis disease and monitor therapy;

- support medical and surgical treatment planning; and

- guide medical personnel as they insert catheters, stents, or other devices inside the body, treat tumors, or remove blood clots or other blockages.

Risks

As in many aspects of medicine, there are risks associated with the use of X-ray imaging, which uses ionizing radiation to generate images of the body. Ionizing radiation is a form of radiation that has enough energy to potentially cause damage to DNA. Risks from exposure to ionizing radiation include:

- a small increase in the possibility that a person exposed to X-rays will develop cancer later in life. (General information for patients and healthcare providers on cancer detection and treatment is available from the National Cancer Institute.)

- tissue effects such as cataracts, skin reddening, and hair loss, which occur at relatively high levels of radiation exposure and are rare for many types of imaging exams. For example, the typical use of a CT scanner or conventional radiography equipment should not result in tissue effects, but the dose to the skin from some long, complex interventional fluoroscopy procedures might, in some circumstances, be high enough to result in such effects.

Another risk of X-ray imaging is possible reactions associated with an intravenously injected contrast agent, or "dye," that is sometimes used to improve visualization.

The risk of developing cancer from medical imaging radiation exposure is generally very small, and it depends on:

- radiation dose—The lifetime risk of cancer increases the larger the dose and the more X-ray exams a patient undergoes.

- patient's age—The lifetime risk of cancer is larger for a patient who receives X-rays at a younger age than for one who receives them at an older age.

- patient's sex—Women are at a somewhat higher lifetime risk than men for developing radiation-associated cancer after receiving the same exposures at the same ages.

- body region—Some organs are more radiosensitive than others.

The above statements are generalizations based on scientific analyses of large population data sets, such as survivors exposed to radiation from the atomic bomb. One of the reports of such analyses is Health Risks from Exposure to Low Levels of Ionizing Radiation: BEIR VII Phase 2 (Committee to Assess Health Risks from Exposure to Low Levels of Ionizing Radiation, National Research Council). While specific individuals or cases may not fit into such generalizations, they are still useful in developing an overall approach to medical imaging radiation safety by identifying at-risk populations or higher-risk procedures.

Because radiation risks are dependent on exposure to radiation, an awareness of the typical radiation exposures involved in different imaging exams is useful for communication between the physician and patient. (For a comparison of radiation doses associated with different imaging procedures.

The medical community has emphasized radiation dose reduction in CT because of the relatively high radiation dose for CT exams (as compared to radiography) and their increased use, as reported in the National Council on Radiation Protection and Measurements (NCRP) Report No. 160. Because tissue effects are extremely rare for typical use of many X-ray imaging devices (including CT), the primary radiation risk concern for most imaging studies is cancer; however, the long exposure times needed for complex interventional fluoroscopy exams and resulting high skin doses may result in tissue effects, even when the equipment is used appropriately.

Balancing Benefits and Risks

While the benefit of a clinically appropriate X-ray imaging exam generally far outweighs the risk, efforts should be made to minimize this risk by reducing unnecessary exposure to ionizing radiation. To help reduce risk to the patient, all exams using ionizing radiation should be performed only when necessary to answer a medical question, treat a disease, or guide a procedure. If there is a medical need for a particular imaging procedure and other exams using no or less radiation are less appropriate, then the benefits exceed the risks, and radiation risk considerations should not influence the physician's decision to perform the study or the patient's decision to have the procedure. However, the "As Low as Reasonably Achievable" (ALARA) principle should always be followed when choosing equipment settings to minimize radiation exposure to the patient.

Patient factors are important to consider in this balance of benefits and risks. For example:

- Because younger patients are more sensitive to radiation, special care should be taken in reducing radiation exposure to pediatric patients for all types of X-ray imaging exams.

- Special care should also be taken in imaging pregnant patients due to possible effects of radiation exposure to the developing fetus.

- The benefit of possible disease detection should be carefully balanced against the risks of an imaging screening study on healthy, asymptomatic patients.

575

Information for Patients

X-ray imaging (CT, fluoroscopy, and radiography) exams should be performed only after careful consideration of the patient's health needs. They should be performed only when the referring physician judges them to be necessary to answer a clinical question or to guide treatment of a disease. The clinical benefit of a medically appropriate X-ray imaging exam outweighs the small radiation risk. However, efforts should be made to help minimize this risk.

Questions to Ask Your Healthcare Provider

Patients and parents of children undergoing X-ray imaging exams should be well informed and prepared by:

- Keeping track of medical-imaging histories as part of a discussion with the referring physician when a new exam is recommended.

- Informing their physician if they are pregnant or think they might be pregnant.

- Asking the referring physician about the benefits and risks of imaging procedures, such as:

  - How will the results of the exam be used to evaluate my condition or guide my treatment (or that of my child)?

  - Are there alternative exams that do not use ionizing radiation that are equally useful?

- Asking the imaging facility:

  - If it uses techniques to reduce radiation dose, especially to sensitive populations such as children.

  - About any additional steps that may be necessary to perform the imaging study (e.g., administration of oral or intravenous contrast agent to improve visualization, sedation, or advanced preparation).

  - If the facility is accredited. (Accreditation may only be available for specific types of X-ray imaging such as CT.)

Section 42.3

Magnetic Resonance Imaging (MRI)

This section includes text excerpted from "MRI
(Magnetic Resonance Imaging)," U.S. Food and
Drug Administration (FDA), November 7, 2016.

Magnetic Resonance Imaging (MRI) is a medical imaging procedure for making images of the internal structures of the body. MRI scanners use strong magnetic fields and radio waves (radio frequency energy) to make images. The signal in an MR image comes mainly from the protons in fat and water molecules in the body.

During an MRI exam, an electric current is passed through coiled wires to create a temporary magnetic field in a patient's body. Radio waves are sent from and received by a transmitter/receiver in the machine, and these signals are used to make digital images of the scanned area of the body. A typical MRI scan last from 20–90 minutes, depending on the part of the body being imaged.

For some MRI exams, intravenous (IV) drugs, such as gadolinium-based contrast agents (GBCAs) are used to change the contrast of the MR image. Gadolinium-based contrast agents are rare earth metals that are usually given through an IV in the arm.

Uses

MRI gives healthcare providers useful information about a variety of conditions and diagnostic procedures including:

- abnormalities of the brain and spinal cord

- abnormalities in various parts of the body such as breast, prostate, and liver

- injuries or abnormalities of the joints

- the structure and function of the heart (cardiac imaging)

- areas of activation within the brain (functional MRI or fMRI)

- blood flow through blood vessels and arteries (angiography)

577

- the chemical composition of tissues (spectroscopy)

In addition to these diagnostic uses, MRI may also be used to guide certain interventional procedures.

Benefits and Risks

Benefits

An MRI scanner can be used to take images of any part of the body (e.g., head, joints, abdomen, legs, etc.), in any imaging direction. MRI provides better soft tissue contrast than CT and can differentiate better between fat, water, muscle, and other soft tissue than CT (CT is usually better at imaging bones). These images provide information to physicians and can be useful in diagnosing a wide variety of diseases and conditions.

Risks

MR images are made without using any ionizing radiation, so patients are not exposed to the harmful effects of ionizing radiation. But while there are no known health hazards from temporary exposure to the MR environment, the MR environment involves a strong, static magnetic field, a magnetic field that changes with time (pulsed gradient field), and radiofrequency energy, each of which carry specific safety concerns:

- The strong, static magnetic field will attract magnetic objects (from small items such as keys and cell phones, to large, heavy items such as oxygen tanks and floor buffers) and may cause damage to the scanner or injury to the patient or medical professionals if those objects become projectiles. Careful screening of people and objects entering the MR environment is critical to ensure nothing enters the magnet area that may become a projectile.

- The magnetic fields that change with time create loud knocking noises which may harm hearing if adequate ear protection is not used. They may also cause peripheral muscle or nerve stimulation that may feel like a twitching sensation.

- The radiofrequency energy used during the MRI scan could lead to heating of the body. The potential for heating is greater during long MRI examinations.

The use of gadolinium-based contrast agents (GBCAs) also carries some risk, including side effects such as allergic reactions to the contrast agent.

Some patients find the inside of the MRI scanner to be uncomfortably small and may experience claustrophobia. Imaging in an open MRI scanner may be an option for some patients, but not all MRI systems can perform all examinations, so you should discuss these options with your doctor. Your doctor may also be able to prescribe medication to make the experience easier for you.

To produce good quality images, patients must generally remain very still throughout the entire MRI procedure. Infants, small children, and other patients who are unable to lay still may need to be sedated or anesthetized for the procedure. Sedation and anesthesia carry risks not specific to the MRI procedure, such as slowed or difficult breathing, and low blood pressure.

Patients with Implants, External, and Accessory Devices

The MR environment presents unique safety hazards for patients with implants, external devices and accessory medical devices. Examples of implanted devices include artificial joints, stents, cochlear implants, and pacemakers. An external device is a device that may touch the patient like an external insulin pump, a leg brace, or a wound dressing. An accessory device is a non-implanted medical device (such as a ventilator, patient monitor) that is used to monitor or support the patient.

- The strong, static magnetic field of the MRI scanner will pull on magnetic materials and may cause unwanted movement of the medical device.

- The radiofrequency energy and magnetic fields that change with time may cause heating of the implanted medical device and the surrounding tissue, which could lead to burns.

- The magnetic fields and radiofrequency energy produced by an MRI scanner may also cause electrically active medical devices to malfunction, which can result in a failure of the device to deliver the intended therapy.

- The presence of the medical device will degrade the quality of the MR image, which may make the MRI scan uninformative or may lead to an inaccurate clinical diagnosis, potentially resulting in inappropriate medical treatment.

Therefore patients with implanted medical devices should not receive an MRI exam unless the implanted medical device has been positively identified as MR Safe or MR Conditional. An MR Safe device is nonmagnetic, contains no metal, does not conduct electricity and poses no known hazards in all MR environments. An MR Conditional device may be used safely only within an MR environment that matches its conditions of safe use. Any device with an unknown MRI safety status should be assumed to be MR Unsafe.

Adverse Events

Adverse events for MRI scans are very rare. Millions of MRI scans are performed in the U.S. every year, and the FDA receives around 300 adverse event reports for MRI scanners and coils each year from manufacturers, distributors, user facilities, and patients. The majority of these reports describe heating and/or burns (thermal injuries). Second degree burns are the most commonly reported patient problem. Other reported problems include injuries from projectile events (objects being drawn toward the MRI scanner), crushed and pinched fingers from the patient table, patient falls, and hearing loss or a ringing in the ear (tinnitus). The FDA has also received reports concerning the inadequate display or quality of the MR images.

Section 42.4

Electromyograms and Nerve Conduction Studies

This section contains text excerpted from the following sources: Text under the heading "What Are Electrodiagnostic Tests?" is excerpted from "Questionable Billing for Medicare Electrodiagnostic Tests," U.S. Department of Health and Human Services (HHS), April 2014; Text under the heading "What Can EMG/NCS Detect?" is excerpted from "Peripheral Neuropathy Fact Sheet," National Institute of Neurological Disorders and Stroke (NINDS), December 2014; Text under the heading "Preparing for an Electrodiagnostic Test" is excerpted from "Electrodiagnostic Testing Information Sheet," U.S. Department of Veterans Affairs (VA), June 13, 2016.

What Are Electrodiagnostic Tests?

Electrodiagnostic tests are used to evaluate patients who may have nerve damage. These specialized tests measure the electrical activity of the muscles and nerves and detect abnormalities of the peripheral nervous system (i.e., nerves outside the brain and spinal cord). Several conditions, including diabetes and carpal tunnel syndrome, can cause peripheral nerve damage.

Two common electrodiagnostic tests to assess nerve damage are needle electromyography tests (EMG) and nerve conduction tests (NCT).

- Electromyography, or EMG, is used to diagnose nerve and muscle dysfunction and spinal cord disease. It records the electrical activity from the brain and/or spinal cord to a peripheral nerve root (found in the arms and legs) that controls muscles during contraction and at rest.

- During an EMG, very fine wire electrodes are inserted into a muscle to assess changes in electrical voltage that occur during movement and when the muscle is at rest. The electrodes are attached through a series of wires to a recording instrument. Testing usually takes place at a testing facility and lasts about an hour but may take longer, depending on the number of muscles and nerves to be tested. Most patients find this test to be somewhat uncomfortable.

- Nerve conduction tests, or nerve conduction velocity (NCV)

- An EMG is usually done in conjunction with a nerve conduction velocity (NCV) test, which measures electrical energy by assessing the nerve's ability to send a signal. This two-part test is conducted most often in a hospital. A technician tapes two sets of flat electrodes on the skin over the muscles. The first set of electrodes is used to send small pulses of electricity (similar to the sensation of static electricity) to stimulate the nerve that directs a particular muscle. The second set of electrodes transmits the responding electrical signal to a recording machine. The physician then reviews the response to verify any nerve damage or muscle disease. Patients who are preparing to take an EMG or NCV test may be asked to avoid caffeine and not smoke for 2 to 3 hours prior to the test, as well as to avoid aspirin and non-steroidal anti-inflammatory drugs for 24 hours before the EMG. There is no discomfort or risk associated with this test.

Electromyography, or EMG, is used to diagnose nerve and muscle dysfunction and spinal cord disease. It records the electrical activity from the brain and/or spinal cord to a peripheral nerve root (found in the arms and legs) that controls muscles during contraction and at rest.

During an EMG, very fine wire electrodes are inserted into a muscle to assess changes in electrical voltage that occur during movement and when the muscle is at rest. The electrodes are attached through a series of wires to a recording instrument. Testing usually takes place at a testing facility and lasts about an hour but may take longer, depending on the number of muscles and nerves to be tested. Most patients find this test to be somewhat uncomfortable.

Nerve conduction tests, or nerve conduction velocity (NCV)

An EMG is usually done in conjunction with a *nerve conduction velocity (NCV)* test, which measures electrical energy by assessing the nerve's ability to send a signal. This two-part test is conducted most often in a hospital. A technician tapes two sets of flat electrodes on the skin over the muscles. The first set of electrodes is used to send small pulses of electricity (similar to the sensation of static electricity) to stimulate the nerve that directs a particular muscle. The second set of electrodes transmits the responding electrical signal to a recording machine. The physician then reviews the response to verify any nerve damage or muscle disease. Patients who are preparing to take an EMG or NCV test may be asked to avoid caffeine and not smoke for 2 to 3 hours prior to the test, as well as to avoid aspirin and non-steroidal anti-inflammatory drugs for 24 hours before the EMG. There is no discomfort or risk associated with this test.

What Can EMG/NCS Detect?

Peripheral Neuropathy

An estimated 20 million people in the United States have some form of peripheral neuropathy, a condition that develops as a result of damage to the peripheral nervous system—the vast communications network that transmits information between the central nervous system (the brain and spinal cord) and every other part of the body. (Neuropathy means nerve disease or damage.) Symptoms can range from numbness or tingling, to pricking sensations (paresthesia), or muscle weakness. Areas of the body may become abnormally sensitive leading to an exaggeratedly intense or distorted experience of touch (allodynia). In such cases, pain may occur in response to a stimulus that does not normally provoke pain. Severe symptoms may include burning pain (especially at night), muscle wasting, paralysis, or organ or gland dysfunction. Damage to nerves that supply internal organs may impair digestion, sweating, sexual function, and urination. In the most extreme cases, breathing may become difficult, or organ failure may occur.

Peripheral nerves send sensory information back to the brain and spinal cord, such as a message that the feet are cold. Peripheral nerves also carry signals from the brain and spinal cord to the muscles to generate movement. Damage to the peripheral nervous system interferes with these vital connections. Like static on a telephone line, peripheral neuropathy distorts and sometimes interrupts messages between the brain and spinal cord and the rest of the body.

More than 100 types of peripheral neuropathy have been identified, each with its own symptoms and prognosis. In general, peripheral neuropathies are classified according to the type of damage to the nerves. Some forms of neuropathy involve damage to only one nerve and are called mononeuropathies. More frequently however, multiple nerves are affected, called polyneuropathy.

Some peripheral neuropathies are due to damage to the axons (the long, threadlike portion of the nerve cell), while others are due to damage to the myelin sheath, the fatty protein that coats and insulates the axon. Peripheral neuropathies may also be caused by a combination of both axonal damage and demyelination. Electrodiagnostic studies can help healthcare providers determine the type of damage involved.

Preparing for an Electrodiagnostic Test

Preparing for an Electrodiagnostic Test

On The Day of Your Test:

- Bath or shower to remove excess body oils

- Do not use any oils, lotions or creams as these can interfere with your test

- Wear loose, comfortable clothing but be aware that you may have to change into a hospital gown

- Be sure to inform the physician if you are taking blood thinning medication such as Coumadin, have hemophilia or a cardiac pacemaker

- There are no meal or activity restrictions before or after the test

About The Test:

Nerve Conduction Studies: To perform this test the physician tapes small metal electrodes to the surface of your skin and applies an electrical pulse to one portion of the nerve being tested.

EMG (Electromyographic): A sterile fine "acupuncture-like" needle electrode is gently inserted into the muscle. Needle insertion may cause mild temporary discomfort. The needle is not used for injections and no shocks are given. The needle itself serves as a small microphone that allows the physician to detect if there may be abnormalities The study takes approximately 60-90 minutes.

Chapter 43

Conventional and Integrative Approaches to Pain Management

Chapter Contents

Section 43.1

Chronic Pain Treatment Plans

This section includes text excerpted from "Chronic Pain:
Symptoms, Diagnosis, and Treatment," U.S. National Library of
Medicine (NLM), National Institutes of Health (NIH),
April 28, 2011. Reviewed June 2017.

Symptoms

Chronic pain is often defined as any pain lasting more than 12 weeks. Whereas acute pain is a normal sensation that alerts us to possible injury, chronic pain is very different. Chronic pain persists—often for months or even longer.

Chronic pain may arise from an initial injury, such as a back sprain, or there may be an ongoing cause, such as illness. However, there may also be no clear cause. Other health problems, such as fatigue, sleep disturbance, decreased appetite, and mood changes, often accompany chronic pain. Chronic pain may limit a person's movements, which can reduce flexibility, strength, and stamina. This difficulty in carrying out important and enjoyable activities can lead to disability and despair.

Diagnosis

Pain is a very personal and subjective experience. There is no test that can measure and locate pain with precision. So, health professionals rely on the patient's own description of the type, timing, and location of pain. Defining pain as sharp or dull, constant or on-and-off, or burning or aching may give the best clues to the cause of the pain. These descriptions are part of what is called the pain history, taken during the start of the evaluation of a patient with pain.

Since chronic pain may occur in a variety of locations in the body and for many different reasons, patients and their health professionals need to work together to identify the causes and symptoms of that pain and how it can be relieved.

Although technology can help health professionals form a diagnosis, the best treatment plans are tailored to the person, with input from healthcare team members, who each have different training backgrounds and understand chronic pain. The person with pain and his or her loved ones also must be actively involved in the treatment.

Treatment

With chronic pain, the goal of treatment is to reduce pain and improve function, so the person can resume day-to-day activities. Patients and their healthcare providers have a number of options for the treatment of pain. Some are more effective than others. Whatever the treatment plan, it is important to remember that chronic pain usually cannot be cured, but it can be managed. The following treatments are among the most common ways to manage pain.

Medications, acupuncture, electrical stimulation, nerve blocks, or surgery are some treatments used for chronic pain. Less invasive psychotherapy, relaxation therapies, biofeedback, and behavior modification may also be used to treat chronic pain. These methods can be powerful and effective in some people. When it comes to chronic pain treatment, many people find adding complementary or alternative medicine (CAM) approaches can provide additional relief. These may include tai chi, acupuncture, meditation, massage therapies, and similar treatments.

Self-management of chronic pain holds great promise as a treatment approach. In self-management programs, the individual patient becomes an active participant in his or her pain treatment—engaging in problem-solving, pacing, decision-making, and taking actions to manage their pain. Although self-management programs can differ, they have some common features. Their approach is that the person living with pain needs help learning to think, feel, and do better, despite the persistence of pain. Improving communication with the healthcare provider is part of that empowerment.

Through National Institutes of Health (NIH)-supported research, starting successful self-management programs has reduced many barriers to effective pain management, regardless of the underlying conditions. Individuals who participate in these programs have significantly increased their ability to cope with pain. They improve their ability to be active, healthy, and involved members of their communities. In fact, new research suggests that the best self-management programs teach people different ways of thinking about and responding to pain, making their actions to relieve it more effective.

Section 43.2

Pain Management Therapies

This section contains text excerpted from the following
sources: Text in this section begins with excerpts from "Pain:
You Can Get Help," National Institute on Aging (NIA), National
Institutes of Health (NIH), May 2015; Text beginning with
the heading "When to Taper" is excerpted from "Pocket Guide:
Tapering Opioids for Chronic Pain," Centers for Disease Control
and Prevention (CDC), August 17, 2016; Text beginning with the
heading "Principles of Chronic Pain Treatment" is excerpted from
"Alternative Treatments Fact Sheet," National Heart, Lung, and
Blood Institute (NHLBI), April 27, 2016.

In addition to drugs, there are a variety of complementary and
alternative approaches that may provide relief. Talk to your doctor
about these treatments. It may take both medicine and other treatments to feel better.

- **Acupuncture** uses hair-thin needles to stimulate specific points
  on the body to relieve pain.

- **Biofeedback** helps you learn to control your heart rate, blood
  pressure, and muscle tension. This may help reduce your pain
  and stress level.

- **Cognitive behavioral therapy** is a form of short-term counseling that may help reduce your reaction to pain.

- **Distraction** can help you cope with pain by learning new skills
  that may take your mind off your discomfort.

- **Electrical nerve stimulation** uses electrical impulses in order
  to relieve pain.

- **Guided imagery** uses directed thoughts to create mental pictures that may help you relax, manage anxiety, sleep better, and
  have less pain.

- **Hypnosis** uses focused attention to help manage pain.

- **Massage therapy** can release tension in tight muscles.

- **Physical therapy** uses a variety of techniques to help manage everyday activities with less pain and teaches you ways to improve flexibility and strength.

Helping Yourself

There are things you can do yourself that might help you feel better. Try to:

- Keep a healthy weight. Putting on extra pounds can slow healing and make some pain worse. Keeping a healthy weight might help with knee pain, or pain in the back, hips, or feet.

- Be active. Try to keep moving. Pain might make you inactive, which can lead to a cycle of more pain and loss of function. Mild activity can help.

- Get enough sleep. It will improve healing and your mood.

- Avoid tobacco, caffeine, and alcohol. They can get in the way of your treatment and increase your pain.

- Join a pain support group. Sometimes, it can help to talk to other people about how they deal with pain. You can share your ideas and thoughts while learning from others.

- Participate in activities you enjoy. Taking part in activities that you find relaxing, like listening to music or doing art, might help take your mind off of some of the pain.

When to Taper

Consider tapering to a reduced opioid dosage or tapering and discontinuing opioid therapy when your patient:

- requests dosage reduction

- does not have clinically meaningful improvement in pain and function (e.g., at least 30% improvement on the 3-item Pain, Enjoyment, General Activity Scale (PEG) scale)

- is on dosages $\geq$ 50 Morphine milligram equivalents (MME)/day without benefit or opioids are combined with benzodiazepines

- shows signs of substance use disorder (e.g., work or family problems related to opioid use, difficulty controlling use)

- experiences overdose or other serious adverse event

- shows early warning signs for overdose risk such as confusion, sedation, or slurred speech

How to Taper

Tapering plans should be individualized and should minimize symptoms of opioid withdrawal while maximizing pain treatment with nonpharmacologic therapies and nonopioid medications. In general:

Go Slow

A decrease of 10 percent of the original dose per week is a reasonable starting point. Some patients who have taken opioids for a long time might find even slower tapers (e.g., 10% per month) easier.

Discuss the increased risk for overdose if patients quickly return to a previously prescribed higher dose.

Consult

Coordinate with specialists and treatment experts as needed — especially for patients at high risk of harm such as pregnant women or patients with an opioid use disorder.

Use extra caution during pregnancy due to possible risk to the pregnant patient and to the fetus if the patient goes into withdrawal.

Support

Make sure patients receive appropriate psychosocial support. If needed, work with mental health providers, arrange for treatment of opioid use disorder, and offer naloxone for overdose prevention.

Watch for signs of anxiety, depression, and opioid use disorder during the taper and offer support or referral as needed.

Encourage

Let patients know that most people have improved function without worse pain after tapering opioids. Some patients even have improved pain after a taper, even though pain might briefly get worse at first.

Tell patients "I know you can do this" or "I'll stick by you through this."

Considerations

1. Adjust the rate and duration of the taper according to the patient's response.

2. Don't reverse the taper; however, the rate may be slowed or paused while monitoring and managing withdrawal symptoms.

3. Once the smallest available dose is reached, the interval between doses can be extended and opioids may be stopped when taken less than once a day.

Principles of Chronic Pain Treatment

Patients with pain should receive treatment that provides the greatest benefit. Opioids are not the first-line therapy for chronic pain outside of active cancer treatment, palliative care, and end-of-life care. Evidence suggests that nonopioid treatments, including nonopioid medications and nonpharmacological therapies can provide relief to those suffering from chronic pain, and are safer. Effective approaches to chronic pain should:

- Use nonopioid therapies to the extent possible

- Identify and address co-existing mental health conditions (e.g., depression, anxiety, Posttraumatic stress disorder (PTSD))

- Focus on functional goals and improvement, engaging patients actively in their pain management

- Use disease-specific treatments when available (e.g., triptans for migraines, gabapentin/pregabalin/duloxetine for neuropathic pain)

- Use first-line medication options preferentially

- Consider interventional therapies (e.g., corticosteroid injections) in patients who fail standard non-invasive therapies

- Use multimodal approaches, including interdisciplinary rehabilitation for patients who have failed standard treatments, have severe functional deficits, or psychosocial risk factors

Table 43.1. Nonopioid Medications

Medication	Magnitude of Benefits	Harms	Comments
Acetaminophen	Small-moderate	Hepatotoxic, particularly at higher doses	First-line analgesic, probably less effective than NSAIDs
NSAIDs	Small-moderate	Cardiac, GI, renal	First-line analgesic, COX-2 selective NSAIDs less GI toxicity
Gabapentin/pregabalin	Small-moderate	Sedation, dizziness, ataxia	First-line agent for neuropathic pain; pregabalin approved for fibromyalgia
Tricyclic antidepressants and serotonin/norephinephrine reuptake inhibitors	Small-moderate	TCAs have anticholinergic and cardiac toxicities; SNRIs safer and better tolerated	First-line for neuropathic pain; TCAs and SNRIs for fibromyalgia, TCAs for headaches
Topical agents (lidocaine, capsaicin, NSAIDs)	Small-moderate	Capsaicin initial flare/ burning, irritation of mucus membranes	Consider as alternative first-line, thought to be safer than systemic medications. Lidocaine for neuropathic pain, topical NSAIDs for localized osteoarthritis, topical capsaicin for musculoskeletal and neuropathic pain

Recommended Treatments for Common Chronic Pain Conditions

Low Back Pain

Self-care and education in all patients. Advise patients to remain active and limit bedrest

Nonpharmacological treatments. Exercise, cognitive behavioral therapy, interdisciplinary rehabilitation

Medications

- **First-line**. Acetaminophen, non-steroidal anti inflammatory drugs (NSAIDs)
- **Second-line**. Serotonin and norepinephrine reuptake inhibitors (SNRIs)/tricyclic antidepressants (TCAs)

Migraine

Preventive treatments

- Beta-blockers
- TCAs
- Antiseizure medications
- Calcium channel blockers
- Non-pharmacological treatments (Cognitive behavioral therapy, relaxation, biofeedback, exercise therapy)
- Avoid migraine triggers

Acute treatments

Aspirin, acetaminophen, NSAIDs (may be combined with caffeine)

- Antinausea medication
- Triptans-migraine-specific

Neuropathic Pain

Medications. TCAs, SNRIs, gabapentin/pregabalin, topical lidocaine

Osteoarthritis

Nonpharmacological treatments. Exercise, weight loss, patient education

Medications

- **First-line**. Acetamionphen, oral NSAIDs, topical NSAIDs

- **Second-line**. Intra-articular hyaluronic acid, capsaicin (limited number of intra-articular glucocorticoid injections if acetaminophen and NSAIDs insufficient)

Fibromyalgia

Patient education. Address diagnosis, treatment, and the patient's role in treatment

Nonpharmacological treatments. Low-impact aerobic exercise (e.g., brisk walking, swimming, water aerobics, or bicycling), cognitive behavioral therapy, biofeedback, interdisciplinary rehabilitation

Medications

U.S. Food and Drug Administration (FDA)-approved. Pregabalin, duloxetine, milnacipran

- **Other options**. TCAs, gabapentin

Chapter 44

Complementary and Alternative Medicine (CAM) Therapies for Pain

Chapter Contents

Section 44.1

Research on Pain Management through CAM

This section includes text excerpted from "Complementary Health Approaches: Research on Pain Management," NIHSeniorHealth, National Institute on Aging (NIA), June 2016.

How Many Have Chronic Pain?

Chronic pain is pain that lasts a long time. It's a very common problem. Results from the 2012 National Health Interview Survey (NHIS) show that:

- about 25.3 million U.S. adults (11.2 percent) had pain every day for the previous 3 months

- nearly 40 million adults (17.6 percent) had severe pain

- individuals with severe pain had worse health, used more healthcare, and had more disability than those with less severe pain

The annual economic cost of chronic pain in the United States, including both treatment and lost productivity, has been estimated at approximately $600 billion.

Chronic Pain and Aging

Chronic pain is more common among women than men, and it becomes more common with increasing age. Experts expect the number of people with pain to increase, in part because the U.S. population is aging. Some painful conditions, such as arthritis, become more common as people get older.

Use of Complementary Approaches

The use of complementary health approaches is common among adults with painful conditions. For example, in a national survey, 47 percent of people who had migraine or back pain with sciatica used complementary approaches, as did 41 percent of those who had headaches regularly.

The most common reasons why adults use complementary approaches are conditions that involve pain. Back pain is the number one reason why adults use complementary approaches, neck pain is second, and joint pain or stiffness is third, according to 2012 national survey data.

What the Research Shows

Research has shown that some complementary health approaches may help people with some types of pain. Here are examples of complementary approaches that may be helpful for certain conditions.

- **Low-back pain.** Acupuncture, progressive relaxation, spinal manipulation, and yoga may be helpful.

- **Neck pain.** Acupuncture and spinal manipulation may be helpful.

- **Osteoarthritis pain.** Acupuncture, massage, and tai chi may be helpful.

- **Rheumatoid arthritis pain.** Omega-3 fatty acids (fish oil) may help to a modest extent.

- **Headaches:** Acupuncture may be helpful. According to the American Academy of Neurology (AAN) and the American Headache Society, butterbur is effective for preventing migraines; feverfew, magnesium, and riboflavin are probably effective; and coenzyme Q10 is possibly effective.

- **Fibromyalgia.** Some studies of tai chi, yoga, mindfulness meditation, and biofeedback have had promising results, but there isn't enough evidence to be certain that any of these methods is helpful.

Pain Research at NIH

NIH (National Institutes of Health) has established a Pain Consortium to enhance research on pain and promote collaboration among researchers from the many NIH agencies that have programs and activities related to pain.

The National Center for Complementary and Integrative Health (NCCIH), which is National Institutes of Health's lead agency for complementary health approaches, is part of the consortium and is working to improve the evidence on the effectiveness and safety of complementary approaches for pain. In addition, National Center for Complementary and Alternative Medicine (NCCAM) has a research program that focuses on the role of the brain in perceiving, modifying, and managing pain.

NIH-Sponsored Research on Complementary Health Approaches for Pain

Examples of NIH-sponsored research on complementary health approaches for pain include the following:

- **Yoga for low-back pain.** Two NIH-sponsored studies showed that participating in yoga classes may be helpful in reducing symptoms of low-back pain.

- **Massage therapy for back or neck pain.** NIH-sponsored studies of back pain and neck pain indicated that massage therapy may be helpful for both of these problems.

- **Mindfulness-based stress reduction for low-back pain.** An NIH-sponsored study found that both mindfulness-based stress reduction and cognitive behavioral therapy (CBT) (a type of conventional psychotherapy) were more effective than usual care for chronic low-back pain.

- **How mindfulness may help relieve pain.** In an NIH-sponsored study, researchers found that the mechanism by which mindfulness meditation relieves pain is different from the mechanism by which opioid drugs achieve the same effect.

- **Spinal manipulation for neck pain and low-back.** Either spinal manipulation therapy or home exercise instruction was more effective than medication for neck pain, according to an NIH-sponsored study. Another study showed that a type of spinal manipulation commonly used by chiropractors was helpful in reducing pain and disability in people with acute or sub-acute low-back pain.

- **Acupuncture for pain.** A group of researchers supported by NIH analyzed data from 29 studies of acupuncture for various types of pain (back and neck pain, osteoarthritis, shoulder pain, or headache). They found that when acupuncture was compared with simulated (fake) acupuncture, true acupuncture was more effective, but the difference in the pain relief produced by the two procedures was small. When acupuncture was compared with no acupuncture, a larger difference was seen.

- **How acupuncture may affect the brain during the treatment of pain.** Several NIH-supported studies have investigated how acupuncture may affect the brain in people with pain. For example, a study in women with fibromyalgia found differences in the brain's responses to acupuncture and simulated (fake) acupuncture.

- **Tai chi for fibromyalgia and knee osteoarthritis.** A preliminary NIH-supported study indicated that tai chi may help to relieve symptoms of fibromyalgia; a larger follow up study is comparing the effects of tai chi to those of aerobic exercise in people with fibromyalgia. Another preliminary study showed that tai chi may be helpful for pain in knee osteoarthritis; a followup study showed that tai chi classes were as helpful as physical therapy for knee osteoarthritis pain.

Section 44.2

Acupuncture

This section includes text excerpted from "Acupuncture: In Depth," National Center for Complementary and Integrative Health (NCCIH), January 2016.

What Is Acupuncture?

Acupuncture is a technique in which practitioners stimulate specific points on the body—most often by inserting thin needles through the skin. It is one of the practices used in traditional Chinese medicine.

What the Science Says about the Effectiveness of Acupuncture

Results from a number of studies suggest that acupuncture may help ease types of pain that are often chronic such as low-back pain, neck pain, and osteoarthritis/knee pain. It also may help reduce the frequency of tension headaches and prevent migraine headaches. Therefore, acupuncture appears to be a reasonable option for people with chronic pain to consider. However, clinical practice guidelines are inconsistent in recommendations about acupuncture.

The effects of acupuncture on the brain and body and how best to measure them are only beginning to be understood. Evidences suggests that many factors—like expectation and belief—that are unrelated to acupuncture needling may play important roles in the beneficial effects of acupuncture on pain.

What the Science Says about Safety and Side Effects of Acupuncture

- Relatively few complications from using acupuncture have been reported. Still, complications have resulted from use of nonsterile needles and improper delivery of treatments.

- When not delivered properly, acupuncture can cause serious adverse effects, including infections, punctured organs, collapsed lungs, and injury to the central nervous system.

What's the Bottom Line?

How Much Do We Know about Acupuncture?

There have been extensive studies conducted on acupuncture, especially for back and neck pain, osteoarthritis/knee pain, and headache. However, researchers are only beginning to understand whether acupuncture can be helpful for various health conditions.

What Do We Know about the Effectiveness of Acupuncture?

Research suggests that acupuncture can help manage certain pain conditions, but evidence about its value for other health issues is uncertain.

What Do We Know about the Safety of Acupuncture?

Acupuncture is generally considered safe when performed by an experienced, well-trained practitioner using sterile needles. Improperly performed acupuncture can cause serious side effects.

Section 44.3

Chiropractic

This section includes text excerpted from "Chiropractic: In Depth," National Center for Complementary and Integrative Health (NCCIH), February 2012. Reviewed June 2017.

Chiropractic is a healthcare profession that focuses on the relationship between the body's structure—mainly the spine—and its functioning. Although practitioners may use a variety of treatment approaches, they primarily perform adjustments (manipulations) to the spine or other parts of the body with the goal of correcting alignment problems, alleviating pain, improving function, and supporting the body's natural ability to heal itself.

Key Points

- Most research on chiropractic has focused on spinal manipulation. Spinal manipulation appears to benefit some people with low-back pain and may also be helpful for headaches, neck pain, upper- and lower-extremity joint conditions, and whiplash-associated disorders.

- Side effects from spinal manipulation can include temporary headaches, tiredness, or discomfort in the parts of the body that were treated. There have been rare reports of serious complications such as stroke, but whether spinal manipulation actually causes these complications is unclear. Safety remains an important focus of ongoing research.

- Tell all your healthcare providers about any complementary health approaches you use. Give them a full picture of what you do to manage your health. This will help ensure coordinated and safe care.

Overview and History

The term "chiropractic" combines the Greek words cheir (hand) and praxis (practice) to describe a treatment done by hand. Hands-on therapy—especially adjustment of the spine—is central to chiropractic care. Chiropractic is based on the notion that the relationship between the body's structure (primarily that of the spine) and its function (as coordinated by the nervous system) affects health.

Spinal adjustment/manipulation is a core treatment in chiropractic care, but it is not synonymous with chiropractic. Chiropractors commonly use other treatments in addition to spinal manipulation, and other healthcare providers (e.g., physical therapists or some osteopathic physicians) may use spinal manipulation.

Use in the United States

In the United States, chiropractic is often considered a complementary health approach. According to a National Health Interview Survey (NHIS), which included a comprehensive survey of the use of complementary health approaches by Americans, about 8 percent of adults (more than 18 million) and nearly 3 percent of children (more than 2 million) had received chiropractic or osteopathic manipulation in the past 12 months. Additionally, an analysis of NHIS cost data found that adults in the United States spent approximately $11.9 billion out-of-pocket on visits to complementary health practitioners—$3.9 billion of which was spent on visits to practitioners for chiropractic or osteopathic manipulation.

Many people who seek chiropractic care have low-back pain. People also commonly seek chiropractic care for other kinds of musculoskeletal pain (e.g., neck, shoulder), headaches, and extremity (e.g., hand or foot) problems.

An analysis of the use of complementary health approaches for back pain, based on data from the 2002 NHIS, found that chiropractic was by far the most commonly used therapy. Among survey respondents who had used any of these therapies for their back pain, 74 percent (approximately 4 million Americans) had used chiropractic. Among those who had used chiropractic for back pain, 66 percent perceived "great benefit" from their treatments.

Treatment

During the initial visit, chiropractors typically take a health history and perform a physical examination, with a special emphasis on the spine. Other examinations or tests such as X-rays may also be performed. If chiropractic treatment is considered appropriate, a treatment plan will be developed.

During follow up visits, practitioners may perform one or more of the many different types of adjustments and other manual therapies used in chiropractic care. Given mainly to the spine, a chiropractic adjustment involves using the hands or a device to apply a controlled, rapid force to a joint. The goal is to increase the range and quality of motion in the area being treated and to aid in restoring health. Joint mobilization is another type of manual therapy that may be used.

Chiropractors may combine the use of spinal adjustments and other manual therapies with several other treatments and approaches such as:

- Heat and ice
- Electrical stimulation
- Relaxation techniques
- Rehabilitative and general exercise
- Counseling about diet, weight loss, and other lifestyle factors
- Dietary supplements

What the Science Says

Researchers have studied spinal manipulation for a number of conditions ranging from back, neck, and shoulder pain to asthma, carpal tunnel syndrome, fibromyalgia, and headaches. Much of the research has focused on low-back pain, and has shown that spinal manipulation appears to benefit some people with this condition.

A 2010 review of scientific evidence on manual therapies for a range of conditions concluded that spinal manipulation/mobilization may be helpful for several conditions in addition to back pain, including migraine and cervicogenic (neck-related) headaches, neck pain, upper- and lower-extremity joint conditions, and whiplash-associated disorders. The review also identified a number of conditions for which spinal manipulation/mobilization appears not to be helpful (including asthma, hypertension, and menstrual pain) or the evidence is inconclusive (e.g., fibromyalgia, mid-back pain, premenstrual syndrome, sciatica, and temporomandibular disorders (TMD)).

Safety

- Side effects from spinal manipulation can include temporary headaches, tiredness, or discomfort in the parts of the body that were treated.

- There have been rare reports of serious complications such as stroke, cauda equina syndrome (a condition involving pinched nerves in the lower part of the spinal canal), and worsening of herniated discs, although cause and effect are unclear.

- Safety remains an important focus of ongoing research:

  - A study of treatment outcomes for 19,722 chiropractic patients in the United Kingdom concluded that minor side effects (such as temporary soreness) after cervical spine manipulation were relatively common, but that the risk of a serious adverse event was "low to very low" immediately or up to 7 days after treatment.

  - A study that drew on 9 years of hospitalization records for the population of Ontario, Canada analyzed 818 cases of vertebrobasilar artery (VBA) stroke (involving the arteries that supply blood to the back of the brain). The study found an association between visits to a healthcare practitioner and subsequent VBA stroke, but there was no evidence that visiting a chiropractor put people at greater risk than visiting a primary care physician. The researchers attributed the association between healthcare visits and VBA stroke to the likelihood that people with VBA dissection (torn arteries) seek care for related headache and neck pain before their stroke.

If You Are Thinking about Seeking Chiropractic Care

- Ask about the chiropractor's education and licensure.

- Mention any medical conditions you have, and ask whether the chiropractor has specialized training or experience in the condition for which you are seeking care.

- Ask about typical out-of-pocket costs and insurance coverage. (Chiropractic is covered by many health maintenance organizations and private health plans, Medicare, and state workers' compensation systems.)

- Tell the chiropractor about any medications (prescription or over-the-counter) and dietary supplements you take. If the chiropractor suggests a dietary supplement, ask about potential interactions with your medications or other supplements.

- Tell all of your healthcare providers about any complementary health approaches you use. Give them a full picture of what you do to manage your health. This will help ensure coordinated and safe care.

Section 44.4

Dietary Supplements

This section includes text excerpted from "Dietary Supplements: What You Need to Know," U.S. Food and Drug Administration (FDA), May 4, 2017.

You've heard about them, may have used them, and may have even recommended them to friends or family. While some dietary supplements are well understood and established, others need further study.

Before making decisions about whether to take a supplement, talk to your healthcare provider. They can help you achieve a balance between the foods and nutrients you personally need.

What Are Dietary Supplements?

Dietary supplements include such ingredients as vitamins, minerals, herbs, amino acids, and enzymes. Dietary supplements are marketed in forms such as tablets, capsules, softgels, gelcaps, powders, and liquids.

What Are the Benefits of Dietary Supplements?

Some supplements can help assure that you get enough of the vital substances the body needs to function; others may help reduce the risk of disease. But supplements should not replace complete meals which are necessary for a healthful diet—so, be sure you eat a variety of foods as well.

Unlike drugs, **supplements are not permitted to be marketed for the purpose of treating, diagnosing, preventing, or curing diseases.** That means supplements should not make disease claims, such as "lowers high cholesterol" or "treats heart disease." Claims like these cannot be legitimately made for dietary supplements.

Are There Any Risks in Taking Supplements?

Yes. Many supplements contain active ingredients that have strong biological effects in the body. This could make them unsafe in some situations and hurt or complicate your health. For example, the following actions could lead to harmful—even life-threatening—consequences.

- Combining supplements.

- Using supplements with medicines (whether prescription or over-the-counter).

- Substituting supplements for prescription medicines.

- Taking too much of some supplements, such as vitamin A, vitamin D, or iron. Some supplements can also have unwanted effects before, during, and after surgery. So, be sure to inform your healthcare provider, including your pharmacist about any supplements you are taking.

Some Common Dietary Supplements

- Calcium
- Echinacea
- Fish Oil
- Ginseng
- Glucosamine and/or
- Chondroitin Sulphate

- Garlic
- Vitamin D
- St. John's Wort
- Saw Palmetto
- Ginkgo
- Green Tea

Note: These examples do not represent either an endorsement or approval by U.S. Food and Drug Administration (FDA).

Who Is Responsible for the Safety of Dietary Supplements?

FDA is not authorized to review dietary supplement products for safety and effectiveness before they are marketed.

The manufacturers and distributors of dietary supplements are responsible for making sure their products are safe before they go to market.

If the dietary supplement contains a new ingredient, manufacturers must notify FDA about that ingredient prior to marketing. However, the notification will only be reviewed by FDA (not approved) and only for safety, not effectiveness.

Manufacturers are required to produce dietary supplements in a quality manner and ensure that they do not contain contaminants or impurities, and are accurately labeled according to current Good Manufacturing Practice (cGMP) and labeling regulations.

If a serious problem associated with a dietary supplement occurs, manufacturers must report it to FDA as an adverse event. FDA can take dietary supplements off the market if they are found to be unsafe or if the claims on the products are false and misleading.

How Can I Find out More about the Dietary Supplement I'm Taking?

Dietary supplement labels must include name and location information for the manufacturer or distributor.

If you want to know more about the product that you are taking, check with the manufacturer or distributor about:

- Information to support the claims of the product

- Information on the safety and effectiveness of the ingredients in the product

How Can I Be a Smart Supplement Shopper?

Be a savvy supplement user. Here's how:

- When searching for supplements on the internet, use noncommercial sites (e.g., National Institutes of Health (NIH), FDA, United States Department of Agriculture (USDA)) rather than depending on information from sellers.

- If claims sound too good to be true, they probably are. Be mindful of product claims such as "works better than [a prescription drug]," "totally safe," or has "no side effects."

- Be aware that the term natural doesn't always means safe.

- Ask your healthcare provider if the supplement you're considering would be safe and beneficial for you.

- Always remember—safety first!

Section 44.5

Spinal Manipulation

This section includes text excerpted from "Spinal Manipulation for
Low-Back Pain," National Center for Complementary and Integrative
Health (NCCIH), April 2013. Reviewed June 2017.

Low-back pain (often referred to as "lower back pain") is a common
condition that usually improves with self-care (practices that people
can do by themselves, such as remaining active, applying heat, and
taking pain-relieving medications). However, it is occasionally difficult
to treat. Some healthcare professionals are trained to use a technique
called spinal manipulation to relieve low-back pain and improve physical function (the ability to walk and move). This section provides basic
information about low-back pain and summarizes research on spinal
manipulation for low-back pain.

Key Points

- Spinal manipulation is one of several options—including
  exercise, massage, and physical therapy—that can provide
  mild-to-moderate relief from low-back pain. Spinal manipulation appears to work as well as conventional treatments such as
  applying heat, using a firm mattress, and taking pain-relieving
  medications.

- Spinal manipulation appears to be a generally safe treatment
  for low-back pain when performed by a trained and licensed
  practitioner. The most common side effects (e.g., discomfort in
  the treated area) are minor and go away within 1 to 2 days. Serious complications are very rare.

- Cauda equina syndrome (CES), a significant narrowing of the
  lower part of the spinal canal in which nerves become pinched
  and may cause pain, weakness, loss of feeling in one or both legs,
  and bowel or bladder problems, may be an extremely rare complication of spinal manipulation. However, it is unclear if there
  is actually an association between spinal manipulation and CES.

- Tell all your healthcare providers about any complementary health practices you use. Give them a full picture of what you do to manage your health. This will help ensure coordinated and safe care.

About Low-Back Pain

Back pain is one of the most common health complaints, affecting 8 out of 10 people at some point during their lives. The lower back is the area most often affected. For many people, back pain goes away on its own after a few days or weeks. But for others, the pain becomes chronic and lasts for months or years. Low-back pain can be debilitating, and it is a challenging condition to diagnose, treat, and study. The total annual costs of low-back pain in the United States—including lost wages and reduced productivity—are more than $100 billion.

About Spinal Manipulation

Spinal manipulation—sometimes called "spinal manipulative therapy"—is practiced by healthcare professionals such as chiropractors, osteopathic physicians, naturopathic physicians, physical therapists, and some medical doctors. Practitioners perform spinal manipulation by using their hands or a device to apply a controlled force to a joint of the spine. The amount of force applied depends on the form of manipulation used. The goal of the treatment is to relieve pain and improve physical functioning.

Side Effects and Risks

Reviews have concluded that spinal manipulation for low-back pain is relatively safe when performed by a trained and licensed practitioner. The most common side effects are generally minor and include feeling tired or temporary soreness.

Reports indicate that cauda equina syndrome (CES), a significant narrowing of the lower part of the spinal canal in which nerves become pinched and may cause pain, weakness, loss of feeling in one or both legs, and bowel or bladder problems, may be an extremely rare complication of spinal manipulation. However, it is unclear if there is actually an association between spinal manipulation and CES, since CES usually occurs without spinal manipulation. In people whose pain is caused by a herniated disc, manipulation of the low back appears to have a very low chance of worsening the herniation.

609

What the Science Says about Spinal Manipulation for Low-Back Pain

Overall, studies have shown that spinal manipulation is one of several options—including exercise, massage, and physical therapy—that can provide mild-to-moderate relief from low-back pain. Spinal manipulation also appears to work as well as conventional treatments such as applying heat, using a firm mattress, and taking pain-relieving medications.

Researchers are investigating whether the effects of spinal manipulation depend on the length and frequency of treatment. In one study funded by National Center for Complementary and Integrative Health (NCCIH) that examined long-term effects in more than 600 people with low-back pain, results suggested that chiropractic care involving spinal manipulation was at least as effective as conventional medical care for up to 18 months. However, less than 20 percent of participants in this study were pain free at 18 months, regardless of the type of treatment used.

Researchers are also exploring how spinal manipulation affects the body. In an NCCIH-funded study of a small group of people with low-back pain, spinal manipulation affected pain perception in specific ways that other therapies (stationary bicycle and low-back extension exercises) did not.

Managing Low-Back Pain

A review of evidence-based clinical guidelines for managing low-back pain resulted in several recommendations for primary care physicians and pointed to potential benefits of nondrug therapies including spinal manipulation, as well as exercise, massage, and physical therapy:

- Acute low-back pain. Routine imaging (X-rays or magnetic resonance imaging (MRI)) generally is not necessary for patients who have had nonspecific low-back pain for a short time. These patients often improve on their own and usually should remain active, learn about back pain and self-care options, and consider nondrug therapies, including spinal manipulation, if pain persists longer than 4 weeks.

- Chronic low-back pain. Long-term use of opioid drugs usually does not improve functioning for patients with chronic low-back pain. However, these patients may benefit from nondrug therapies, including spinal manipulation. Psychological and social factors also may play a role in chronic low-back pain. Most patients will not become pain free; a realistic outlook focuses on improving function in addition to reducing pain.

Section 44.6

Massage Therapy

This section includes text excerpted from "Massage Therapy for Health Purposes," National Center for Complementary and Integrative Health (NCCIH), June 2016.

What Is Massage Therapy?

The term "massage therapy" includes many techniques, and the type of massage given usually depends on your needs and physical condition.

What the Science Says about the Effectiveness of Massage

A lot of the scientific research on massage therapy is preliminary or conflicting, but much of the evidence points toward beneficial effects on pain and other symptoms associated with a number of different conditions. Much of the evidence suggests that these effects are short term and that people need to keep getting massages for the benefits to continue.

Researchers have studied the effects of massage for many conditions. Some that they have studied more extensively are the following:

- Pain

- Cancer

  Numerous research reviews and clinical studies have suggested that at least for the short term, massage therapy for cancer patients may reduce pain, promote relaxation, and boost mood.

However, the National Cancer Institute (NCI) urges massage therapists to take specific precautions with cancer patients and avoid massaging:

- Open wounds, bruises, or areas with skin breakdown
- Directly over the tumor site
- Areas with a blood clot in a vein
- Sensitive areas following radiation therapy
- Mental health
- Fibromyalgia
- Headaches
- HIV/AIDS
- Infant care
- Other Conditions

Researchers have studied massage for the following but it's still unclear if it helps:

- Behavior of children with autism or autism spectrum disorders (ASD)
- Immune function in women with breast cancer
- Anxiety and pain in patients following heart surgery
- Quality of life and glucose levels in people with diabetes
- Lung function in children with asthma

What the Science Says about the Safety and Side Effects of Massage Therapy

Massage therapy appears to have few risks when performed by a trained practitioner. However, massage therapists should take some precautions in people with certain health conditions.

What's the Bottom Line?

How Much Do We Know about Massage?

A lot of research on the effects of massage therapy has been carried out.

What Do We Know about the Effectiveness of Massage?

While often preliminary or conflicting, there is scientific evidence that massage may help with back pain and may improve quality of life for people with depression, cancer, and Human immunodeficiency virus infection and acquired immune deficiency syndrome (HIV/AIDS).

What Do We Know about the Safety of Massage?

Massage therapy appears to have few risks if it's used appropriately and provided by a trained massage professional.

Section 44.7

Yoga

This section includes text excerpted from "Yoga: In Depth,"
National Center for Complementary and Integrative
Health (NCCIH), June 2013. Reviewed June 2017.

Yoga is a mind and body practice with historical origins in ancient Indian philosophy. Like other meditative movement practices used for health purposes, various styles of yoga typically combine physical postures, breathing techniques, and meditation or relaxation. This section provides basic information about yoga and summarizes scientific research on effectiveness and safety.

Key Facts

• Studies in people with chronic low-back pain suggest that a carefully adapted set of yoga poses may help reduce pain and improve function (the ability to walk and move). It also suggests that practicing yoga (as well as other forms of regular exercise) might have other health benefits such as reducing heart rate and blood pressure, and may also help relieve anxiety and depression. Other research suggests yoga is not helpful for asthma, and studies looking at yoga and arthritis have had mixed results.

- People with high blood pressure, glaucoma, or sciatica, and women who are pregnant should modify or avoid some yoga poses.

- Ask a trusted source (such as a healthcare provider or local hospital) to recommend a yoga practitioner. Contact professional organizations for the names of practitioners who have completed an acceptable training program.

- Tell all your healthcare providers about any complementary health approaches you use. Give them a full picture of what you do to manage your health. This will help ensure coordinated and safe care.

About Yoga

Yoga in its full form combines physical postures, breathing exercises, meditation, and a distinct philosophy. There are numerous styles of yoga. Hatha yoga, commonly practiced in the United States and Europe, emphasizes postures, breathing exercises, and meditation. Hatha yoga styles include Ananda, Anusara, Ashtanga, Bikram, Iyengar, Kripalu, Kundalini, Viniyoga, and others.

Side Effects and Risks

- Yoga is generally low-impact and safe for healthy people **when practiced appropriately under the guidance of a well-trained instructor.**

- Overall, those who practice yoga have a low rate of side effects, and the risk of serious injury from yoga is quite low. However, certain types of stroke as well as pain from nerve damage are among the rare possible side effects of practicing yoga.

- Women who are pregnant and people with certain medical conditions, such as high blood pressure, glaucoma (a condition in which fluid pressure within the eye slowly increases and may damage the eye's optic nerve), and sciatica (pain, weakness, numbness, or tingling that may extend from the lower back to the calf, foot, or even the toes), should modify or avoid some yoga poses.

Use of Yoga for Health in the United States

According to the 2007 National Health Interview Survey (NHIS), which included a comprehensive survey on the use of complementary health approaches by Americans, yoga is the sixth most commonly used complementary health practice among adults. More than 13 million adults practiced yoga in the year 2006, and between the 2002 and 2007 NHIS, use of yoga among adults increased by 1 percent (or approximately 3 million people). The 2007 survey also found that more than 1.5 million children practiced yoga in the previous year.

Many people who practice yoga do so to maintain their health and well-being, improve physical fitness, relieve stress, and enhance quality of life. In addition, they may be addressing specific health conditions, such as back pain, neck pain, arthritis, and anxiety.

What the Science Says about Yoga

Research suggests that a carefully adapted set of yoga poses may reduce low-back pain and improve function. Other studies also suggest that practicing yoga (as well as other forms of regular exercise) might improve quality of life; reduce stress; lower heart rate and blood pressure; help relieve anxiety, depression, and insomnia; and improve overall physical fitness, strength, and flexibility. But some research suggests yoga may not improve asthma, and studies looking at yoga and arthritis have had mixed results.

If You Are Considering Practicing Yoga

- Do not use yoga to replace conventional medical care or to postpone seeing a healthcare provider about pain or any other medical condition.

- If you have a medical condition, talk to your healthcare provider before starting yoga.

- Ask a trusted source (such as your healthcare provider or a nearby hospital) to recommend a yoga practitioner. Find out about the training and experience of any practitioner you are considering.

- Everyone's body is different, and yoga postures should be modified based on individual abilities. Carefully selecting an instructor who is experienced with and attentive to your needs is an important step toward helping you practice yoga safely. Ask about the physical demands of the type of yoga in which you are interested and inform your yoga instructor about any medical issues you have.

- Carefully think about the type of yoga you are interested in. For example, hot yoga (such as Bikram yoga) may involve standing and moving in humid environments with temperatures as high as 105°F. Because such settings may be physically stressful, people who practice hot yoga should take certain precautions. These include drinking water before, during, and after a hot yoga practice and wearing suitable clothing. People with conditions that may be affected by excessive heat, such as heart disease, lung disease, and a prior history of heatstroke may want to avoid this form of yoga. Women who are pregnant may want to check with their healthcare providers before starting hot yoga.

- Tell all your healthcare providers about any complementary health approaches you use. Give them a full picture of what you do to manage your health. This will help ensure coordinated and safe care.

Chapter 45

Understanding Pain Medicine

If you've ever been treated for severe pain from surgery, an injury, or an illness, you know just how vital pain relief medications can be.

Pain relief treatments come in many forms and potencies, are available by prescription or over-the-counter (OTC), and treat all sorts of physical pain—including that brought on by chronic conditions, sudden trauma, and cancer.

Pain relief medicines (also known as "analgesics" and "painkillers") are regulated by the U.S. Food and Drug Administration (FDA). Some analgesics, including opioid analgesics, act on the body's peripheral and central nervous systems to block or decrease sensitivity to pain. Others act by inhibiting the formation of certain chemicals in the body.

Among the factors healthcare professionals consider in recommending or prescribing them are the cause and severity of the pain.

Types of Pain Relievers

OTC Medications

These relieve the minor aches and pains associated with conditions such as headaches, fever, colds, flu, arthritis, toothaches, and menstrual cramps.

This chapter includes text excerpted from "A Guide to Safe Use of Pain Medicine," U.S. Food and Drug Administration (FDA), June 16, 2016.

There are basically two types of OTC pain relievers: acetaminophen and nonsteroidal anti-inflammatory drugs (NSAIDs).

Acetaminophen is an active ingredient found in more than 600 OTC and prescription medicines, including pain relievers, cough suppressants, and cold medications.

NSAIDs are common medications used to relieve fever and minor aches and pains. They include aspirin, naproxen, and ibuprofen, as well as many medicines taken for colds, sinus pressure, and allergies. They act by inhibiting an enzyme that helps make a specific chemical.

Prescription Medications

Typical prescription pain relief medicines include opioids and non-opioid medications.

Derived from opium, opioid drugs are very powerful products. They act by attaching to a specific "receptor" in the brain, spinal cord, and gastrointestinal tract. Opioids can change the way a person experiences pain.

Types of prescription opioid medications include:

- **morphine**, which is often used before and after surgical procedures to alleviate severe pain

- **oxycodone**, which is also often prescribed for moderate to severe pain

- **codeine**, which comes in combination with acetaminophen or other non-opioid pain relief medications and is often prescribed for mild to moderate pain

- **hydrocodone**, which comes in combination with acetaminophen or other non-opioid pain relief medications and is prescribed for moderate to moderately severe pain

FDA has notified makers of certain opioid drugs that these products will need to have a Risk Evaluation and Mitigation Strategy (REMS) to ensure that the benefits continue to outweigh the risks.

Affected opioid drugs, which include brand name and generic products, are formulated with the active ingredients fentanyl, hydromorphone, methadone, morphine, oxycodone, and oxymorphone.

FDA has authority to require a REMS under the Food and Drug Administration Amendments Act of 2007.

Types of non-opioid prescription medications include ibuprofen and diclofenac, which treat mild to moderate pain.

Use as Directed

Pain medications are safe and effective when used as directed. However, misuse of these products can be extremely harmful and even deadly.

Consumers who take pain relief medications must follow their healthcare professional's instructions carefully. If a measuring tool is provided with your medicine, use it as directed.

Do not change the dose of your pain relief medication without talking to your doctor first.

Also, pain medications should never be shared with anyone else. Only your healthcare professional can decide if a prescription pain medication is safe for someone.

Here are other key points to remember.

With Acetaminophen:

- Taking a higher dose than recommended will not provide more relief and can be dangerous.

- Too much can lead to liver damage and death. Risk for liver damage may be increased in people who drink three or more alcoholic beverages a day while using acetaminophen-containing medicines.

- Be cautious when giving acetaminophen to children. Infant drop medications can be significantly stronger than regular children's medications. Read and follow the directions on the label every time you use a medicine. Be sure that your infant is getting the infants' pain formula and your older child is getting the children's pain formula.

With NSAIDs:

- Too much can cause stomach bleeding. This risk increases in people who are over 60 years of age, are taking prescription blood thinners, are taking steroids, have a history of stomach bleeding or ulcers, and/or have other bleeding problems.

- Use of NSAIDs can also cause kidney damage. This risk may increase in people who are over 60 years of age, are taking a diuretic (a drug that increases the excretion of urine), have high blood pressure, heart disease, or pre-existing kidney disease.

With opioids:

- Use of opioids can lead to drowsiness. Do not drive or use any machinery that may injure you, especially when you first start the medication.

619

- The dose of an opioid pain medication that is safe for you could be high enough to cause an overdose and death in someone else, especially children.

Know the Active Ingredients

A specific area of concern with OTC pain medicines is when products sold for different uses have the same active ingredient. A cold and cough remedy may have the same active ingredient as a headache remedy or a prescription pain reliever.

To minimize the risks of an accidental overdose, consumers should avoid taking multiple medications with the same active ingredient at the same time.

All OTC medicines must have all of their active ingredients listed on the package. For prescription drugs, the active ingredients are listed on the container label.

Talk with your pharmacist or another healthcare professional if you have questions about using OTC medicines, and especially before using them in combination with dietary supplements or other OTC or prescription medicines.

Misuse and Abuse

Misuse and abuse of pain medications can be extremely dangerous. This is especially so in regard to opioids. These medications should be stored in a place where they cannot be stolen.

According to the National Institutes of Health (NIH), studies have shown that properly managed medical use of opioid analgesic compounds (taken exactly as prescribed) is safe, can manage pain effectively, and rarely causes addiction.

But the abuse of opioids is a significant public safety concern. Abusers ingest these drugs orally, and also crush the pills in order to snort or inject them.

Commonly abused opioid pain medicines include prescription drugs such as codeine, and the brand-name products Oxycontin (oxycodone), Vicodin (hydrocodone with acetaminophen), and Demerol (meperidine).

Addiction is just one serious danger of opioid abuse. A number of overdose deaths have resulted from snorting and injecting opioids, particularly the drug OxyContin, which was designed to be a slow-release formulation.

Use Opioids Safely: 3 Key Steps

1. **Keep your doctor informed.** Inform your healthcare professional about any past history of substance abuse. All patients treated with opioids for pain require careful monitoring by their healthcare professional for signs of abuse and addiction, and to determine when these analgesics are no longer needed.

2. **Follow directions carefully.** Opioids are associated with significant side effects, including drowsiness, constipation, and depressed breathing depending on the amount taken. Taking too much could cause severe respiratory depression or death. Do not crush or break pills. This can alter the rate at which the medication is absorbed and lead to overdose and death.

3. **Reduce the risk of drug interactions.** Don't mix opioids with alcohol, antihistamines, barbiturates, or benzodiazepines. All of these substances slow breathing and their combined effects could lead to life-threatening respiratory depression.

Chapter 46

Over-the-Counter Pain Relievers

Chapter Contents

Section 46.1

Way to Take Your Over-the-Counter Pain Reliever

This section includes text excerpted from "Resources for You—The Best Way to Take Your Over-the-Counter Pain Reliever? Seriously," U.S. Food and Drug Administration (FDA), October 23, 2015.

Over-the-counter (OTC) pain relievers/fever reducers (the kind you can buy without a prescription) are safe and effective when used as directed. However, they can cause serious problems when used by people with certain conditions or taking specific medicines. They can also cause problems in people who take too much, or use them for a longer period of time than the product's Drug Facts Label recommends. That is why it is important to follow label directions carefully. If you have questions, talk to a pharmacist or healthcare professional.

What Are Pain Relievers/Fever Reducers?

There are two categories of over-the-counter pain relievers/fever reducers: acetaminophen and nonsteroidal anti-inflammatory drugs (NSAIDs). Acetaminophen is used to relieve headaches, muscle aches and fever. It is also found in many other medicines, such as cough syrup and cold and sinus medicines. OTC NSAIDs are used to help relieve pain and reduce fever. NSAIDs include aspirin, naproxen, ketoprofen and ibuprofen, and are also found in many medicines taken for colds, sinus pressure and allergies.

How Do I Use Pain Relievers/Fever Reducers Safely?

These products, when used occasionally and taken as directed, are safe and effective. Read the labels of all your over-the-counter medicines so you are aware of the correct recommended dosage. If a measuring tool is provided with your medicine, use it as directed.

What Can Happen If I Do Not Use Pain Relievers/Fever Reducers Correctly?

Using too much acetaminophen can cause serious liver damage, which may not be noticed for several days. NSAIDs, for some people with certain medical problems, can lead to the development of stomach bleeding and kidney disease.

What If I Need to Take More than One Medicine?

There are many OTC medicines that contain the same active ingredient. If you take several medicines that happen to contain the same active ingredient, for example a pain reliever along with a cough-cold-fever medicine, you might be taking two times the normal dose and not know it. So read the label and avoid taking multiple medicines that contain the same active ingredient or talk to your pharmacist or healthcare professional.

Before using any medicine, remember to think SAFER:

- **S**peak up
- **A**sk questions
- **F**ind the facts
- **E**valuate your choices
- **R**ead the label

Section 46.2

Use Caution with Over-the-Counter Pain Reliever

This section includes text excerpted from "Resources for You—
Health Hints: Use Caution with Pain Relievers," U.S. Food and Drug
Administration (FDA), March 25, 2016.

Pain relievers, when used correctly, are safe and effective. Millions of people use these medicines everyday. Not using them according to the label directions can have serious consequences.

The U.S. Food and Drug Administration (FDA) wants you to benefit from your medicines and not be hurt by them. You should know the active ingredients and directions of all your medicines before you use them.

Over-the-counter (OTC) medicines list all their active ingredients on the package. For prescription drugs, the leaflet that comes with your prescription lists the active ingredients contained in the medicine.

Many OTC medicines sold for different uses have the same active ingredient. Also, active ingredients in OTC medicines can be ingredients in prescription medicines. For example, a cold-and-cough remedy may have the same active ingredient as a headache remedy or a prescription pain reliever.

There are basically two types of OTC pain relievers. Some contain acetaminophen and others contain non-steroidal anti-inflammatory drugs (NSAIDs). These medicines are used to relieve the minor aches and pains associated with:

- headaches
- colds
- flu
- arthritis
- toothaches
- menstrual cramps

These medicines are also used to treat migraine headaches, and to reduce fever.

Acetaminophen is a very common pain reliever and fever reducer. Taking too much of this active ingredient can lead to liver damage. The risk for liver damage may be increased if you drink three or more alcoholic drinks while using acetaminophen-containing medicines.

NSAIDs are common pain relievers and fever reducers. Examples of OTC NSAIDs are aspirin, ibuprofen, naproxen sodium, and ketoprofen. There are some factors that can increase your risk for stomach bleeding:

- if you are over 60
- taking prescription blood thinners
- have previous stomach ulcers or
- other bleeding problems

If you have any of these factors, you should talk to your Doctor before using NSAIDS.

NSAIDs can also cause reversible damage to the kidneys. The risk of kidney damage may increase in:

- people who are over 60

- people who have high blood pressure, heart disease or pre-existing kidney disease

- people who are taking a diuretic

The FDA recommends that you talk with your healthcare professional if you have questions about using an OTC medicine before using it in combination with other medicines—either OTC or prescription medicine.

You can learn more about what medicines are right for you by reading the label carefully and talking to your healthcare professional or pharmacist.

Chapter 47

Topical Pain Relievers

If you've ever rubbed a topical pain reliever—a cream, gel or other product applied to the skin—on a sore muscle or joint, you're familiar with the sensation of warmth or coolness that soon follows.

But if, instead, you experience burning pain or blistering, you must seek medical attention immediately.

The U.S. Food and Drug Administration (FDA) is warning that some consumers have reported receiving serious skin injuries while using certain over-the-counter (OTC) pain relievers applied to the skin to relieve mild muscle and joint pain.

The injuries, while rare, have ranged from mild to severe chemical burns with use of such brand-name topical muscle and joint pain relievers as Icy Hot, Bengay, Capzasin, Flexall, and Mentholatum.

OTC topical pain relievers for muscles and joints include creams, lotions, ointments and patches. In many cases, burns where the product was applied occurred after just one application, with severe burning or blistering occurring within 24 hours. Some had complications serious enough to require hospitalization.

"There's no way to predict who will have this kind of reaction to a topical pain reliever for muscles and joints," says Jane Filie, M.D., a medical officer in FDA's Division of Nonprescription Regulation Development (DNRD).

This chapter includes text excerpted from "Consumer Updates—Topical Pain Relievers May Cause Burns," U.S. Food and Drug Administration (FDA), September 13, 2012. Reviewed June 2017.

More than 40 Reported Cases

According to an FDA chemist Reynold Tan, Ph.D., there have been 43 reported cases of burns associated with the use of OTC topical muscle and joint pain relievers containing the active ingredients menthol, methyl salicylate and capsaicin. These cases were uncovered by FDA scientists during safety surveillance of U.S. Food and Drug Administration's adverse event reporting database and the medical literature.

This is a very small number of cases when compared to the number of people who purchase these products, Tan notes.

Menthol, methyl salicylate and capsaicin create sensations of local warmth or coolness, but should not burn.

According to the available data, a majority of the more severe burns occurred with the use of a menthol or menthol/methyl salicylate combination product. Most of these cases involved products that contain higher concentrations of menthol and methyl salicylate (greater than 3% menthol or 10% methyl salicylate). Few of the cases involved capsaicin.

Safety Do's and Don'ts

FDA has the following advice for consumers using OTC topical muscle and joint pain relievers:

- Don't apply these products onto damaged or irritated skin.

- Don't apply bandages to the area where you've applied a topical muscle and joint pain reliever.

- Don't apply heat to the area in the form of heating pads, hot water bottles or lamps. Doing so increases the risk of serious burns.

- Don't allow these products to come in contact with eyes and mucous membranes (such as the skin inside your nose, mouth or genitals).

- It's normal for these products to produce a warming or cooling sensation where you've applied them. But if you feel actual pain after applying them, look for signs of blistering or burning. If you see any of these signs, stop using the product and seek medical attention.

- If you have any concerns about using one of these products, talk to a medical professional first.

- Report unexpected side effects from the use of OTC topical pain reliever to the FDA MedWatch program.

Chapter 48

Non-Opioid Analgesic Pain Relievers

Chapter Contents

Section 48.1

Aspirin

This section includes text excerpted from "Aspirin: Questions and Answers," U.S. Food and Drug Administration (FDA), December 18, 2015.

What Are the Different Uses for Aspirin?

- **Strokes.** Aspirin use recommended in both men and women to treat mini-strokes (transient ischemic attack—TIA) or ischemic stroke to prevent subsequent cardiovascular events or death.

- **Heart attacks.** Aspirin:

  - reduces the risk of death in patients with suspected acute heart attacks (myocardial infarctions)

  - prevents recurrent heart attacks and

  - reduces the risk of heart attacks or sudden death in patients with unstable and chronic stable angina pectoris (chest pain)

- **Other coronary conditions.** Aspirin can be used to treat patients who have had certain revascularization procedures such as angioplasty, and coronary bypass operations—if they have a vascular condition for which aspirin is already indicated.

- **Rheumatologic diseases.** Aspirin is indicated for relief of the signs and symptoms of rheumatoid arthritis, juvenile rheumatoid arthritis, osteoarthritis, spondylarthropathies, and arthritis and pleurisy associated with systemic lupus erythematosus.

- **Pain relief.** Aspirin is indicated for the temporary relief of minor aches and pains.

What Is the Basis for the Prescribing Information?

The information on the uses of aspirin is based on scientific studies that support treatment with aspirin for heart attacks, strokes, and some related conditions in patients who have cardiovascular disease or who have already had a heart attack or stroke. Convincing data support these uses in lower doses than previously believed to be effective in treating heart attacks and strokes in both men and women.

What Does This Mean for Patients?

Physicians will be better able to prescribe the proper doses for these uses for male and female patients with these medical conditions. Dose-related adverse events for patients with stroke and cardiovascular conditions should be minimized because lower dosages are recommended. The full prescribing information now provided for physicians who treat rheumatologic diseases will enhance the safe and effective prescribing of aspirin to these patients as well.

Is U.S. Food and Drug Administration (FDA) Concerned That Some Patients May Self-Treat?

U.S. Food and Drug Administration (FDA) emphasizes that consumers should not self-medicate for these serious conditions because it is very important to make sure that aspirin is their best treatment. In these conditions, the risk and benefit of each available treatment for each patient must be carefully weighed. Patients with these conditions should be under the care and supervision of a doctor.

If a Consumer Is Interested in Using Aspirin to Prevent or Treat Symptoms of Heart Problems, What Should He or She Do?

Consumers should always first ask their doctor. In fact, aspirin products are labeled this way: "Important: See your doctor before taking this product for other new uses of aspirin because serious side effects could occur with self treatment."

Do the Data on Treatment or Prevention of Cardiovascular Effects Pertain Only to Aspirin?

Yes. Although acetaminophen, ibuprofen, naproxen sodium and ketoprofen are good drugs for pain and fever, as is aspirin, only aspirin has demonstrated a beneficial effect for preventing another heart attack or stroke in patients who have cardiovascular disease or who have already had a heart attack or stroke.

What Should Consumers Be Made Aware Of?

Consumers should be informed that these professional uses of aspirin may be lifesaving when used upon the recommendation and under the supervision of a doctor. However, they must also be informed that even familiar and readily available products like aspirin may have important risks when used in new ways. For example, because aspirin can cause bleeding; in rare cases bleeding in the brain may occur in people who are using aspirin to prevent stroke. Therefore these uses should be recommended and monitored by a physician.

What Should Consumers Do If They Are Taking Other Pain Medications Such as Ibuprofen?

Consumers who have been told by their doctor to take aspirin to help prevent a heart attack, should know that taking ibuprofen at the same time, for pain relief, may interfere with the benefits of aspirin for the heart. It is alright to use them together, but the FDA recommends that consumers contact their doctor for more information on the timing of when to take these two medicines, so that both medicines can be effective.

What Should Consumers Who Are Taking Low Dose Aspirin for Disease Maintenance or Prevention Know about Alcohol Use?

Patients who consume 3 or more alcoholic drinks every day should be counseled about the bleeding risks involved with chronic, heavy alcohol use while taking aspirin.

Can Consumers Safely Use Aspirin to Treat Suspected Acute Heart Attacks?

If consumers suspect they are having a heart attack, their most important action must be to seek emergency medical care immediately. The advice and supervision of a doctor should direct this use of aspirin and patients are encouraged to speak with their doctor about this use.

What Do We Know about How Aspirin Works for Heart Conditions and Stroke?

The mechanism by which aspirin works in the treatment of heart attack and stroke is not completely understood. However, as an antiplatelet drug, we do know that aspirin help reduce platelet clumping which helps cause blockage in blood vessels.

Who Should Not Take Aspirin?

Generally, people who have:

- allergy to aspirin or other salicylates
- asthma
- uncontrolled high blood pressure
- severe liver or kidney disease
- bleeding disorders

Always check first with your doctor to determine whether the benefit of these professional uses of aspirin is greater than the risks to you.

What Other Side Effects Are Associated with Aspirin?

There is a wide range of adverse reactions that may result from aspirin use including effects on the body as a whole, or on specific body systems and functions.

High doses can cause hearing loss or tinnitus—ringing in the ears. (Note that this usually only occurs with large doses as prescribed in rheumatologic diseases and is rare in treatment with low doses used for cardiovascular purposes.)

What Is Key Message for Consumers?

The results of studies of people with a history of coronary artery disease and those in the immediate phases of a heart attack have proven to be of tremendous importance in the prevention and treatment of cardiovascular and cerebrovascular diseases.

Studies showed that aspirin substantially reduces the risk of death and/or non-fatal heart attacks in patients with a previous myocardial infarction (MI) or unstable angina pectoris which often occur before a heart attack. Patients with these conditions should be under the care and supervision of a doctor.

Aspirin has potential risks as well as benefits, like any drug. Patients should be careful to ask their doctor or healthcare professional before deciding whether aspirin is right for them and how much aspirin they should take.

Section 48.2

Acetaminophen

This section contains text excerpted from the following sources:
Text in this section begins with excerpts from "Information by
Drug Class—Acetaminophen Information," U.S. Food and Drug
Administration (FDA), April 13, 2016; Text beginning with the
heading "Reducing Fever in Children: Safe Use of Acetaminophen"
is excerpted from "Consumer Updates—Reducing Fever in Children:
Safe Use of Acetaminophen," U.S. Food and Drug Administration
(FDA), July 21, 2011. Reviewed June 2017; Text beginning with the
heading "Safety Announcement" is excerpted from "Drug Safety and
Availability—FDA Drug Safety Communication: FDA Has Reviewed
Possible Risks of Pain Medicine Use during Pregnancy," U.S. Food
and Drug Administration (FDA), January 9, 2015.

Acetaminophen is an active ingredient in hundreds of over-the-
counter (OTC) and prescription medicines. It relieves pain and fever.
And, it is also combined with other active ingredients in medicines
that treat allergy, cough, colds, flu, and sleeplessness. In prescription
medicines, acetaminophen is found with other active ingredients to
treat moderate to severe pain. Acetaminophen can cause serious liver
damage if more than directed is used. The U.S. Food and Drug Administration (FDA) has taken action to improve the safety of consumers
when using acetaminophen.

Reducing Fever in Children: Safe Use of Acetaminophen

You're in the drug store, looking for a fever-reducing medicine for
your children. They range in age from 6 months to 7 years, and you
want to buy one product you can use for all of them. So you buy liquid
acetaminophen in concentrated drops for infants, figuring you can use
the dropper for the baby and a teaspoon for the oldest.

This could be a dangerous mistake.

This use of concentrated drops in much larger amounts—as would
be given with a teaspoon—can cause fatal overdoses, says Sandra
Kweder, M.D., deputy director of the U.S. Food and Drug Administration's Office of New Drugs (OND).

You can't just give an older child more of an infant's medicine, adds Kweder. "Improper dosing is one of the biggest problems in giving acetaminophen to children."

Confusion about dosing is partly caused by the availability of different formulas, strengths, and dosage instructions for different ages of children.

Sold as a single active ingredient under such brand names as Tylenol, acetaminophen is commonly used to reduce fever and relieve pain. It is also used in combination with other ingredients in products to relieve multiple symptoms, such as cough and cold medicines. Acetaminophen can be found in more than 600 over-the-counter (OTC, or non-prescription) and prescription medicines.

Acetaminophen is generally safe and effective if you follow the directions on the package, but if you give a child even a little more than directed or give more than one medicine that contains acetaminophen, it can cause nausea and vomiting, says Kweder.

In some cases—in both adults and children—it can cause liver failure and death. In fact, acetaminophen poisoning is a leading cause of liver failure in the United States.

Advice from outside Experts

An FDA Advisory Panel of outside experts met May 17–18, 2011, to discuss how to minimize medication errors and make children's OTC medicines that contain acetaminophen safer to use.

The panel recommended:

- That liquid, chewable, and tablet forms be made in just one strength. Currently, there are seven strengths available for these forms combined.

- That dosing instructions to reduce fever be developed for children as young as 6 months. Current instructions apply to children ages 2 to 12 years and for those under 2, only state "consult a doctor."

- That dosing instructions be based on weight, not just age.

- Setting standards for dosing devices, such as spoons and cups, for children's medicines. Currently, some use milliliters (mL) while others use cubic centimeters (cc) or teaspoons (tsp).

"FDA is considering these recommendations," says Kweder, and for those that the agency adopts, "we will work with manufacturers to try to get them in place on a voluntary basis." The process of getting a regulation finalized could take several years, she adds, so having the drug industry act voluntarily would help make acetaminophen safer sooner.

Drug makers have already agreed to phase out the concentrated infant drops to reduce confusion for parents who try to use them for older children. In 2011, the Consumer Healthcare Products Association (CHPA), a trade group representing the makers of OTC medicines, announced plans to convert liquid acetaminophen products for children to just one strength (160 mg/5 mL). In addition, the industry is voluntarily standardizing the unit of measurement "mL" on dosing devices for these products.

Safety Announcement

The U.S. Food and Drug Administration (FDA) is aware of and understands the concerns arising from recent reports questioning the safety of prescription and over-the-counter (OTC) pain medicines when used during pregnancy. As a result, FDA evaluated research studies published in the medical literature and determined they are too limited to make any recommendations based on these studies at this time. Because of this uncertainty, the use of pain medicines during pregnancy should be carefully considered. FDA urges pregnant women to always discuss all medicines with their healthcare professionals before using them.

Severe and persistent pain that is not effectively treated during pregnancy can result in depression, anxiety, and high blood pressure in the mother. Medicines including nonsteroidal anti-inflammatory drugs (NSAIDs), opioids, and acetaminophen can help treat severe and persistent pain. However, it is important to carefully weigh the benefits and risks of using prescription and OTC pain medicines during pregnancy.

The published studies FDA reviewed reported on the potential risks associated with the following three types of pain medicines used during pregnancy:

- Prescription NSAIDs and the risk of miscarriage in the first half of pregnancy. Examples of prescription NSAIDs include ibuprofen, naproxen, diclofenac, and celecoxib.

- Opioids, which are available only by prescription, and the risk of birth defects of the brain, spine, or spinal cord in babies born to women who took these products during the first trimester of pregnancy. Examples of opioids include oxycodone, hydrocodone, hydromorphone, morphine, and codeine.

- Acetaminophen in both OTC and prescription products and the risk of attention deficit hyperactivity disorder (ADHD) in children born to women who took this medicine at any time during pregnancy. Acetaminophen is a common pain reducer and fever reducer found in hundreds of medicines including those used for colds, flu, allergies, and sleep.

FDA found all of the studies they reviewed to have potential limitations in their designs; sometimes the accumulated studies on a topic contained conflicting results that prevented them from drawing reliable conclusions. As a result, their recommendations on how pain medicines are used during pregnancy will remain the same at this time.

Pregnant women should always consult with their healthcare professional before taking any prescription or OTC medicine. Women taking pain medicines who are considering becoming pregnant should also consult with their healthcare professionals to discuss the risks and benefits of pain medicine use. Healthcare professionals should continue to follow the recommendations in the drug labels when prescribing pain medicines to pregnant patients.

FDA will continue to monitor and evaluate the use of pain medicines during pregnancy and will update the public as new safety information becomes available.

Facts about Pain Medicines during Pregnancy

- A variety of medicines are prescribed to treat pain, including severe and persistent pain in pregnant women. These include nonsteroidal anti-inflammatory drugs (NSAIDs), opioids, and acetaminophen.

- NSAIDs are available by prescription and over-the-counter (OTC). They are used to relieve fever and pain, such as those associated with headaches, colds, flu, and arthritis. Examples of prescription NSAIDs include ibuprofen, naproxen, diclofenac, and celecoxib. Ibuprofen and naproxen are also available OTC at lower strengths.

- Findings from two U.S. studies indicate that approximately 18–25 percent of pregnancies are exposed to OTC ibuprofen and 4 percent of pregnancies are exposed to OTC naproxen.

- Opioids are a class of pain medicines available only by prescription. During each trimester of pregnancy, approximately six percent of pregnant women in the United States are exposed to opioids. Examples of opioids include oxycodone, hydrocodone, hydromorphone, morphine, and codeine.

- Acetaminophen is used in prescription combination products to reduce pain and in OTC products to reduce pain and fever. Acetaminophen is found in hundreds of medicines including those used for colds, flu, allergies, and sleep.

- Findings from two U.S. studies indicate that 65–70 percent of pregnant U.S. women reported using acetaminophen anytime during pregnancy.

More Information for Pregnant Women

- Always consult your healthcare professional about the use of all prescription and over-the-counter (OTC) medicines during pregnancy.

- Avoid using nonsteroidal anti-inflammatory drugs (NSAIDs) in the third trimester of pregnancy because these drugs may cause a blood vessel in the fetus to close prematurely.

- Do not stop taking any prescribed medicines without first talking to your healthcare professional.

- Talk to your healthcare professional if you have any questions or concerns about medicines you are taking.

Tips for Giving Acetaminophen to Children

- Never give your child more than one medicine containing acetaminophen at a time. To find out if an OTC medicine contains acetaminophen, look for "acetaminophen" on the Drug Facts label under the section called "Active Ingredient." For prescription pain relievers, ask the pharmacist if the medicine contains acetaminophen.

- Choose the right OTC medicine based on your child's weight and age. The "Directions" section of the Drug Facts label tells you if the medicine is right for your child and how much to give. If a dose for your child's weight or age is not listed on the label or you can't tell how much to give, ask your pharmacist or doctor what to do.

- Never give more of an acetaminophen-containing medicine than directed. If the medicine doesn't help your child feel better, talk to your doctor, nurse, or pharmacist.

- If the medicine is a liquid, use the measuring tool that comes with the medicine—not a kitchen spoon.

- Keep a daily record of the medicines you give to your child. Share this information with anyone who is helping care for your child.

- If your child swallows too much acetaminophen, get medical help right away, even if your child doesn't feel sick. For immediate help, call the 24-hour Poison Control Center at 800-222-1222, or call 911.

Section 48.3

Ibuprofen

This section includes text excerpted from "Postmarket Drug Safety Information for Patients and Providers—Ibuprofen Drug Facts Label," U.S. Food and Drug Administration (FDA), April 6, 2016.

Drug Facts

Active ingredient (in each tablet or capsule)
Ibuprofen 200 mg (NSAID)*
*nonsteroidal anti-inflammatory drug
Purpose. Pain reliever/fever
Uses. Temporarily relieves minor aches and pains due to:

- headache

- minor pain of arthritis

- the common cold

- muscular aches

- temporarily reduces fever

- backache

- toothache

- menstrual cramps

Warnings

Allergy alert. Ibuprofen may cause a severe allergic reaction, especially in people allergic to aspirin. Symptoms may include:

- hives
- facial swelling
- asthma (wheezing)
- shock
- skin reddening
- rash
- blister

If an allergic reaction occurs, stop use and seek medical help right away.

Stomach bleeding warning. This product contains a nonsteroidal anti-inflammatory drug (NSAID), which may cause stomach bleeding. The chance is higher if you:

- are age 60 or older
- have had stomach ulcers or bleeding problems
- take a blood thinning (anticoagulant) or steroid drug
- take other drugs containing an NSAID [aspirin, ibuprofen, naproxen, or others]
- have 3 or more alcoholic drinks every day while using this product
- take more or for a longer time than directed

Do not use:

- if you have ever had an allergic reaction to any other pain reliever/fever reducer
- right before or after heart surgery

Ask a doctor before use if you have:

- problems or serious side effects from taking pain relievers or fever reducers
- stomach problems that last or come back, such as heartburn, upset stomach, or stomach pain

- ulcers

- bleeding problems

- high blood pressure

- heart or kidney disease

- taken a diuretic

- reached age 60 or older

Ask a doctor or pharmacist before use if you are:

- taking any other drug containing an NSAID (prescription or nonprescription)

- taking a blood thinning (anticoagulant) or steroid drug

- under a doctor's care for any serious condition

- taking any other drug

When using this product:

- take with food or milk if stomach upset occurs

- long term continuous use may increase the risk of heart attack or stroke

Stop use and ask a doctor if:

- you feel faint, vomit blood, or have bloody or black stools. These are signs of stomach bleeding

- pain gets worse or lasts more than 10 days

- fever gets worse or lasts more than 3 days

- stomach pain or upset gets worse or lasts

- redness or swelling is present in the painful area

- any new symptoms appear

If pregnant or breast-feeding, ask a health professional before use. It is especially important not to use ibuprofen during the last 3 months of pregnancy unless definitely directed to do so by a doctor because it may cause problems in the unborn child or complications during delivery.

Keep out of reach of children. In case of overdose, get medical help or contact a Poison Control Center right away.

Directions

- do not take more than directed
- the smallest effective dose should be used
- do not take longer than 10 days, unless directed by a doctor
- Refer to the product container for additional directions

Other information. Refer to the specific product container for this information.

Inactive Ingredients. The specific product container has an alphabetical list of the inactive ingredients included in the product.

Chapter 49

Opioid Pain Relievers

Chapter Contents

Section 49.1

Commonly Prescribed Opioid Medications

This section includes text excerpted from
"Prescription Pain Medications (Opioids)," National
Institute on Drug Abuse (NIDA) for Teens, May 14, 2017.

Prescription opioids are medications that are chemically similar to endorphins—opioids that our body makes naturally to relieve pain—and also similar to the illegal drug heroin. In nature, opioids are found in the seed pod of the opium poppy plant.

Opioid medications can be natural (made from the plant), semi-synthetic (modified in a lab from the plant), and fully synthetic (completely made by people).

Prescription opioids usually come in pill form and are given to treat severe pain—for example, pain from dental surgery, serious sports injuries, or cancer. Opioids are also commonly prescribed to treat other kinds of pain that lasts a long time (chronic pain), but it is unclear if they are effective for long term pain.

For most people, when opioids are taken as prescribed by a medical professional for a short time, they are relatively safe and can reduce pain effectively. However, dependence and addiction are still potential risks when taking prescription opioids. Dependence means you feel withdrawal symptoms when not taking the drug. Continued use can can lead to addiction, where you continue to use despite negative consequences. These risks increase when these medications are misused. Prescription medications are some of the most commonly misused drugs by teens, after tobacco, alcohol, and marijuana.

Common opioids and their medical uses are listed below.

Table 49.1. Common Opioids and Their Medical Uses

Opioid Types	Conditions They Treat
• oxycodone (OxyContin, Percodan, Percocet)	• severe pain, often after surgery
• hydrocodone (Vicodin, Lortab, Lorcet)	• acute (severe) pain

Table 49.1. Continued

Opioid Types	Conditions They Treat
• diphenoxylate (Lomotil)	• some forms of chronic pain (severe)
• morphine (Kadian, Avinza, MS Contin)	• cough and diarrhea
• codeine	
• fentanyl (Duragesic)	
• propoxyphene (Darvon)	
• hydromorphone (Dilaudid)	
• meperidine (Demerol)	
• methadone	

Fentanyl has been in the news. It is a powerful opioid prescribed for extreme pain that is 50 to 100 times more potent than morphine. It is extremely dangerous if misused, and is sometimes added to illicit drugs sold by drug dealers.

Table 49.2. Types of Opioids

Type of Opioid	How Are They Derived	Examples
Natural opioids (sometimes called opiates)	nitrogen-containing base chemical compounds, called alkaloids, that occur in plants such as the opium poppy	morphine, codeine, thebaine
Semi-synthetic/ man-made opioids	created in labs from natural opioids	hydromorphone, hydrocodone, and oxycodone (the prescription drug OxyContin), heroin (which is made from morphine)
Fully synthetic/ man-made opioids	completely man-made	fentanyl, pethidine, levorphanol, methadone, tramadol, dextropropoxyphene

How Prescription Opioids Are Misused

People misuse prescription opioid medications by taking them in a way that is not intended, such as:

- **Taking someone else's prescription**, even if it is for a legitimate medical purpose like relieving pain.

- **Taking an opioid medication in a way other than prescribed**—for instance, taking more than your prescribed dose or taking it more often, or crushing pills into powder to snort or inject the drug.

- **Taking the opioid prescription to get high**.

- **Mixing them with alcohol or certain other drugs**. Your pharmacist can tell you what other drugs are safe to use with prescription pain relievers.

What Happens to Your Brain When You Use Prescription Opioids?

Opioids attach to specific proteins, called opioid receptors, on nerve cells in the brain, spinal cord, gut, and other organs. When these drugs attach to their receptors, they block pain messages sent from the body through the spinal cord to the brain. They can also reduce or stop other essential functions like breathing.

Opioid receptors are also located in the brain's reward center, where they cause a large release of the neurotransmitter dopamine. This causes a strong feeling of relaxation and euphoria (extreme good feelings). Repeated surges of dopamine in the reward center from drug-taking can lead to addiction.

What Happens to Your Body When You Use Prescription Opioids?

In addition to pain relief and euphoria, other effects of opioids include:

- sleepiness
- confusion
- nausea (feeling sick to the stomach)
- constipation
- slowed or stopped breathing

Can You Overdose or Die If You Use Prescription Opioids?

Yes, you can overdose and die from prescription opioid misuse. In fact, taking just one large dose could cause the body to stop breathing.

Deaths from overdoses of prescription drugs have been increasing since the early 1990s, largely due to the increase in misuse of prescription opioid pain relievers. Nearly 23,000 people died from an overdose of a prescription pain medication in 2015, with alarming increases among young people ages 15 to 24.

The risk of overdose and death increase if you combine opioids with alcohol or other medications that also slow breathing, such as Benzodiazepines (e.g., Xanax).

Signs of Overdose

Signs of a possible prescription opioid overdose are:

- slow breathing
- blue lips and fingernails
- cold damp skin
- shaking
- vomiting or gurgling noise

People who are showing symptoms of overdose need urgent medical help (call 911 immediately). A drug called naloxone can be given to reverse the effects of an opioid overdose and prevent death—but only if it is given in time.

Naloxone is available as an easy-to-use nasal spray or autoinjector. It is often carried by emergency first responders, including police officers and emergency medical services. In some states, doctors can now prescribe naloxone in advance to people who use prescription opioids or to their family members, so that in the event of an overdose, it can be given right away without waiting for emergency personnel (who may not arrive in time).

Are Prescription Opioids Addictive?

Yes, prescription opioids can be addictive. People who misuse prescription opioids are at greater risk of becoming addicted to opioids than people who take them as prescribed by a doctor.

Opioid withdrawal can cause:

- restlessness
- muscle and bone pain
- sleep problems
- diarrhea
- vomiting (throwing up)

- cold flashes with goosebumps ("cold turkey")

- involuntary leg movements

Carefully following the doctor's instructions for taking a medication can make it less likely that someone will develop dependence or addiction, because the medication is prescribed in amounts and forms that are considered appropriate for that person.

Doctors should always weigh the risks of opioid dependence and addiction against the benefits of the medication, and patients should communicate any issues or concerns to their doctor as soon as they arise. The earlier a problem is identified, the better the chances are for long term recovery.

How Many Teens Use Prescription Opioids?

Below is a chart showing the percentage of teens who misuse prescription opioid pain medicines.

Table 49.3. Monitoring the Future Study: Trends in Prevalence of Various Drugs for 8th Graders, 10th Graders, and 12th Graders; 2016 (in Percent)*

Drug	Time Period	8th Graders	10th Graders	12th Graders
Vicodin	Past Year	0.8	1.7	[2.90]
OxyContin	Past Year	0.9	2.1	3.4

Data in brackets indicate statistically significant change from the previous year.

What Should I Do If Someone I Know Needs Help?

If you see or hear about someone misusing steroids, talk to a coach, teacher, or other trusted adult.

If you, or a friend, are in crisis and need to speak with someone now, please call:

- **National Suicide Prevention Lifeline at 1-800-273-8255 (1-800-273-TALK)** (they don't just talk about suicide—they cover a lot of issues and will help put you in touch with someone close by).

If you need information on treatment and where you can find it, you can call:

- **Substance Abuse Treatment Facility Locator at 1-800-662-4357 (1-800-662-HELP)** or visit www.findtreatment.samhsa.gov.

Section 49.2

What to Ask Your Doctor before Taking Opioids

This section includes text excerpted from "Consumer Updates—What to Ask Your Doctor before Taking Opioids," U.S. Food and Drug Administration (FDA), November 21, 2016.

Every patient should ask questions when getting a new prescription. This is especially important when your doctor, dentist or other healthcare professional prescribes you an opioid, such as hydrocodone, oxycodone, codeine, and morphine.

Questions to Ask Your Doctor before Taking Opioids

Why Do I Need This Medication—Is It Right for Me?

This conversation could begin like this: "My condition is causing pain. How long do you expect it to last? What medication are you giving me? If it's an opioid, are there non-opioid options that could help with pain relief while I recover?"

Opioids approved by the U.S. Food and Drug Administration (FDA) can be used to treat certain kinds of acute and chronic pain. They also can have some very serious side effects.

If your doctor thinks your pain is best managed with a prescription opioid, then ask:

How Long Should I Take This Medication?

Find out when and how to stop using, or taper off, opioids. Ask that your doctor prescribe the lowest dose and the smallest quantity you may need and find out when to call to follow up on how well it is working. Other questions to consider:

How Can I Reduce the Risk of Potential Side Effects from This Medication?

Take your medicine exactly as prescribed by your healthcare provider. If you are still feeling pain, call your healthcare provider; do not take an extra dose. Learn to identify serious side effects (such as excessive sleepiness or a feeling of craving more of the medication) so you and your family will know when to call a doctor or go to the hospital. Ask your pharmacist if your prescription comes with a Medication Guide (paper handouts that come with many prescription medicines) for more information.

What If I Have a History of Addiction?

Tell your healthcare provider about any history you have had with substance misuse or addiction to drugs or alcohol and if you have a history of smoking cigarettes. You should also tell your healthcare provider if anyone in your family has had a problem with substance misuse, alcoholism or drug addiction.

What about the Other Medications I'm Taking?

It is also very important that you tell your healthcare provider about all of the medicines you are taking, especially those prescribed to treat anxiety, sleeping problems, or seizure. Even medicines you take only occasionally could interact with the opioid pain medicine. Ask your healthcare provider about possible interactions.

How Should I Store My Opioid Medicine?

If you have children at home—from a toddler to a teenager—consider a lockbox for your medications. Even one accidental dose of an opioid pain medicine meant for an adult can cause a fatal overdose in a child. Also, teenagers and others in the home or who are visiting may seek out opioid pain medicines for nonmedical use. They may look in bathroom medicine cabinets for a chance to steal these medicines.

What Should I Do with Unused Opioid Medicine?

Don't store it in case you have more pain later. Your leftover opioids can be targeted by people who you'd never expect to take it: friends, relatives, and even your kids and their friends. If there is no drug take-back program near you, FDA has created a list of opioid pain medicines they recommend you flush down the toilet when they're no longer needed. This way there can be no accidental exposures or mistakes in the home.

Can I Share This Medication with Someone Else?

No. Your prescription is for you. Your doctor considers many factors when prescribing opioids. What's safe for you might lead to an overdose for someone else.

Can I Have an Rx for Naloxone?

You should discuss with your doctor whether you should also receive a prescription for naloxone, a drug that can reverse the effects of an opioid overdose and could save lives. In many cases it makes sense to be prepared for potential problems by keeping naloxone in your home.

Play it safe. It doesn't matter who is writing the prescription, ask these questions before taking opioids.

Chapter 50

Other Medications Used for Pain Management

Overview of Nonopioid Pain Medication

Several nonopioid pharmacologic therapies (including acetamino-phen, NSAIDs, and selected antidepressants and anticonvulsants) are effective for chronic pain. In particular, acetaminophen and NSAIDs can be useful for arthritis and low back pain. Selected anticonvul-sants such as pregabalin and gabapentin can improve pain in diabetic neuropathy and post-herpetic neuralgia. Pregabalin, gabapentin, and carbamazepine are FDA-approved for treatment of certain neuropathic pain conditions, and pregabalin is FDA approved for fibromyalgia management. In patients with or without depression, tricyclic antide-pressants and SNRIs provide effective analgesia for neuropathic pain conditions including diabetic neuropathy and post-herpetic neuralgia, often at lower dosages and with a shorter time to onset of effect than for treatment of depression. Tricyclics and SNRIs can also relieve fibromyalgia symptoms. The SNRI duloxetine is FDA-approved for the

This chapter contains text excerpted from the following sources: Text under the heading "Overview of Nonopioid Pain Medication" is excerpted from "CDC Guideline for Prescribing Opioids for Chronic Pain—United States, 2016," Centers for Disease Control and Prevention (CDC), March 18, 2016; Text under the head-ing "Classes of Nonopioid Medications," is excerpted from "Cognitive Behavioral Therapy for Chronic Pain," U.S. Department of Veterans Affairs (VA), 2014.

treatment of diabetic neuropathy and fibromyalgia. Because patients with chronic pain often suffer from concurrent depression, and depression can exacerbate physical symptoms including pain, patients with co-occurring pain and depression are especially likely to benefit from antidepressant medication. Nonopioid pharmacologic therapies are not generally associated with substance use disorder, and the numbers of fatal overdoses associated with nonopioid medications are a fraction of those associated with opioid medications. For example, acetaminophen, NSAIDs, and opioid pain medication were involved in 881, 228, and 16,651 pharmaceutical overdose deaths in the United States in 2010. However, nonopioid pharmacologic therapies are associated with certain risks, particularly in older patients, pregnant patients, and patients with certain co-morbidities such as cardiovascular, renal, gastrointestinal, and liver disease. For example, acetaminophen can be hepatotoxic at dosages of > 3-4 grams/day and at lower dosages in patients with chronic alcohol use or liver disease. NSAID use has been associated with gastritis, peptic ulcer disease, cardiovascular events and fluid d retention, and most NSAIDs (choline magnesium trilisate and selective COX-2 inhibitors are exceptions) interfere with platelet aggregation.

Classes of Nonopioid Medications

Nonsteroidal Anti-Inflammatory Drugs (NSAIDs)

Aspirin and other related compounds constitute a class of drugs known as nonsteroidal anti-inflammatory drugs (NSAIDs). This class of medication produces three desirable effects including anti-inflammatory, analgesic, and antipyretic (fever reducing). Commonly used medications in this category include aspirin, ibuprofren, naproxen, etolodac, meloxicam, and piroxicam. The most common adverse effects of NSAIDs are gastrointestinal and renal (kidney). Acetaminophen is also a non-opioid analgesic but is not an NSAID because, though possessing pain relieving and antipyretic properties, it lacks an anti-inflammatory effect.

Tramadol

Tramadol does not fit neatly into a single category because it is dual acting. It interferes with the transmission of pain signals like an opioid, but it also releases norepinephrine and serotonin like an antidepressant. It is used for moderate to severe chronic pain and the most common side effects are dizziness, sedation, constipation, nausea, and headaches. Because it is not a pure opioid, risk of physiological dependence is lower but is still present.

Topical Analgesic

Topical analgesics are applied to the skin for delivery of medication to targeted pain areas. They block the generation and transmission of nerve signals to the brain through a local numbing effect. Topical products are available in various creams, gels, lotions, patches, and plasters. Since they are applied to a localized area externally, topical agents afford a lower risk for systemic adverse events and side effects. They are frequently used in the VA and the most commonly prescribed topicals are capsaicin, lidocaine, diclofenac, and menthol-methylsalcilate.

Muscle Relaxants

Muscle relaxants (or spasmolytics, antispasmodic) are most commonly prescribed for LBP, neck pain, fibromyalgia, and tension headaches in situations where muscular contractions appear to be a prominent component of pain. Muscle relaxants used most commonly in VA include cyclobenzaprine, tizanidine, baclofen, and methocarbamol. Muscle relaxants work by inhibiting the central nervous system, which contributes to the commonly reported side effect of sedation and the recommendation against driving or operating heavy machinery. Other common side effects include dizziness, headache, nausea, irritability, and nervousness. Muscle relaxants also pose a risk of physiological dependence.

Adjuvant Analgesics

Adjuvant analgesics, or co-analgesics, are medications that were originally developed and marketed for uses other than analgesia and are also used in pain management. The two most common classes of medications that fall into this category are certain types of antidepressants and anticonvulsants. Antidepressants commonly used for analgesic purposes include duloxetine, venlafaxine, and nortriptyline. Anticonvulsants, primarily used to relieve neuropathic pain, include gabapentin, pregablin, topiramate, and lamotrigine. Common side effects of antidepressants include nausea, vomiting, insomnia, decreased sex drive, and constipation. Common side effects of anticonvulsant medications include dizziness, fatigue, weight gain, and drowsiness.

Headache Analgesics

Analgesics used to treat headaches vary widely and do not fall into a neat class. Migraine medications are generally categorized by nature of their action into those that are preventative (e.g., propranolol, topiramate or Topamax), abortive (e.g., sumatriptan or Maxalt), and rescue (butalbital/acetaminophen/caffeine or Fioricet). Of note, medication overuse headaches, or rebound headaches, may occur when excessive analgesics are taken for headache relief, leading to chronic daily headaches of a different type.

OnabotulinnumtoxinA (Brand name: Botox)*

Botox is a drug made from a toxin produced by the bacterium Clostridium botulinum. It's the same toxin that causes a life-threatening type of food poisoning called botulism. Doctors use it in small doses to treat health problems, including pain. Botox injections work by weakening or paralyzing certain muscles or by blocking certain nerves. The effects last about three to twelve months, depending on what you are treating. The most common side effects are pain, swelling, or bruising at the injection site. You could also have flu-like symptoms, headache, and upset stomach. Injections in the face may also cause temporary drooping eyelids. You should not use Botox if you are pregnant or breastfeeding.

(*Source: "Botox," U.S. National Library of Medicine (NLM), National Institutes of Health (NIH), January 24, 2017.)

Chapter 51

Corticosteroid Injections for Relieving Pain

The corticosteroids are a group of chemically related natural hormones and synthetic agents that resemble the human adrenal hormone cortisol and have potent antiinflammatory and immunosuppressive properties and are widely used in medicine. Corticosteroid therapy is associated with several forms of liver injury, some due to exacerbation of an underlying liver disease and some that appear to be caused directly by corticosteroid therapy. This chapter will cover eight agents: betamethasone, cortisone, dexamethasone, hydrocortisone, methylprednisolone, prednisolone, prednisone, and triamcinolone.

Background

The corticosteroids are hormones that have glucocorticoid (cortisol-like) and/or mineralocorticoid (aldosterone-like) activities and which are synthesized predominantly by the adrenal cortex. In clinical practice, the term "corticosteroids" usually refers to the

---

This chapter contains text excerpted from the following sources: Text in this chapter begins with excerpts from "Corticosteroids," National Institutes of Health (NIH), April 11, 2012. Reviewed June 2017; Text beginning with the heading "Injectable Corticosteroids" is excerpted from "FDA Drug Safety Communication: FDA Requires Label Changes to Warn of Rare but Serious Neurologic Problems after Epidural Corticosteroid Injections for Pain," U.S. Food and Drug Administration (FDA), January 15, 2016.

glucocorticoids and are represented by a large group of natural or synthetic steroid compounds that have varying potency, durations of action and relative glucocorticoid (measured by antiinflammatory activity) vs mineralocorticoid (measured by sodium retention) activities. Cortisol and the corticosteroids act by engagement of the intracellular glucocorticoid receptor, which then is translocated to the cell nucleus where the receptor-ligand complex binds to specific glucocorticoid-response elements on DNA, thus activating genes that mediate glucocorticoid responses. The number of genes modulated by corticosteroids are many and the effects are multiple and interactive with other intracellular pathways. Thus, the effects of corticosteroids on inflammation and the immune system cannot be attributed to a single gene or pathway. The potent antiinflammatory and immuno-suppressive qualities of the corticosteroids have made them important agents in the therapy of many diseases. Corticosteroids are available in multiple forms, including oral tablets and capsules; powders and solutions for parenteral administration; topical creams and lotions for skin disease; eye, ear and nose liquid drops for local application; aerosol solutions for inhalation and liquids or foams for rectal application. Representative corticosteroids (and the year of their approval for use in the United States) include cortisone (1950), prednisone (1955), prednisolone (1955), methylprednisolone (1957), dexamethasone (1958), betamethasone (1961), and hydrocortisone (1983). All are available in generic forms. In this website, only the oral and intravenous formulations of corticosteroids are described and they are discussed together with common list of references and representative case reports.

The corticosteroids are used widely in medicine largely for their potent antiinflammatory and immunosuppressive activities. The clinical conditions for which corticosteroids are used include, but are not limited to: asthma, systemic lupus erythematosis, rheumatoid arthritis, psoriasis, inflammatory bowel disease, nephritic syndrome, cancer, leukemia, organ transplantation, autoimmune hepatitis, hypersensitivity reactions, cardiogenic and septic shock, and, of course, glucocorticoid deficiency diseases such as in Addison's disease and panhypopituitarism.

Corticosteroids are used in several liver diseases, most commonly in autoimmune hepatitis for which they have been shown to improve outcome and survival. Corticosteroids are also used after liver transplantation to prevent rejection. An important element in managing these liver diseases and conditions is to maintain the dose of corticosteroids at the lowest effective level. The adverse effects of long term corticosteroid therapy (which are rarely hepatic) are still major causes of morbidity and even mortality in these conditions.

Prednisone, prednisolone, methylprednisone and triamcinolone are the most commonly used oral agents as they are inexpensive, rapid in onset, intermediate in duration of action and have potent glucocorticoid with minimal mineralocorticoid activities, at least as compared to cortisone and hydrocortisone. Betamethasone and dexamethasone have greater glucocorticoid potency and less aldosterone-like activity than prednisone, but have a longer duration of action, and they are mostly used in topical or liquid forms for local application and in injectable forms for severe hypersensitivity reactions and inflammation. Methylprednisone and hydrocortisone are most commonly used for intravenous administration, typically given in emergency or critical situations in which rapid and profound immunosuppression or anti-inflammatory activity is needed.

Major Forms of Corticosteroids

Cortisone is a short acting glucocorticoid that is used for therapy of adrenal insufficiency and for treatment of allergic and inflammatory conditions. Cortisone is available in generic forms in tablets of 25 mg, which is considered a daily physiologic dose in adults. Cortisone has both glucocorticoid and mineralocorticoid properties.

Hydrocortisone is a rapid and short acting glucocorticoid that is used for therapy of adrenal insufficiency and in treatment of allergic and inflammatory conditions. Hydrocortisone has the same chemical structure as cortisol and thus most closely resembles the human adrenal hormone. Hydrocortisone is available in generic forms in tablets of 5, 10 and 20 mg, with 20 mg being considered a daily physiologic dose in adults. Hydrocortisone is also available in multiple forms in solution for oral, rectal, topical or parenteral administration. A major use of intravenous hydrocortisone is in the acute therapy of severe hypersensitivity reactions and shock. Hydrocortisone has both glucocorticoid and mineralocorticoid properties.

Prednisone is a synthetic, intermediate acting glucocorticoid that is widely used in the therapy of severe inflammation, autoimmune conditions, hypersensitivity reactions and organ rejection. Prednisone is converted to prednisolone, its active form, in the liver. Prednisone is available in multiple generic forms in tablets of 1, 2.5, 5, 10, 20 and 50 mg and as oral solutions. Four times more potent that cortisol, prednisone is used in varying doses, with 5 mg daily being considered physiologic doses in adults.

Prednisolone is a synthetic, intermediate acting glucocorticoid that is widely used in the therapy of severe inflammation, autoimmune conditions, hypersensitivity reactions and organ rejection. Prednisolone is available in multiple generic forms in tablets of 5, 10, 15 and 30 mg and in several forms for systemic administration. Four times more potent that cortisol, prednisolone is used in varying doses, with 5 mg daily being considered physiologic doses in adults.

Methylprednisolone is a synthetic, intermediate acting glucocorticoid that widely used in the therapy of severe inflammation, autoimmune conditions, hypersensitivity reactions and organ rejection. Methylprednisolone is available in multiple forms in tablets of 2, 4, 8, 16 and 32 mg generically and under the brand name of Medrol and in Medrol Dosepaks (21 tablets of 4 mg each). Injectable forms of methylprednisolone are also available generically and under brand names of Solu-Medrol and Depo-Medrol. Five times more potent that cortisol, methylprednisolone is used in varying doses, with 4 mg daily being considered physiologic doses in adults. Methylprednisolone has minimal mineralocorticoid activity.

Triamcinolone is a synthetic, long acting glucocorticoid that is used in topical solutions and aerosols for therapy of allergic and hypersensitivity reactions and control of inflammation as well as in parenteral formulations for therapy of hypersensitivity reactions, shock and severe inflammation. Oral forms of triamcinolone include tablets of 4 and 8 mg and oral syrups. Parenteral forms for injection are available under various generic and trade names including Aristocort and Kenacort. Triamcinolone is five times more potent than cortisol in its glucocorticoid activity, but has minimal mineralocorticoid activity.

Dexamethasone is a synthetic, long acting glucocorticoid that is used parenterally as therapy of severe hypersensitivity reactions, shock and control of severe inflammation as well as in topical, otic, ophthalmologic solutions, aerosols and lotions or creams for local therapy of allergic reactions and inflammation. Dexamethasone is available in multiple forms for injection under various generic and trade names including Decadron. Dexamethasone is 25 times more potent than cortisol in its glucocorticoid activity, but has minimal mineralocorticoid activity.

Betamethasone is a synthetic, long acting glucocorticoid that used in parenteral forms for therapy of allergic and hypersensitivity reactions and control of severe inflammation. Betamethasone is available in solution for injection under the trade name of Celestone and in multiple generic forms as syrups and effervescent tablets for oral use, edemas and foams for rectal use, aerosols for nasal and respiratory use, and creams and lotions for topical use. Betamethasone is 25 times more potent than cortisol in glucocorticoid activity, but has minimal mineralocorticoid activity.

Injectable Corticosteroids

Injectable corticosteroids are commonly used to reduce swelling or inflammation. Injecting corticosteroids into the epidural space of the spine has been a widespread practice for many decades; however, the effectiveness and safety of the drugs for this use have not been established, and FDA has not approved corticosteroids for such use. FDA started investigating this safety issue when they became aware of medical professionals' concerns about epidural corticosteroid injections and the risk of serious neurologic adverse events. This concern prompted them to review cases in the FDA Adverse Event Reporting System (FAERS) database and in the medical literature.

To raise awareness of the risks of epidural corticosteroid injections in the medical community, FDA's Safe Use Initiative convened a panel of experts, including pain management experts to help define the techniques for such injections which would reduce preventable harm. The expert panel's recommendations will be released when they are finalized.

As part of FDA's ongoing effort to investigate this issue, they plan to convene an Advisory Committee meeting of external experts in late 2014 to discuss the benefits and risks of epidural corticosteroid injections and to determine if further FDA actions are needed.

Injectable corticosteroids include methylprednisolone, hydrocortisone, triamcinolone, betamethasone, and dexamethasone. This safety issue is unrelated to the contamination of compounded corticosteroid injection products reported in 2012.

Facts about Corticosteroids

- A class of drugs commonly used to reduce swelling or inflammation

- Injectable corticosteroids include methylprednisolone, hydrocortisone, triamcinolone, betamethasone, and dexamethasone

- Corticosteroids are not approved by FDA for injection into the epidural space of the spine.

Additional Information for Patients

- Rare but serious problems have occurred after injection of corticosteroids into the epidural space of the spine to treat neck and back pain, and radiating pain in the arms and legs.

- These serious problems include loss of vision, stroke, paralysis, and death.

- The effectiveness and safety of injection of corticosteroids into the epidural space of the spine have not been established, and FDA has not approved corticosteroids for this use.

- Discuss the benefits and risks of epidural corticosteroid injections with your healthcare professional, along with the benefits and risks associated with other possible treatments.

- Seek emergency medical attention immediately if you experience any unusual symptoms after receiving an epidural corticosteroid injection, such as loss of vision or vision changes; tingling in your arms or legs; sudden weakness or numbness of your face, arm, or leg on one or both sides of the body; dizziness; severe headache; or seizures.

- Report any side effects from epidural corticosteroid injections to the FDA MedWatch program.

Chapter 52

Invasive and Implanted Pain Interventions

Epidural Steroid Injections

Epidural steroid injections (ESIs) are used for back pain complaints associated with conditions such as spinal stenosis or spinal disc herniation. ESIs include a combination of corticosteroids and local anesthesia that is injected into the epidural space around the spinal cord and nerves. The injection may be guided by fluoroscopy or X-ray. The effects of the injection last from one week to six months.

Nerve Blocks

Nerve blocks (aka, regional nerve blockade) are used for pain in the neck, back, feet or even the head. Nerve blocks may include local anesthetic and epinephrine, with corticosteroids, and/or opioids that are injected directly into the nerve group associated with reported pain. Nerve blocks can be used to treat painful conditions, to determine sources of pain, or to judge the benefits of more permanent treatments such as surgery.

This chapter includes text excerpted from "Cognitive Behavioral Therapy for Chronic Pain," U.S. Department of Veterans Affairs (VA), 2014.

Trigger Point Injections

Trigger point injections (TPI) are used to relieve muscles where knots form when muscles do not relax. TPI is used in many muscle groups ranging from arms, legs, low back, and neck and is most associated with treatment of fibromyalgia and tension headache. The injection contains a local anesthetic that may include a corticosteroid.

Facet Injections

Facet injections are used for those with chronic neck or back pain caused by inflamed facet joints, which are located between each set of vertebrae in the spine from the neck to the tailbone. A mixture of local anesthetic and corticosteroid medication is injected into the facet joint to reduce swelling and inflammation around the facet joint space.

Radiofrequency Ablation

Radiofrequency ablation (RFA) is used to treat severe chronic low back pain. Radiofrequency waves produce high heat on specifically identified nerves surrounding the facet joints in the lumbar spine, ablating the nerves and destroying their ability to transmit pain signals. RFA is an outpatient procedure using local anesthesia. While the procedure may provide pain relief, in most patients the nerves regenerate.

OnabotulinnumtoxinA (Brand Name: Botox)

Botox injections are typically used for relief of frequent migraine headaches. Botox received approval from the FDA as a treatment for chronic migraines in 2010.

Spinal Cord Stimulator

The most common use of spinal cord stimulators (SCS) is with patients diagnosed with failed back syndrome (see definition under Surgery below). A SCS includes electrodes implanted in the epidural space, an electrical pulse generator implanted in the lower abdominal area of gluteal region, connecting wires to the generator, and a generator remote control.

Intrathecal Pump

An intrathecal pump is an implantable device that delivers pain medication directly to the spinal fluid. Common medications used in pumps include baclofen or morphine. The pumps deliver medications at higher dosages than possible with oral medications.

Surgery

Surgery may be offered for various pain locations such as back, neck, knee, shoulder, or ankle. Surgery for chronic pain is usually considered only after conservative treatments have failed or if seen as medically necessary. Individuals who have undergone one or more unsuccessful back surgeries may receive the diagnosis or label of "failed back syndrome" or "failed back surgery syndrome." Causes for failure of surgery vary but the results can lead to frustration and distrust of medical providers, increased depression, and increased perceptions of disability.

Chapter 53

Surgical Procedures for Pain Relief

Chapter Contents

Section 53.1

Types of Back Surgery

This section includes text excerpted from "Handout on
Health: Back Pain," National Institute of Arthritis and
Musculoskeletal and Skin Diseases (NIAMS), August 2016.

Surgical Treatments

Depending on the diagnosis, surgery may either be the first treatment of choice—although this is rare—or it is reserved for chronic back pain for which other treatments have failed. If you are in constant pain or if pain reoccurs frequently and interferes with your ability to sleep, to function at your job, or to perform daily activities, you may be a candidate for surgery.

Some of the diagnoses that may need surgery include:

Herniated disks: In this potentially painful problem, the hard outer coating of the disks, which are the circular pieces of connective tissue that cushion the bones of the spine, are damaged, allowing the disks' jelly-like center to leak, irritating nearby nerves. This causes severe sciatica and nerve pain down the leg. A herniated disk is sometimes called a ruptured disk.

Spinal stenosis: Spinal stenosis is the narrowing of the spinal canal, through which the spinal cord and spinal nerves run. It is often caused by the overgrowth of bone caused by osteoarthritis of the spine. Compression of the nerves caused by spinal stenosis can lead not only to pain, but also to numbness in the legs and the loss of bladder or bowel control. Patients may have difficulty walking any distance and may have severe pain in their legs along with numbness and tingling.

Spondylolisthesis: In this condition, a vertebra of the lumbar spine slips out of place. As the spine tries to stabilize itself, the joints between the slipped vertebra and adjacent vertebrae can become enlarged, pinching nerves as they exit the spinal column. Spondylolisthesis may cause not only low back pain but also severe sciatica leg pain.

Vertebral fractures: These fractures are caused by trauma to the vertebrae of the spine or by crumbling of the vertebrae resulting from osteoporosis. This causes mostly mechanical back pain, but it may also put pressure on the nerves, creating leg pain.

Diskogenic low back pain (degenerative disk disease): Most people's disks degenerate over a lifetime, but in some, this aging process can become chronically painful, severely interfering with their quality of life.

Following are some of the most commonly performed back surgeries:

Surgical Treatments for Herniated Disks

Laminectomy/diskectomy: In this operation, part of the lamina, a portion of the bone on the back of the vertebrae, is removed, as well as a portion of a ligament. The herniated disk is then removed through the incision, which may extend two or more inches.

Microdiskectomy: As with traditional diskectomy, this procedure involves removing a herniated disk or damaged portion of a disk through an incision in the back. The difference is that the incision is much smaller and the doctor uses a magnifying microscope or lenses to locate the disk through the incision. The smaller incision may reduce pain and the disruption of tissues, and it reduces the size of the surgical scar.

Laser surgery: Technological advances in recent decades have led to the use of lasers for operating on patients with herniated disks accompanied by lower back and leg pain. During this procedure, the surgeon inserts a needle in the disk that delivers a few bursts of laser energy to vaporize the tissue in the disk. This reduces its size and relieves pressure on the nerves. Although many patients return to daily activities within 3 to 5 days after laser surgery, pain relief may not be apparent until several weeks or even months after the surgery. The usefulness of laser diskectomy is still being debated.

For Spinal Stenosis

Laminectomy: When narrowing of the spine compresses the nerve roots, causing pain or affecting sensation, doctors sometimes open up the spinal column with a procedure called a laminectomy. In a laminectomy, the doctor makes a large incision down the affected area of the spine and removes the lamina and any bone spurs, which are overgrowths of bone that may have formed in the spinal canal as the result of osteoarthritis. The procedure is major surgery that requires a short hospital stay and physical therapy afterwards to help regain strength and mobility.

For Spondylolisthesis

Spinal fusion: When a slipped vertebra leads to the enlargement of adjacent facet joints, surgical treatment generally involves both laminectomy (as described above) and spinal fusion. In spinal fusion, two or more vertebrae are joined together using bone grafts, screws, and rods to stop slippage of the affected vertebrae. Bone used for grafting comes from another area of the body, usually the hip or pelvis. In some cases, donor bone is used.

Although the surgery is generally successful, either type of graft has its drawbacks. Using your own bone means surgery at a second site on your body. With donor bone, there is a slight risk of disease transmission or tissue rejection, which happens when your immune system attacks the donor tissue. In recent years, a new development has eliminated those risks for some people undergoing spinal fusion: proteins called bone morphogenic proteins are being used to stimulate bone generation, eliminating the need for grafts. The proteins are placed in the affected area of the spine, often in collagen putty or sponges.

Regardless of how spinal fusion is performed, the fused area of the spine becomes immobilized.

For Vertebral Osteoporotic Fractures

Vertebroplasty: When back pain is caused by a compression fracture of a vertebra caused by osteoporosis or trauma, doctors may make a small incision in the skin over the affected area and inject a cement-like mixture called polymethylacrylate into the fractured vertebra to relieve pain and stabilize the spine.[3] The procedure is generally performed on an outpatient basis under a mild anesthetic.

Kyphoplasty: Much like vertebroplasty, kyphoplasty is used to relieve pain and stabilize the spine following fractures caused by osteoporosis. Kyphoplasty is a twostep process. In the first step, the doctor inserts a balloon device to help restore the height and shape of the spine. In the second step, he or she injects polymethylacrylate to repair the fractured vertebra. The procedure is done under anesthesia, and in some cases it is performed on an outpatient basis.

For Diskogenic Low Back Pain (Degenerative Disk Disease)

Intradiskal electrothermal therapy (IDET): One of the least invasive therapies for low back pain involves inserting a heating wire through a small incision in the back and into a disk. An electrical current is then passed through the wire to strengthen the collagen fibers that hold the disk together. The procedure is done on an outpatient basis, often under local anesthesia. The effectiveness of IDET is not clear.

Spinal fusion: When the degenerated disk is painful, the surgeon may recommend removing it and fusing the disk to help with the pain. This fusion can be done through the abdomen, a procedure known as anterior lumbar interbody fusion, or through the back, called posterior fusion. Fusion for low back pain or any spinal surgeries should only be done as a last resort, and the patient should be fully informed of risks.

Disk replacement: When a disk is herniated, one alternative to a diskectomy, in which the disk is simply removed, is removing the disk and replacing it with a synthetic disk. Replacing the damaged one with an artificial one restores disk height and movement between the vertebrae. Artificial disks come in several designs.

Section 53.2

Minimally Invasive Spine Surgery

This section contains text excerpted from the following sources: Text in this section begins with excerpts from "Summary: Position Statement for Endoscopic Discectomy," Centers for Medicare and Medicaid Services (CMS), n.d. Reviewed June 2017; Text beginning with the heading "Surgical Treatments for Herniated Disks" is excerpted from "Handout on Health: Back Pain," National Institute of Arthritis and Musculoskeletal and Skin Diseases (NIAMS), August 2016.

Conventional spine surgery has been associated with good results but the innate invasiveness associated with surgery, even microsurgery may result in significant tissue damage. Surgical techniques may be associated with blood loss; risks related to general anesthesia (especially in the elderly), failed back surgery syndrome (FBSS); soft tissue scarring, bone resection; and iatrogenic instability. Additionally, the amount of tissue damage also relates to the amount of postoperative pain and speed of recovery. While microsurgical techniques have reduced damage to the tissues, they too are associated with more trauma than less invasive approaches such as full endoscopic transforaminal and interlaminar lumbar discectomy. The length of the incision and the amount of muscle damage will contribute to the amount of blood loss, the amount of postoperative pain (and the need for pain medications). It will also affect the time that is required for healing and recovery, and return to work and everyday activities.

Clinical Equivalence of Open Surgical and Full Endoscopic Approaches

Physicians who perform endoscopic procedures take the position that, except for the approach, they are accomplishing the exact same surgical goal as those surgeons practicing open techniques. For example, they are removing the same fragment of herniated nucleus with an endoscope as other surgeons would with a microdiscectomy procedure. The only difference is that the surgeon performing a full endoscopic procedure makes a very small incision and accesses the anatomy through a 7mm working sleeve causing minimal trauma to the patient. By contrast, a surgeon performing a microdiscectomy will make a 20mm, or larger, incision, and likely cut muscles, bone and ligaments to reach and remove the same herniation, in order to achieve the same decompression of the nerve.

Advantages of Full Endoscopic Techniques

Further, in the literature and in surgeons' experience, the full endoscopic techniques have demonstrated clinical outcomes equivalent to microdiscectomy, and have demonstrated several advantages over microdiscectomy:

- Smaller incision with less soft tissue damage and less scar tissue formation
- Less bone and ligament resection
- Less intracanal disruption and epidural fibrosis
- Less postoperative pain, and less need for pain medication

- Faster recovery and earlier return to work and ADLs
- Fewer surgical complications
- Visualizes anatomy not visible with a microscope (endoscope "sees around corners")
- Less operative blood loss
- Shorter operating time
- Does not require general anesthesia
- Feedback from awake patient helps monitor for neurological complications

Surgical Treatments for Herniated Disks

Microdiskectomy

As with traditional diskectomy, this procedure involves removing a herniated disk or damaged portion of a disk through an incision in the back. The difference is that the incision is much smaller and the doctor uses a magnifying microscope or lenses to locate the disk through the incision. The smaller incision may reduce pain and the disruption of tissues, and it reduces the size of the surgical scar.

Vertebroplasty

When back pain is caused by a compression fracture of a vertebra caused by osteoporosis or trauma, doctors may make a small incision in the skin over the affected area and inject a cement-like mixture called polymethylacrylate into the fractured vertebra to relieve pain and stabilize the spine. The procedure is generally performed on an outpatient basis under a mild anesthetic.

Intradiskal electrothermal therapy (IDET)

One of the least invasive therapies for low back pain involves inserting a heating wire through a small incision in the back and into a disk. An electrical current is then passed through the wire to strengthen the collagen fibers that hold the disk together. The procedure is done on an outpatient basis, often under local anesthesia.

Foraminotomy*

Foraminotomy is an operation that "cleans out" or enlarges the bony hole (foramen) where a nerve root exits the spinal canal. Bulging discs or joints thickened with age can cause narrowing of the space through which the spinal nerve exits and can press on the nerve, resulting in pain, numbness, and weakness in an arm or leg. Small pieces of bone over the nerve are removed through a small slit, allowing the surgeon to cut away the blockage and relieve pressure on the nerve.

(*Source: "Low Back Pain Fact Sheet," National Institute of Neurological Disorders and Stroke (NINDS), December 2014.)

Section 53.3

Nerve Blocks, Traction, and TENS

This section includes text excerpted from "Managing
Pain from a Broken Hip: A Guide for Adults and Their
Caregivers," Agency for Healthcare Research and Quality (AHRQ),
U.S. Department of Health and Human Services (HHS),
May 17, 2011. Reviewed June 2017.

Nerve Blocks

What Is a Nerve Block?

A nerve block uses a medicine called an "anesthetic" to numb the nerves so that you do not feel pain for a little while. Anesthetics are the same kind of medicine dentists use to numb teeth and gums. The nerve block will make a part of your body numb for a little while.

Your doctor might use a nerve block to help ease your pain if you cannot take medicines like nonsteroidal antiinflammatory drugs (NSAIDs) or opioids. Nerve blocks may be used before, during, or after an operation.

There are many types of nerve blocks. They are named for the part of the body where the doctor injects the anesthetic. Your doctor (or anesthesiologist or nurse anesthetist) may inject these medicines into more than one place in your body to give you the most pain relief. For a broken hip, injections are often given around the hip and groin area.

What Are the Benefits of Using a Nerve Block?

Some research shows that nerve blocks used before, during, or after an operation may ease short-term pain more than the usual treatment of opioid or NSAID pain medication. Nerve blocks may help you avoid "delirium," or confusion and cloudy thinking, which can be caused by pain or by opioid pain medicines.

Are There Any Side Effects from Using a Nerve Block?

Researchers cannot say if nerve blocks cause more or less side effects than other treatments for the pain from a broken hip.

Traction

Traction is a treatment where a part of the body is pulled into a certain position. Traction is usually used before an operation.

There have been only a few studies on traction. They show that traction before an operation does not help relieve pain more than using pain medicines alone, but there is not enough research to know for sure.

Traction may be needed for reasons other than pain.

Researchers do not know if using both traction and medicines for pain increases your risks of serious side effects compared to taking only medicines.

Acupressure, Muscle-Relaxation Therapy, and Neurostimulation (TENS)

Although some studies show that these methods might help, there is not enough research to say if these options can lessen pain from a broken hip. These therapies can be used before or after an operation.

What Is Acupressure?

"Acupressure" is when a trained therapist presses on specific parts of the body to relieve pain in other body parts.

What Is Muscle-Relaxation Therapy?

"Muscle-relaxation therapy" involves breathing and relaxation routines to reduce muscle tension.

What Is Neurostimulation?

"Neurostimulation," also known as "TENS," involves giving small amounts of electricity to excite the nerves around the painful area.

Will Acupressure, Muscle-Relaxation Therapy, or TENS Help Relieve My Pain?

Doctors do not know if the pain from your broken hip will be improved or relieved by acupressure, relaxation therapy, or TENS more than by medicines like opioid and NSAID medicines.

What Are the Risks of Acupressure, Muscle-Relaxation Therapy, and TENS?

There is not enough research to say if these options have any risks or can cause any side effects for people with a broken hip.

Section 53.4

Joint Replacement Surgery

This section includes text excerpted from "Joint Replacement Surgery: Health Information Basics for You and Your Family," National Institute of Arthritis and Musculoskeletal and Skin Diseases (NIAMS), August 2016.

What Is Joint Replacement Surgery?

Joint replacement surgery is removing a damaged joint and putting in a new one. A joint is where two or more bones come together, like the knee, hip, and shoulder. The surgery is usually done by a doctor called an orthopaedic surgeon. Sometimes, the surgeon will not remove the whole joint, but will only replace or fix the damaged parts.

The doctor may suggest a joint replacement to improve how you live. Replacing a joint can relieve pain and help you move and feel better. Hips and knees are replaced most often. Other joints that can be replaced include the shoulders, fingers, ankles, and elbows.

What Can Happen to My Joints?

Joints can be damaged by arthritis and other diseases, injuries, or other causes. Arthritis or simply years of use may cause the joint to wear away. This can cause pain, stiffness, and swelling. Diseases and damage inside a joint can limit blood flow, causing problems in the bones, which needs blood to be healthy, grow, and repair themselves.

What Is a New Joint Like?

A new joint, called a prosthesis, can be made of plastic, metal, or ceramic parts. It may be cemented into place or not cemented, so that your bone will grow into it. Both methods may be combined to keep the new joint in place.

A cemented joint is used more often in older people who do not move around as much and in people with "weak" bones. The cement holds the new joint to the bone. An uncemented joint is often recommended for younger, more active people and those with good bone quality. It may take longer to heal, because it takes longer for bone to grow and attach to it.

New joints generally last at least 10 to 15 years. Therefore, younger patients may need to have the same damaged joint replaced more than once.

Do Many People Have Joints Replaced?

Joint replacement is becoming more common. More than 1 million Americans have a hip or knee replaced each year. Research has shown that even if you are older, joint replacement can help you move around and feel better.

Any surgery has risks. Risks of joint surgery will depend on your health of your joints before surgery and the type of surgery done. Many hospitals and doctors have been replacing joints for several decades, and this experience results in better patient outcomes. For answers to their questions, some people talk with their doctor or someone who has had the surgery. A doctor specializing in joints will probably work with you before, during, and after surgery to make sure you heal quickly and recover successfully.

Do I Need to Have My Joint Replaced?

Only a doctor can tell if you need a joint replaced. He or she will look at your joint with an X-ray machine or another machine. The doctor may put a small, lighted tube (arthroscope) into your joint to look for damage. A small sample of your tissue could also be tested.

After looking at your joint, the doctor may say that you should consider exercise, walking aids such as braces or canes, physical therapy, or medicines and vitamin supplements. Medicines for arthritis include drugs that reduce inflammation. Depending on the type of arthritis, the doctor may prescribe corticosteroids or other drugs.

However, all drugs may cause side effects, including bone loss.

If these treatments do not work, the doctor may suggest an operation called an osteotomy, where the surgeon "aligns" the joint. Here, the surgeon cuts the bone or bones around the joint to improve alignment. This may be simpler than replacing a joint, but it may take longer to recover. However, this operation has become less common.

Joint replacement is often the answer if you have constant pain and can't move the joint well—for example, if you have trouble with things such as walking, climbing stairs, and taking a bath.

What Happens during Surgery?

First, the surgical team will give you medicine so you won't feel pain (anesthesia). The medicine may block the pain only in one part of the body (regional), or it may put your whole body to sleep (general). The team will then replace the damaged joint with a new man-made joint.

Each surgery is different. How long it takes depends on how badly the joint is damaged and how the surgery is done. To replace a knee or a hip takes about 2 hours or less, unless there are complicating factors. After surgery, you will be moved to a recovery room for 1 to 2 hours until you are fully awake or the numbness goes away.

What Happens after Surgery?

With knee or hip surgery, you will probably need to stay in the hospital for a few days. If you are elderly or have additional disabilities, you may then need to spend several weeks in an intermediate-care facility before going home. You and your team of doctors will determine how long you stay in the hospital.

After hip or knee replacement, you will often stand or begin walking the day of surgery. At first, you will walk with a walker or crutches. You may have some temporary pain in the new joint because your muscles are weak from not being used. Also, your body is healing. The pain can be helped with medicines and should end in a few weeks or months.

Physical therapy can begin the day after surgery to help strengthen the muscles around the new joint and help you regain motion in the joint. If you have your shoulder joint replaced, you can usually begin exercising the same day of your surgery! A physical therapist will help you with gentle, range-of-motion exercises. Before you leave the hospital, your therapist will show you how to use a pulley device to help bend and extend your arm.

Will My Surgery Be Successful?

The success of your surgery depends a lot on what you do when you go home. Follow your doctor's advice about what to eat, what medicines to take, and how to exercise. Talk with your doctor about any pain or trouble moving.

Joint replacement is usually a success in most people who have it. When problems do occur, most are treatable. Possible problems include:

- **Infection.** Areas in the wound or around the new joint may get infected. It may happen while you're still in the hospital or after you go home. It may even occur years later. Minor infections in the wound are usually treated with drugs. Deep infections may need a second operation to treat the infection or replace the joint.

- **Blood clots.** If your blood moves too slowly, it may begin to form lumps of blood parts called clots. If pain and swelling develop in your legs after hip or knee surgery, blood clots may be the cause. The doctor may suggest drugs to make your blood thin or special stockings, exercises, or boots to help your blood move faster. If swelling, redness, or pain occurs in your leg after you leave the hospital, contact your doctor right away.

- **Loosening.** The new joint may loosen, causing pain. If the loosening is bad, you may need another operation to reattach the joint to the bone.

- **Dislocation.** Sometimes after hip or other joint replacement, the ball of the prosthesis can come out of its socket. In most cases, the hip can be corrected without surgery. A brace may be worn for a while if a dislocation occurs.

- **Wear.** Some wear can be found in all joint replacements. Too much wear may help cause loosening. The doctor may need to operate again if the prosthesis comes loose. Sometimes, the

681

plastic can wear thin, and the doctor may just replace the plastic and not the whole joint.

- **Nerve and blood vessel injury.** Nerves near the replaced joint may be damaged during surgery, but this does not happen often. Over time, the damage often improves and may disappear. Blood vessels may also be injured.

As you move your new joint and let your muscles grow strong again, pain will lessen, flexibility will increase, and movement will improve.

Section 53.5

Hip Replacement Surgery

This section includes text excerpted from "Questions and Answers about Hip Replacement," National Institute of Arthritis and Musculoskeletal and Skin Diseases (NIAMS), July 2016.

What Is a Hip Replacement?

Hip replacement, or arthroplasty, is a surgical procedure in which the diseased parts of the hip joint are removed and replaced with new, artificial parts. These artificial parts are called the prosthesis. The goals of hip replacement surgery include increasing mobility, improving the function of the hip joint, and relieving pain. According to the Centers for Disease Control and Prevention (CDC), 332,000 total hip replacements are performed in the United States each year.

Who Should Have Hip Replacement Surgery?

People with hip joint damage that causes pain and interferes with daily activities despite treatment may be candidates for hip replacement surgery. Osteoarthritis is the most common cause of this type of damage. However, other conditions, such as rheumatoid arthritis (a chronic inflammatory disease that causes joint pain, stiffness, and swelling), osteonecrosis (or avascular necrosis, which is the death of bone caused by insufficient blood supply), injury, fracture, and bone tumors also may lead to breakdown of the hip joint and the need for hip replacement surgery.

In the past, doctors reserved hip replacement surgery primarily for people over 60 years of age. The thinking was that older people typically are less active and put less stress on the artificial hip than do younger people. In more recent years, however, doctors have found that hip replacement surgery can be very successful in younger people as well. New technology has improved the artificial parts, allowing them to withstand more stress and strain and last longer.

Today, a person's overall health and activity level are more important than age in predicting a hip replacement's success. Hip replacement may be problematic for people with some health problems, regardless of their age. For example, people who have chronic disorders such as Parkinson disease, or conditions that result in severe muscle weakness, are more likely than people without chronic diseases to damage or dislocate an artificial hip. People who are at high risk for infections or in poor health are less likely to recover successfully. Therefore, they may not be good candidates for this surgery. Recent studies also suggest that people who elect to have surgery before advanced joint deterioration occurs tend to recover more easily and have better outcomes.

What Are Alternatives to Hip Replacement?

Before considering a total hip replacement, the doctor may try other methods of treatment, such as exercise, walking aids, and medication. An exercise program can strengthen the muscles around the hip joint. Walking aids such as canes and walkers may alleviate some of the stress from painful, damaged hips and help you to avoid or delay surgery.

All medicines can have side effects. Some side effects may be more severe than others. You should review the package insert that comes with your medicine and ask your healthcare provider or pharmacist if you have any questions about the possible side effects.

If exercise and medication do not relieve pain and improve joint function, the doctor may suggest a less complex corrective surgery before proceeding to hip replacement. One common alternative to hip replacement is an osteotomy. This procedure involves cutting and realigning bone, to shift the weight from a damaged and painful bone surface to a healthier one. Recovery from an osteotomy takes several months. Afterward, the function of the hip joint may continue to worsen and additional treatment may be needed. The length of time before another surgery is needed varies greatly and depends on the condition of the joint before the procedure.

What Does Hip Replacement Surgery Involve?

The hip joint is located where the upper end of the femur, or thigh bone, meets the pelvis, or hip bone. A ball at the end of the femur, called the femoral head, fits in a socket (the acetabulum) in the pelvis to allow a wide range of motion.

During a traditional hip replacement, which lasts from 1 to 2 hours, the surgeon makes a 6- to 8-inch incision over the side of the hip through the muscles and removes the diseased bone tissue and cartilage from the hip joint, while leaving the healthy parts of the joint intact. Then the surgeon replaces the head of the femur and acetabulum with new, artificial parts. The new hip is made of materials that allow a natural gliding motion of the joint.

Some surgeons perform what is called a minimally invasive, or mini-incision, hip replacement, which requires smaller incisions and a shorter recovery time than traditional hip replacement. Candidates for this type of surgery are usually age 50 or younger, of normal weight based on body mass index, and healthier than candidates for traditional surgery. Joint resurfacing is also being used.

Regardless of whether you have traditional or minimally invasive surgery, the parts used to replace the joint are the same and come in two general varieties: cemented and uncemented.

Cemented parts are fastened to existing, healthy bone with a special glue or cement. Hip replacement using these parts is referred to as a "cemented" procedure. Uncemented parts rely on a process called biologic fixation, which holds them in place. This means that the parts are made with a porous surface that allows your own bone to grow into the pores and hold the new parts in place. Sometimes a doctor will use a cemented femur part and uncemented acetabular part. This combination is referred to as a hybrid replacement.

Is a Cemented or Uncemented Prosthesis Better?

The answer to this question is different for different people. Because each person's condition is unique, the doctor and you must weigh the advantages and disadvantages.

Cemented replacements are more frequently used for older, less active people and people with weak bones, such as those who have osteoporosis, while uncemented replacements are more frequently used for younger, more active people.

Studies show that cemented and uncemented prostheses have comparable rates of success. Studies also indicate that if you need an additional hip replacement, or revision, the rates of success for cemented and uncemented prostheses are comparable. However, more long-term data are available in the United States for hip replacements with cemented prostheses, because doctors have been using them here since the late 1960s, whereas uncemented prostheses were not introduced until the late 1970s.

The primary disadvantage of an uncemented prosthesis is the extended recovery period. Because it takes a long time for the natural bone to grow and attach to the prosthesis, a person with uncemented replacements must limit activities for up to 3 months to protect the hip joint. Also, it is more common for someone with an uncemented prosthesis to experience thigh pain in the months following the surgery, while the bone is growing into the prosthesis.

What Can Be Expected Immediately after Surgery?

You will be allowed only limited movement immediately after hip replacement surgery. When you are in bed, pillows or a special device are usually used to brace the hip in the correct position. You may receive fluids through an intravenous tube to replace fluids lost during surgery. There also may be a tube located near the incision to drain fluid, and a type of tube called a catheter may be used to drain urine until you are able to use the bathroom. The doctor will prescribe medicine for pain or discomfort.

On the day after surgery or sometimes on the day of surgery, therapists will teach you exercises to improve recovery. A respiratory therapist may ask you to breathe deeply, cough, or blow into a simple device that measures lung capacity. These exercises reduce the collection of fluid in the lungs after surgery.

As early as 1 to 2 days after surgery, you may be able to sit on the edge of the bed, stand, and even walk with assistance. While you are still in the hospital, a physical therapist may teach you exercises such as contracting and relaxing certain muscles, which can strengthen the hip. Because the new, artificial hip has a more limited range of movement than a natural, healthy hip, the physical therapist also will teach you the proper techniques for simple activities of daily living, such as bending and sitting, to prevent injury to your new hip.

How Long Are Recovery and Rehabilitation?

Usually, people do not spend more than 1 to 4 days in the hospital after hip replacement surgery. Full recovery from the surgery takes about 3 to 6 months, depending on the type of surgery, your overall health, and the success of your rehabilitation.

It is important to get instructions from your doctor before leaving the hospital and to follow them carefully once you get home. Doing so will you give you the greatest chance of a successful surgery.

What Are Possible Complications of Hip Replacement Surgery?

New technology and advances in surgical techniques have greatly reduced the risks involved with hip replacements.

The most common problem that may arise soon after hip replacement surgery is hip dislocation. Because the artificial ball and socket are smaller than the normal ones, the ball can become dislodged from the socket if the hip is placed in certain positions. The most dangerous position usually is pulling the knees up to the chest.

The most common later complication of hip replacement surgery is an inflammatory reaction to tiny particles that gradually wear off of the artificial joint surfaces and are absorbed by the surrounding tissues. The inflammation may trigger the action of special cells that eat away some of the bone, causing the implant to loosen. To treat this complication, the doctor may use anti-inflammatory medications or recommend revision surgery (replacement of an artificial joint). Medical scientists are experimenting with new materials that last longer and cause less inflammation. Less common complications of hip replacement surgery include infection, blood clots, and heterotopic bone formation (bone growth beyond the normal edges of bone).

To minimize the risk of complications, it's important to know how to prevent problems and to recognize signs of potential problems early and contact your doctor. For example, tenderness; redness and swelling of your calf; or swelling of your thigh, ankle, or foot could be warning signs of a possible blood clot. Warning signs of infection include fever, chills, tenderness and swelling, or drainage from the wound. You should call your doctor if you experience any of these symptoms.

When Is Revision Surgery Necessary?

Hip replacement is one of the most successful orthopaedic surgeries performed. However, because more people are having hip replacements at a younger age, and wearing away of the joint surface becomes a problem after 15 to 20 years, replacement of an artificial joint, which is also known as revision surgery, is becoming more common. It is more difficult than first-time hip replacement surgery, and the outcome is generally not as good, so it is important to explore all available options before having additional surgery.

Doctors consider revision surgery for two reasons: if medication and lifestyle changes do not relieve pain and disability, or if X-rays of the hip show damage to the bone around the artificial hip that must be corrected before it is too late for a successful revision. This surgery is usually considered only when bone loss, wearing of the joint surfaces, or joint loosening shows up on an X-ray. Other possible reasons for revision surgery include fracture, dislocation of the artificial parts, and infection.

What Types of Exercise Are Most Suitable for Someone with a Total Hip Replacement?

Proper exercise can reduce stiffness and increase flexibility and muscle strength. People who have an artificial hip should talk to their doctor or physical therapist about developing an appropriate exercise program. Most of these programs begin with safe range-of-motion activities and muscle-strengthening exercises. The doctor or therapist will decide when you can move on to more demanding activities. Many doctors recommend avoiding high-impact activities, such as basketball, jogging, and tennis. These activities can damage the new hip or cause loosening of its parts. Some recommended exercises are walking, stationary bicycling, swimming, and cross-country skiing. These exercises can increase muscle strength and cardiovascular fitness without injuring the new hip.

Chapter 54

Palliative Care

Chapter Contents

Section 54.1

Pediatric Palliative Care

This section includes text excerpted from "Pediatric
Palliative Care at a Glance," National Institute of
Nursing Research (NINR), November 2015.

A child's serious illness affects the entire family. Pediatric palliative
care can support everyone. It can help with many serious illnesses,
including genetic disorders, cancer, neurologic disorders, heart and
lung conditions, and others. Whether you are having difficulty managing your child's condition and care or simply want extra support,
palliative care can help.

What Is Pediatric Palliative Care?

Pediatric palliative care is supportive care for children with serious
illnesses and their families. It offers an added layer of support based
on your unique needs. Because you are the expert on your child and
family, palliative care provides services that you consider important.
It can help:

- Ease your child's pain and other symptoms

- Provide emotional support and reduce stress

- Address family concerns

- Communicate with health providers

- Coordinate care and appointments

- Explain complicated terms and care options

- Locate community resources to help your family

Many children need more than relief from symptoms. Palliative
care can also help your child:

- Understand a diagnosis

- Communicate effectively with doctors

- Cope with concerns about school and friends
- Receive services, like art or music therapy
- Find ways to relax and play

When Can Pediatric Palliative Care Start?

Palliative care can help children at any age or stage of a serious illness, from diagnosis forward. It is available at the same time as any other treatments doctors may prescribe and can begin as soon as your child needs it. Care for your child and family can begin when your child's healthcare provider refers you to palliative care services. The provider may suggest a referral, or you can request one.

How Does It Work?

Palliative care surrounds your family with a team of specialists who will listen to your needs and work together to meet them.

Every palliative care team is different. Your team may include:

- Doctors
- Nurses
- Child life specialists
- Respite providers
- Art and music therapists
- Chaplains
- Case managers
- Counselors
- Home health aides
- Social workers
- Nutritionists
- Pharmacists

Where Is Care Provided?

Palliative care can be provided in a hospital, during clinic visits, or at home. If palliative care starts in the hospital, your team can help your child make a successful move to your home or other healthcare setting. Depending on your child's condition and treatment, the care team may be able to find a nursing or community care agency to support care at home.

Who Pays for Palliative Care?

Many insurance plans cover palliative care. Ask your healthcare team to put you in touch with a social worker, case manager, or financial advisor at your hospital or clinic to learn about payment options.

What Next?

Talk to your loved ones, including your child, about how palliative care can support your family. Remember, even young children can express their needs and preferences. Talk to your child's healthcare provider. Prepare by writing down your family's questions about palliative care. It may also help to take notes during the conversation.

Section 54.2

Palliative Care for Adults

This section includes text excerpted from "Palliative Care,"
National Institute of Nursing Research (NINR),
May 2011. Reviewed June 2017.

Dealing with the symptoms of any painful or serious illness is difficult. However, special care is available to make you more comfortable right now. It's called palliative care. You receive palliative care at the same time that you're receiving treatments for your illness. Its primary purpose is to relieve the pain and other symptoms you are experiencing and improve your quality of life. Palliative care is a central part of treatment for serious or life threatening illnesses. The information in this section will help you understand how you or someone close to you can benefit from this type of care.

What Is Palliative Care?

Palliative care is comprehensive treatment of the discomfort, symptoms, and stress of serious illness. It does not replace your primary treatment; palliative care works together with the primary treatment you're receiving. The goal is to prevent and ease suffering and improve your quality of life.

If You Need Palliative Care, Does That Mean You're Dying?

The purpose of palliative care is to address distressing symptoms such as pain, breathing difficulties or nausea, among others. Receiving palliative care does not necessarily mean you're dying.

Palliative Care Gives You a Chance to Live Your Life More Comfortably

Palliative care provides relief from distressing symptoms including pain, shortness of breath, fatigue, constipation, nausea, loss of appetite, problems with sleep and many other symptoms. It can also help you deal with the side effects of the medical treatments you're receiving. Perhaps, most important, palliative care can help improve your quality of life.

Palliative care also provides support for you and your family and can improve communication between you and your healthcare providers. Palliative care strives to provide you with:

- Expert treatment of pain and other symptoms so you can get the best relief possible.

- Open discussion about treatment choices, including treatment for your disease and management of your symptoms.

- Coordination of your care with all of your healthcare providers.

- Emotional support for you and your family.

Palliative Care Can Be Very Effective

Researchers have studied the positive effects palliative care has on patients. Recent studies show that patients who receive palliative care report improvement in:

- Pain and other distressing symptoms, such as nausea or shortness of breath.

- Communication with their healthcare providers and family members.

- Emotional support.

Other studies also show that palliative care:

- Ensures that care is more in line with patients' wishes.

- Meets the emotional and spiritual needs of patients.

Palliative care is comprehensive care designed especially for your needs.

Palliative Care Is Different from Hospice Care

Palliative care is available to you at any time during your illness. Remember that you can receive palliative care at the same time you receive treatments that are meant to cure your illness. Its availability does not depend upon whether or not your condition can be cured. The goal is to make you as comfortable as possible and improve your quality of life.

You don't have to be in hospice or at the end of life to receive palliative care. People in hospice always receive palliative care, but hospice focuses on a person's final months of life. To qualify for some hospice programs, patients must no longer be receiving treatments to cure their illness.

Palliative Care Can Improve Your Quality of Life in a Variety of Ways

Together with your primary healthcare provider, your palliative care team combines vigorous pain and symptom control into every part of your treatment. Team members spend as much time with you and your family as it takes to help you fully understand your condition, care options, and other needs. They also make sure you make a smooth transition between the hospital and other services, such as home care or nursing facilities.

This results in well-planned, complete treatment for all your symptoms throughout your illness—treatment that takes care of you in your present condition and anticipates your future needs.

A Team Approach to Patient-Centered Care

Palliative care is provided by a team of specialists that may include:

- palliative care doctors

- palliative care nurses

- social workers

- chaplains

- pharmacists

- nutritionists

- counselors and others

Special Care That Supports You and Your Wishes

Palliative care supports you and those who love you by maximizing your comfort. It also helps you set goals for the future that lead to a meaningful, enjoyable life while you get treatment for your illness.

How Do You Know If You Need Palliative Care?

Many adults and children living with illnesses such as cancer, heart disease, lung disease, kidney failure, acquired immune deficiency syndrome (AIDS) and cystic fibrosis, among others, experience physical symptoms and emotional distress related to their diseases. Sometimes these symptoms are related to the medical treatments they are receiving.

You may want to consider palliative care if you or your loved one:

- Suffers from pain or other symptoms due to ANY serious illness.

- Experiences physical or emotional pain that is NOT under control.

- Needs help understanding your situation and coordinating your care.

Start Palliative Care as Soon as You Need It

It's never too early to start palliative care. In fact, palliative care occurs at the same time as all other treatments for your illness and does not depend upon the course of your disease.

There is no reason to wait. Serious illnesses and their treatments can cause exhaustion, anxiety and depression. Palliative care teams understand that pain and other symptoms affect your quality of life and can leave you lacking the energy or motivation to pursue the things you enjoy. They also know that the stress of what you're going through can have a big impact on your family. And they can assist you and your loved ones as you cope with the difficult experience.

Working Together as a Team

Patients who are considering palliative care often wonder how it will affect their relationships with their current healthcare providers. Some of their questions include:

- Will I have to give up my primary healthcare provider?

- What do I say if there is resistance to referring me for palliative care services?

- Will I offend my healthcare provider if I ask questions?

Most important, you do NOT give up your own healthcare provider in order to get palliative care. The palliative care team and your healthcare provider work together.

Most clinicians appreciate the extra time and information the palliative care team provides to their patients. Occasionally a clinician may not refer a patient for palliative care services. If this happens to you, ask for an explanation. Let your healthcare provider know why you think palliative care could help you.

Getting Palliative Care Is as Easy as Asking for It

In most cases, palliative care is provided in the hospital. The process begins when either your healthcare provider refers you to the palliative care team or you ask your healthcare provider for a referral. In the hospital, palliative care is provided by a team of professionals, including medical and nursing specialists, social workers, pharmacists, nutritionists, clergy and others.

Insurance Pays for Palliative Care

Most insurance plans cover all or part of the palliative care treatment you receive in the hospital, just as they would other services. Medicare and Medicaid also typically cover palliative care. If you have concerns about the cost of palliative care treatment, a social worker from the palliative care team can help you.

Frequently Asked Questions

What Happens When You Leave the Hospital?

When you leave the hospital, your palliative care team will help you make a successful move to your home, hospice or other healthcare setting.

If Morphine Is Prescribed, Will It Be Dangerous?

If you have an illness causing you pain that is not relieved by drugs such as acetaminophen or ibuprofen, the palliative care team may recommend trying stronger medicines such as morphine.

Simply stated, morphine is an opiate—a strong medicine for treating pain. Like other similar opiate medicines (hydrocodone, oxycodone), it provides safe and effective pain treatment. In fact, almost all pain can be relieved with morphine and similar strong drugs that are available today. So no one should suffer because they or their healthcare provider have concerns about morphine or other drugs in the opiate family.

If I Take Morphine, Will I Become Addicted?

In fact, very few people who use opiates for pain relief ever become addicted or dependent on these medicines. However, it is important to be aware that anyone taking opiates for more than two weeks should not stop doing so abruptly. You should ask your healthcare provider about gradually reducing your dose so that your body is able to adjust.

There is no reason to wait until your pain is unbearable before you begin taking morphine. As your pain increases, your morphine dose can be safely increased to provide the relief you need over time. All opiates can cause nausea, drowsiness and constipation. However, as your body adjusts to the medicine, side effects will generally decrease. Also, side effects such as constipation can easily be managed.

As always, if you have concerns about taking these or any medications, talk to your palliative care team. They can tell you about how various medications work, what their side effects are and how to get the most effective pain relief.

Don't Wait to Get the Help You Deserve. Ask for Palliative Care and Start Feeling Better Now

If you think you need palliative care, ask for it now. Tell your healthcare provider that you'd like to add palliative care specialists to your treatment team and request a consultation.

Chapter 55

Multidisciplinary Pain Management Programs

Chronic pain affects millions of Americans, seriously impacting their quality of life and costing billions of dollars every year in healthcare expenditures and lost productivity. There are currently no definitive cures for the most prevalent chronic pain syndromes. Multidisciplinary Pain Programs (MPPs) follow a model of care that emphasizes, when pain cannot be successfully eliminated, managing the pain to the extent that the patient's independence is restored and overall quality of life improved.

Medical Practice as Related to Management of Chronic Pain

Chronic pain is neither adaptive nor self-limited. By definition, chronic pain has continued past its usefulness—it continues to encourage rest and limits on movement when those limitations impair healing. It persists long enough that the patient may find that side effects and dependence on opioid painkillers limit quality of life. The pain is no longer a signal of new or impending tissue damage—it becomes a disease in itself, sometimes even after the original physical abnormalities

---

This chapter includes text excerpted from "Multidisciplinary Pain Programs for Chronic Noncancer Pain," Agency for Healthcare Research and Quality (AHRQ), September 2011. Reviewed June 2017.

are resolved. Chronic pain that continues after the apparent cause is gone is now thought to be a biopsychosocial phenomenon. Though no one knows exactly how the progression happens, it is thought to be influenced by factors such as acute pain intensity, depressive symptoms, and past trauma or stressful life events.

The progression from acute to chronic pain is common: over 40 percent of people presenting in primary care for pain continue to experience pain a year later. In the case of one disorder—low-back pain— approximately 90 percent of sufferers recover within 3 to 6 months, leaving 10 percent experiencing chronic pain; the majority of those still experiencing pain after 6 months remain disabled after 1 and 2 years.

Multidisciplinary Pain Program

When chronic pain does not fully respond to treatment, patients may be referred to a comprehensive treatment program such as an MPP, if one is available. However, not all chronic pain conditions follow this pattern of acute progressing to chronic pain. Fibromyalgia and some headache syndromes, for example, are not thought to be preceded by a musculoskeletal trauma or other acute event. Even so, these conditions are similar to other chronic pain conditions: they are characterized by patients exhausting more traditional forms of pain treatment, and their prognoses are believed to be influenced by psychological and social factors; for these reasons, conditions like fibromyalgia and chronic headache are believed to be amenable to treatment in the MPP model.

There are currently no definitive cures for the most prevalent chronic pain syndromes, such as back pain, peripheral neuropathies, etc. The goal of chronic pain treatment has evolved from eliminating pain to managing pain to an extent that the patient's physical and emotional functioning is restored and overall quality of life improved. This is the model of care provided by the MPP. There is no single protocol for treatment provided in MPPs, but there is general agreement on some included methods. In addition, and in contrast to other types of pain treatment clinics, MPPs provide interdisciplinary care: providers from each of the components work together to develop the treatment plan.

Components of a Multidisciplinary Pain Program

- Medical therapy
- Responsible for patient's physical wellbeing

700

- Manage medications
- Educational component may be included with medical component (but research study must explicitly state this: e.g., neurophysiology education)
- Behavioral therapy
- Responsible for psychosocial aspects of patients' care
- Cognitive behavioral therapy (CBT)
- Operant behavioral therapy (OBT)
- Stress management training
- Relaxation, progressive muscle relaxation
- Biofeedback
- Comorbidity diagnosis and treatment
- Help patient unlearn maladaptive responses to pain
- Problem solving
- Individual or group psychotherapy
- Educational component is often included with behavioral (but research study must explicitly state this)
- Physical reconditioning
- Physical therapy (PT) and/or occupational therapy (OT)
- Graduated activity exposure (pacing) enabling patients to control exacerbations in pain by learning to regulate the activity and, once a regime of paced activity is established, to gradually increase their activity level
- Graded therapeutic exercises to safely increase functioning (e.g., flexibility, range of motion, posture, body mechanics, ambulation, gait training, core strength/stability, cardiovascular fitness)
- Passive modes (e.g., ultrasound, electrical stimulation, massage) are generally avoided in MPP and focus is teaching patients independent management of pain
- Stretching and strengthening emphasized
- Job analysis and reconditioning
- Educational component is often included with physical reconditioning (but research study must explicitly state this), e.g., back education

- Education

- Improved self management is the focus

- Educational component is sometimes integrated with one or more other components (e.g., by psychologist with behavioral component, by nurse with medical component, by PT with physical reconditioning component)

- Back education

- Home exercise training

- Ergonomic training

- Neurophysiology education provided by a physician or nurse

Other Treatments

Other treatments for chronic pain include partial MPPs, which have some but not all of the components, and procedure-based practices, including such interventions as nerve blocks, discectomy, etc. Though the MPP is often seen as the last resort for intractable pain, it is fundamentally a conservative treatment: other treatments are not necessarily more safe or more effective. Many patients have already exhausted other procedures and less intensive treatment options when they come to the MPP. Even if a patient has not responded to the components when presented separately, advocates of MPP treatment note that there is additional value to providing all four treatment components at once.

Advantages of Integrated Treatment

The MPP is thought to improve on unimodal treatments by simultaneously addressing the multiple influences on chronic pain in the biopsychosocial model. It is also a conservative treatment option that causes few if any adverse effects, especially when compared to surgery or long-term opioid therapy.

Part Five

Additional Help and Information

Chapter 56

Terms Related to Pain and Pain Management

abuse: When another person does something on purpose that causes you mental or physical harm or pain.

acetaminophen: The basic ingredient found in Tylenol® and its many generic equivalents. It is sold over-the-counter, in a prescription-strength preparation, and in combination with codeine (also by prescription).

acupuncture: A form of complementary and alternative medicine that involves inserting thin needles through the skin at specific points on the body to control pain and other symptoms.

anesthesia: The use of medicine to prevent the feeling of pain or another sensation during surgery or other procedures that might be painful.

anesthetic: An agent that causes insensitivity to pain and is used for surgeries and other medical procedures.

angina: A recurring pain or discomfort in the chest that happens when some part of the heart does not receive enough blood. It is a common symptom of coronary heart disease, which occurs when vessels that carry blood to the heart become narrowed and blocked due to atherosclerosis.

This glossary contains terms excerpted from documents produced by several sources deemed reliable.

anticonvulsants: Used to treat seizure disorders because they dampen abnormally fast electrical impulses. They also sometimes are prescribed to treat pain.

anxiety: Fear and anxiety are part of life. You may feel anxious before you take a test or walk down a dark street. This kind of anxiety is useful-it can make you more alert or careful. It usually ends soon after you are out of the situation that caused it. But for millions of people in the United States, the anxiety does not go away, and gets worse over time. They may have chest pains or nightmares. They may even be afraid to leave home.

aromatherapy: A form of complementary and alternative medicine in which the scent of essential oils from flowers, herbs, and trees is inhaled to promote health and well-being.

arthritis: Swelling, redness, warmth, and pain of the joints, the places where two bones meet, such as the elbow or knee. There are more than 100 types of arthritis.

aspirin: May be the most widely used pain-relief agent and has been sold over-the-counter since 1905 as a treatment for fever, headache, and muscle soreness.

bacterial vaginosis: The most common vaginal infection in women of childbearing age, which happens when the normal bacteria (germs) in the vagina get out of balance, such as from douching or from sexual contact.

betablocker: A type of drug that is used to lower blood pressure, treat chest pain (angina) and heart failure, and to help prevent a heart attack.

cannabinoids: Chemicals that bind to cannabinoid receptors in the brain. They are found naturally in the brain (anandamide) and are also chemicals found in marijuana (for example, THC and CBD).

capsaicin: A chemical found in chili peppers that is also a primary ingredient in prescription or over-the-counter pain-relieving creams available as a treatment for a number of pain conditions, such as shingles.

chickenpox: A disease caused by the varicella-zoster virus, which results in a blister-like rash, itching, tiredness, and fever.

chiropractic: An alternative medical system that takes a different approach from standard medicine in treating health problems.

Chiropractic professionals use a type of hands-on therapy called spinal manipulation or adjustment.

chlamydia: A common sexually transmitted disease (STD). Most people have no symptoms, but chlamydia can cause serious damage a women's reproductive organs. When a woman does have symptoms, they may include thin vaginal discharge and other symptoms similar to gonorrhea like burning when urinating. Long-term irritation may cause lower abdominal pain, inflammation of the pelvic organs, and pelvic inflammatory disease (PID).

chronic fatigue syndrome: A complex disorder characterized by extreme fatigue that lasts six months or longer, and does not improve with rest or is worsened by physical or mental activity. Other symptoms can include weakness, muscle pain, impaired memory and/or mental concentration, and insomnia. The cause is unknown.

cognitive-behavioral therapy: Well-established treatment for pain that involves helping the person improve coping skills, address negative thoughts and emotions that can amplify pain, and learn relaxation methods to help prepare for and cope with pain. It is used for chronic pain, postoperative pain, cancer pain, and the pain of childbirth. Many clinical studies provide evidence for the effectiveness of this form of treatment in pain management.

Crohn's disease: chronic medical condition characterized by inflammation of the bowel. Symptoms include abdominal pain, diarrhea, fever, loss of appetite and weight loss. The cause of Crohn's disease is not yet known, but genetic, dietary and infectious factors may play a part.

deep brain (or intracerebral) stimulation: Considered a more extreme treatment and involves surgical stimulation of the brain, usually the thalamus or motor cortex. It is used to treat chronic pain in cases that do not respond to less invasive or conservative treatments.

discectomy: A procedure in which an entire vertebral disc is removed by a surgeon; when microsurgical techniques are used it is called microdiscectomy.

diverticulum: A small sac-like structure that sometimes forms in the walls of the intestines, diverticula can trap particles of food (especially small seeds and undigested grains) and become very inflamed and painful (this condition is called diverticulitis).

endometriosis: A condition in which tissue that normally lines the uterus grows in other areas of the body, usually inside the abdominal cavity, but acts as if it were inside the uterus. Blood shed monthly from the misplaced tissue has no place to go, and tissues surrounding the area of endometriosis may become inflamed or swollen. This can produce scar tissue. Symptoms include painful menstrual cramps that can be felt in the abdomen or lower back, or pain during or after sexual activity, irregular bleeding, and infertility.

epidural: During labor a woman may be offered an epidural, where a needle is inserted into the epidural space at the end of the spine, to numb the lower body and reduce pain. This allows a woman to have more energy and strength for the end stage of labor, when it is time to push the baby out of the birth canal.

fibroids: Fibroids are benign tumors of the uterus and the single most common indication for hysterectomy (a surgical operation to remove the uterus). Fibroids can be present yet undetected. They can cause significant morbidity, including prolonged or heavy menstrual bleeding, pelvic pressure or pain, and, in rare cases, reproductive dysfunction. Fibroids may be removed if they cause discomfort or if they are associated with uterine bleeding.

fibromyalgia: A disorder that causes aches and pain all over the body, and involves tender points on specific places on the neck, shoulders, back, hips, arms, and legs that hurt when pressure is put on them.

gallstone: Solid material that forms in the gallbladder or common bile duct. Gallstones are made of cholesterol or other substances found in the gallbladder. They may occur as one large stone or as many small ones, and they may vary from the size of a grain of sand to a golf ball.

gonorrhea: A sexually transmitted disease that often has no symptoms. However, some women have pain or burning when urinating; yellowish and sometimes bloody vaginal discharge; bleeding between menstrual periods; heavy bleeding with periods; or pain when having sex. Untreated gonorrhea can cause serious and permanent health problems like pelvic inflammatory disease (PID).

Gout: Gout is an inherited disorder where uric acid builds up in the body, often causing painful inflammation of the joints, especially of the feet and hands. Deposits of uric acid can also build up under the skin, forming lumps. Kidney stones may also form from the uric acid buildup.

hemorrhoids: Veins around the anus or lower rectum that are swollen and inflamed.

hypnosis: A focused state of concentration used to reduce pain. With self-hypnosis, you repeat a positive statement over and over. With guided imagery, you create relaxing images in your mind.

ibuprofen: A member of the aspirin family of analgesics, the so-called nonsteroidal anti-inflammatory drugs. It is sold over the counter and also comes in prescription-strength preparations.

inflammation: Used to describe an area on the body that is swollen, red, hot, and in pain.

inflammatory bowel disease: Long-lasting problems that cause irritation and ulcers in the gastrointestinal tract. The most common disorders are ulcerative colitis and Crohn's disease.

influenza: A highly contagious viral infection characterized by sudden onset of fever, severe aches and pains, and inflammation of the mucous membrane.

interstitial cystitis: A long-lasting condition also known as painful bladder syndrome or frequency-urgency-dysuria syndrome. The wall of the bladder becomes inflamed or irritated, which affects the amount of urine the bladder can hold and causes scarring, stiffening, and bleeding in the bladder.

kidney stone: Hard mass developed from crystals that separate from the urine and build up on the inner surfaces of the kidney.

laminectomy: A procedure in which a surgeon removes only a disc fragment, gaining access by entering through the arched portion of a vertebra.

magnets: Increasingly popular with athletes who are convinced of their effectiveness for the control of sports-related pain and other painful conditions. Usually worn as a collar or wristwatch, the use of magnets as a treatment dates back to the ancient Egyptians and Greeks. While it is often dismissed as quackery and pseudoscience by skeptics, proponents offer the theory that magnets may effect changes in cells or body chemistry, thus producing pain relief.

methadone: A long-acting synthetic opioid medication that is effective in treating pain and opioid addiction.

migraine: A medical condition that usually involves a very painful headache, usually felt on one side of the head. Besides intense pain, migraine also can cause nausea and vomiting and sensitivity to light and sound. Some people also may see spots or flashing lights or have a temporary loss of vision.

miscarriage: Miscarriage is the natural or accidental termination of a pregnancy at a stage where the embryo or the fetus is incapable of surviving. Women who experience a miscarriage may bleed for two or more weeks or experience menstrual-like cramps or severe abdominal pain.

nausea: An unpleasant sensation in the stomach usually accompanied by the urge to vomit. Common causes are early pregnancy, sea and motion sickness, emotional stress, intense pain, food poisoning, and various stomach infections.

nerve blocks: Employ the use of drugs, chemical agents, or surgical techniques to interrupt the relay of pain messages between specific areas of the body and the brain. There are many different names for the procedure, depending on the technique or agent used. Types of surgical nerve blocks include neurectomy; spinal dorsal, cranial, and trigeminal rhizotomy; and sympathectomy, also called sympathetic blockade.

neuropathy: A general term for any dysfunction in the peripheral nervous system. Symptoms include pain, muscle weakness, numbness, loss of coordination and paralysis. This condition may result in permanent disability.

nonsteroidal anti-inflammatory drugs (NSAIDs): Including aspirin, ibuprofen and naproxen are widely prescribed and sometimes called non-narcotic or non-opioid analgesics. They work by reducing inflammatory responses in tissues. Many of these drugs irritate the stomach and for that reason are usually taken with food.

opioids (or opiates): Controlled substances most often prescribed for the management of pain. They are natural or synthetic chemicals similar to morphine that work by mimicking the actions of enkephalin and endorphin (endogenous opioids or pain-relieving chemicals produced in the body).

osteoarthritis: A joint disease that mostly affects cartilage, the slippery tissue that covers the ends of bones in a joint. The top layer of cartilage breaks down and wears away. This allows bones under the cartilage to rub together, which causes pain, swelling, and loss of motion of the joint.

osteoporosis: A bone disease that is characterized by progressive loss of bone density and thinning of bone tissue, causing bones to break easily.

pain: A feeling triggered in the nervous system. Pain may be sharp or dull. It may come and go, or it may be constant. Once it is treated, pain usually goes away. However, sometimes pain goes on for weeks, months or even years. This is called chronic pain.

palliative: Palliative means "relief of symptoms." Most often, palliation is the relief of pain.

pelvic inflammatory disease (PID): An infection of the female reproductive organs that are above the cervix, such as the fallopian tubes and ovaries. It is the most common and serious problem caused by sexually transmitted diseases (STDs). PID can cause ectopic pregnancies, infertility, chronic pelvic pain, and other serious problems. Symptoms include fever, foul-smelling vaginal discharge, extreme pain, and vaginal bleeding.

pneumonia: Inflammation of the lungs characterized by fever, chills, muscle stiffness, chest pain, cough, shortness of breath, rapid heart rate and difficulty breathing.

premenstrual syndrome (PMS): A group of symptoms linked to the menstrual cycle that occur in the week or two weeks before menstruation. The symptoms usually go away after menstruation begins and can include acne, breast swelling and tenderness, feeling tired, having trouble sleeping, upset stomach, bloating, constipation or diarrhea, headache or backache, appetite changes or food cravings, joint or muscle pain, trouble concentrating or remembering, tension, irritability, mood swings or crying spells, and anxiety or depression.

psychotherapy: Counseling or talk therapy with a qualified practitioner in which a person can explore difficult, and often painful, emotions and experiences, such as feelings of anxiety, depression, or trauma. It is a process that aims to help the patient become better at making positive choices in his or her life, and to become more self-sufficient. Psychotherapy can be given for an individual or in a group setting.

rheumatoid arthritis: Form of arthritis that causes pain, swelling, stiffness and loss of function in your joints. It can affect any joint but is common in the wrist and fingers. If one hand has RA, the other one usually does too. It's an autoimmune disease. This means the arthritis is caused by your immune system attacking your body's own tissues. RA can affect body parts besides joints, such as your eyes, mouth and lungs.

rhizotomy: A surgical procedure in which a nerve close to the spinal cord is cut.

RICE (rest, ice, compression, and elevation): Four components prescribed by many orthopedists, coaches, trainers, nurses, and other professionals for temporary muscle or joint injuries, such as sprains or strains. Ice is used to reduce the inflammation associated with painful and acute injuries. Ice or heat may be recommended to relieve subacute and chronic pain, allowing for reduced inflammation and increased mobility. While many common orthopedic problems can be controlled with these four simple steps, especially when combined with over-the-counter pain relievers, more serious conditions may require surgery or physical therapy, including exercise, joint movement or manipulation, and stimulation of muscles.

shingles: A disease that occurs when the same virus that causes chicken pox becomes active again. After a person has chicken pox, the virus stays in the body. It may not cause problems for many years. As a person gets older, the virus may come back as shingles. It can cause mild to severe pain, usually on one side of the body or face. Unlike chicken pox, you can't catch shingles from someone who has it. A vaccine can prevent shingles or lessen its effects. The vaccine is for people 60 and older.

sickle cell anemia: A blood disorder passed down from parents to children. It involves problems in the red blood cells. Normal red blood cells are round and smooth and move through blood vessels easily. Sickle cells are hard and have a curved edge. These cells cannot squeeze through small blood vessels. They block the organs from getting blood. Your body destroys sickle red cells quickly, but it can't make new red blood cells fast enough—a condition called anemia.

spinal cord stimulation: Uses electrodes surgically or percutaneously inserted within the epidural space of the spinal cord. The individual is able to deliver a pulse of electricity to the spinal cord using an implanted electrical pulse generator that resembles a cardiac pacemaker.

spinal fusion: A procedure where the entire disc is removed and replaced with a bone graft. In a spinal fusion, the two vertebrae are then fused together. Although the operation can cause the spine to stiffen, resulting in lost flexibility, the procedure serves one critical purpose: protection of the spinal cord.

surgical blocks: Performed on cranial, peripheral, or sympathetic nerves. They are most often done to relieve the pain of cancer and extreme facial pain, such as that experienced with trigeminal neuralgia. There are several different types of surgical nerve blocks and they are not without problems and complications.

tetanus: Toxin-producing bacterial disease marked by painful muscle spasms.

transcutaneous electrical nerve stimulation (TENS): Uses tiny electrical pulses, delivered through the skin to nerve fibers, to cause changes in muscles, such as numbness or contractions. This in turn produces temporary pain relief. There is also evidence that TENS can activate subsets of peripheral nerve fibers that can block pain transmission at the spinal cord level, in much the same way that shaking your hand can reduce pain.

transverse myelitis: The sudden onset of spinal cord disease. Symptoms include general back pain followed by weakness in the feet and legs that moves upward. There is no cure and many patients are left with permanent disabilities or paralysis. Transverse Myelitis is a demyelinating disorder that may be associated with Multiple Sclerosis (MS). Also see demyelinating disorders.

trichomoniasis: A very common STD in both women and men that is caused by a parasite that is passed from one person to another during sexual contact. Symptoms include yellow, green, or gray vaginal discharge (often foamy) with a strong odor; discomfort during sex and when urinating; irritation and itching of the genital area; or lower abdominal pain (rare).

ultrasound: A painless test that uses sound waves to produce images of the organs and structures of the body on a screen. Also called sonography.

uric acid: A chemical created when the body breaks down substances called purines. Purines are found in some foods and drinks, such as liver, anchovies, mackerel, dried beans and peas, beer, and wine. Most uric acid dissolves in blood and passes out of the body in urine. If your body produces too much uric acid or doesn't remove enough of it, you can get sick.

uterine fibroids: Common, benign (noncancerous) tumors that grow in the muscle of the uterus, or womb. Fibroids often cause no symptoms and need no treatment, and they usually shrink after menopause. But sometimes fibroids cause heavy bleeding or pain, and require treatment.

Chapter 57

Resources for More Information about Pain Management

Government Agencies That Provide Information about Pain

Agency for Healthcare Research and Quality (AHRQ)
Office of Communications and Knowledge Transfer
5600 Fishers Ln.
Seventh Fl.
Rockville, MD 20857
Phone: 301-427-1364
Website: www.ahrq.gov

Centers for Disease Control and Prevention (CDC)
1600 Clifton Rd.
Atlanta, GA 30329-4027
Toll-Free: 800-CDC-INFO (800-232-4636)
Toll-Free TTY: 888-232-6348
Website: www.cdc.gov

Resources in this chapter were compiled from several sources deemed reliable; all contact information was verified and updated in June 2017.

Lower Extremity Amputation Prevention (LEAP) Program
Health Resources and Services Administration (HRSA)
5600 Fishers Ln.
Rockville, MD 20857
Toll-Free: 888-ASK-HRSA
(888-275-4772)
Toll-Free TTY: 877-489-4772
Website: www.hrsa.gov/leap
E-mail: comments@hrsa.gov

National Cancer Institute (NCI)
BG 9609 MSC 9760
9609 Medical Center Dr.
Bethesda, MD 20892-9760
Toll-Free: 800-4-CANCER
(800-422-6237)
Website: www.cancer.gov

National Diabetes Education Program
National Institute of Diabetes and Digestive and Kidney Diseases (NIDDK)
1 Diabetes Way
Bethesda, MD 20814-9692
Toll-Free: 888-693-NDEP
(888-693-6337)
Fax: 703-738-4929
Website: www.ndep.nih.gov
E-mail: ndep@mail.nih.gov

National Heart, Lung, and Blood Institute (NHLBI) Health Information Center
P.O. Box 30105
Bethesda, MD 20824-0105
Phone: 301-592-8573
Website: www.nhlbi.nih.gov
E-mail: nhlbiinfo@nhlbi.nih.gov

National Institute for Occupational Safety and Health
Patriots Plaza 1, 395 E. St., S.W. Ste. 9200
Washington, DC 20201
Phone: 202-245-0625
Website: www.cdc.gov/niosh

National Institute of Allergy and Infectious Diseases (NIAID)
5601 Fishers Ln.
MSC 9806
Bethesda, MD 20892-9806
Toll-Free: 866-284-4107
Phone: 301-496-5717
TDD: 800-877-8339
Fax: 301-402-3573
Website: www.niaid.nih.gov
E-mail: ocpostoffice@niaid.nih.gov

National Institute of Arthritis and Musculoskeletal and Skin Diseases (NIAMS)
1 AMS Circle
Bethesda, MD 20892-3675
Toll-Free: 877-22-NIAMS
(877-226-4267)
Phone: 301-495-4484
TTY: 301-565-2966
Fax: 301-718-6366
Website: www.niams.nih.gov
E-mail: NIAMSinfo@mail.nih.gov

National Institute of Child Health and Human Development (NICHD)
P.O. Box 3006
Rockville, MD 20847
Toll-Free: 800-370-2943
TTY: 888-320-6942
Fax: 866-760-5947
Website: www.nichd.nih.gov
E-mail: NICHDInformation-
ResourceCenter@mail.nih.gov

National Institute of Dental and Craniofacial Research (NIDCR)
Bethesda, MD 20892-2190
Toll-Free: 866-232-4528
Phone: 301-496-4261
Website: www.nidcr.nih.gov
E-mail: nidcrinfo@mail.nih.gov

National Institute of Mental Health (NIMH)
6001 Executive Blvd.
Rm. 6200, MSC 9663
Bethesda, MD 20892-9663
Toll-Free: 866-615-6464
Phone: 301-443-4513
TTY: 301-443-8431
Toll-Free TTY: 866-415-8051
Fax: 301-443-4279
Website: www.nimh.nih.gov
E-mail: nimhinfo@nih.gov

National Institute of Neurological Disorders and Stroke (NINDS)
P.O. Box 5801
Bethesda, MD 20824
Toll-Free: 800-352-9424
Phone: 301-496-5751
Website: www.ninds.nih.gov

National Institute of Nursing Research (NINR)
31 Center Dr.
Rm. 5B10
Bethesda, MD 20892-2178
Phone: 301-496-0207
Fax: 301-480-4969
Website: www.ninr.nih.gov
E-mail: info@ninr.nih.gov

National Institute on Aging (NIA)
31 Center Dr., MSC 2292
Bldg. 31, Rm. 5C27
Bethesda, MD 20892
Toll-Free: 800-222-2225
TTY: 800-222-4225
Website: www.nia.nih.gov
E-mail: niaic@nia.nih.gov

National Kidney and Urologic Diseases Information Clearinghouse (NKUDIC)
3 Information Way
Bethesda, MD 20892-3580
Toll-Free: 800-891-5390
TTY: 866-569-1162
Fax: 703-738-4929
Website: www.kidney.niddk.nih.gov
E-mail: nkudic@info.niddk.nih.gov

717

National Women's Health Information Center (NWHIC)
Office on Women's Health (OWH), Department of Health and Human Services (HHS)
200 Independence Ave. S.W.
Rm. 712E
Washington, DC 20201
Toll-Free: 800-994-9662
Phone: 202-690-7650
Fax: 202-205-2631
Website: www.womenshealth.gov

NIH Osteoporosis and Related Bone Diseases— National Resource Center
2 AMS Cir.
Bethesda, MD 20892-3676
Toll-Free: 800-624-BONE
(800-624-2663)
Phone: 202-223-0344
TTY: 202-466-4315
Fax: 202-293-2356
Website: www.bones.nih.gov
E-mail: NIHBoneInfo@mail.nih.gov

NIH Pain Consortium
Website: painconsortium.nih.gov
E-mail: NIHPainInfo@mail.nih.gov

Occupational Safety and Health Administration (OSHA)
U.S. Department of Labor (DOL)
200 Constitution Ave. N.W.
Rm. Number N3626
Washington, DC 20210
Toll-Free: 800-321-OSHA
(800-321-6742)
Toll-Free TTY: 877-889-5627
Website: www.osha.gov

U.S. Department of Veterans Affairs (VA)
810 Vermont Ave. N.W.
Washington, DC 20420
Toll-Free: 800-827-1000
Website: www.va.gov

U.S. Food and Drug Administration (FDA)
10903 New Hampshire Ave.
Silver Spring, MD 20993
Toll-Free: 888-INFO-FDA
(888-463-6332)
Website: www.fda.gov

Private Agencies That Provide Information about Pain

American Academy of Orthopaedic Surgeons (AAOS)
9400 W. Higgins Rd.
Rosemont, IL 60018
Toll-Free: 800-626-6726
Phone: 847-823-7186
Fax: 847-823-8125
Website: www.aaos.org
Email: customerservice@aaos.org

The American Academy of Pain Medicine (AAPM)
8735 W. Higgins Rd.
Ste. 300
Chicago, IL 60631-2738
Phone: 847-375-4731
Fax: 847-375-6477
Website: www.painmed.org
E-mail: info@painmed.org

The American Academy of Pediatrics (AAP)
141 N.W. Pt. Blvd.
Elk Grove Village, IL
60007-1098
Toll-Free: 800-433-9016
Phone: 847-434-4000
Fax: 847-434-8000
Website: www.aap.org

American Association of Endodontists (AAE)
211 E. Chicago Ave.
Ste. 1100
Chicago, IL 60611-2691
Toll-Free: 800-872-3636
Phone: 312-266-7255
Fax: 312-266-9867
Toll-Free Fax: 866-451-9020
Website: www.aae.org
E-mail: info@aae.org

American Association of Neurological Surgeons (AANS)
5550 Meadowbrook Dr.
Rolling Meadows, IL 60008-3852
Toll-Free: 888-566-AANS
(888-566-2267)
Phone: 847-378-0500
Fax: 847-378-0600
Website: www.aans.org
E-mail: info@aans.org

American Board of Pain Medicine (ABPM)
85 W. Algonquin Rd., Ste. 550
Arlington Heights, IL 60005
Phone: 847-981-8905
Fax: 847-427-9656
Website: www.abpm.org
E-mail: info@abpm.org

American Burn Association (ABA)
311 S. Wacker Dr.
Ste. 4150
Chicago, IL 60606
Phone: 312-642-9260
Website: www.ameriburn.org
E-mail: info@ameriburn.org

American Chiropractic Association (ACA)
1701 Clarendon Blvd.
Ste. 220
Arlington, VA 22209
Phone: 703-276-8800
Fax: 703-243-2593
Website: www.acatoday.org

The American Chronic Pain Association (ACPA)
P.O. Box 850
Rocklin, CA 95677
Toll-Free: 800-533-3231
Fax: 916-652-8190
Website: www.theacpa.org
E-mail: ACPA@theacpa.org

American College of Rheumatology (ACR)
Association of Rheumatology
Health Professionals
Rheumatology Research
Foundation
2200 Lake Blvd. N.E.
Atlanta, GA 30319
Phone: 404-633-3777
Fax: 404-633-1870
Website: www.rheumatology.org

719

American College of Sports Medicine (ACSM)
401 W. Michigan St.
Indianapolis, IN 46202-3233
Phone: 317-637-9200
Fax: 317-634-7817
Website: www.acsm.org

American Diabetes Association (ADA)
2451 Crystal Dr.
Arlington, VA 22202
Toll-Free: 800-DIABETES
(800-342-2383)
Phone: 703-549-1500
Fax: 703-549-6294
Website: www.diabetes.org
E-mail: webmaster@diabetes.org

American Gastroenterological Association (AGA)
4930 Del Ray Ave.
Bethesda, MD 20814
Phone: 301-654-2055
Fax: 301-654-5920
Website: www.gastro.org
E-mail: member@gastro.org

American Industrial Hygiene Association (AIHA)
3141 Fairview Park Dr.
Ste. 777
Falls Church, VA 22042
Phone: 703-849-8888
Fax: 703-207-3561
Website: www.aiha.org
E-mail: infonet@aiha.org

American Medical Society for Sports Medicine (AMSSM)
4000 W. 114th St.
Ste. 100
Leawood, KS 66211
Phone: 913-327-1415
Fax: 913-327-1491
Website: www.amssm.org
E-mail: office@amssm.org

American Migraine Foundation (AMF)
19 Mantua Rd.
Mt. Royal, NJ 08061
Phone: 856-423-0043
Fax: 856-423-0082
Website: www.achenet.org
E-mail: amf@talley.com

The American Orthopaedic Society for Sports Medicine (AOSSM)
9400 W. Higgins Rd.
Ste. 300
Rosemont, IL 60018
Toll-Free: 877-321-3500
Phone: 847-292-4900
Fax: 847-292-4905
Website: www.sportsmed.org

American Osteopathic Association (AOA)
142 E. Ontario St.
Chicago, IL 60611-2864
Toll-Free: 888-62-MYAOA
(888-626-9262)
Phone: 312-202-8000
Fax: 312-202-8202
Website: www.osteopathic.org
E-mail: crc@osteopathic.org

American Physical Therapy Association (APTA)
1111 N. Fairfax St.
Alexandria, VA 22314-1488
Toll-Free: 800-999-APTA
(800-999-2782)
Phone: 703-684-APTA
(703-684-2782)
TDD: 703-683-6748
Fax: 703-684-7343
Website: www.apta.org
E-mail: memberservices@apta.org

American Podiatric Medical Association (APMA)
9312 Old Georgetown Rd.
Bethesda, MD 20814-1621
Toll-Free: 800-FOOTCARE
(800-366-8227)
Phone: 301-581-9200
Fax: 301-530-2752
Website: www.apma.org
E-mail: membership_ask_
apma@apma.org

American Psychological Association (APA)
750 First St. N.E.
Washington, DC 20002-4242
Toll-Free: 800-374-2721
Phone: 202-336-5500
TDD/TTY: 202-336-6123
Website: www.apa.org

American Society for Bone and Mineral Research (ASBMR)
2025 M St. N.W.
Ste. 800
Washington, DC 20036-3309
Phone: 202-367-1161
Fax: 202-367-2161
Website: www.asbmr.org
E-mail: asbmr@asbmr.org

American Society of Interventional Pain Physicians (ASIPP)
81 Lakeview Dr.
Paducah, KY 42001
Phone 270-554-9412
Fax 270-554-5394
Website: www.asipp.org
E-mail: asipp@asipp.org

Anxiety and Depression Association of America (ADAA)
8701 Georgia Ave.
Ste. 412
Silver Spring, MD 20910
Phone: 240-485-1001
Fax: 240-485-1035
Website: www.adaa.org
E-mail: information@adaa.org

Arthritis Foundation
1355 Peachtree St. N.E.
Ste. 600
Atlanta, GA 30309
Toll-Free: 800-283-7800
Phone: 404-872-7100
Website: www.arthritis.org

*Charcot-Marie-Tooth
Association (CMTA)*
P.O. Box 105
Glenolden, PA 19036
Toll-Free: 800-606-CMTA
(800-606-2682)
Phone: 610-499-9264
Fax: 610-499-9267
Website: www.cmtausa.org
E-mail: info@cmtausa.org

Cleveland Clinic
9500 Euclid Ave.
Cleveland, OH 44195
Toll-Free: 800-223-2273
TTY: 216-444-0261
Website: my.clevelandclinic.org

The Ehlers-Danlos Society
P.O. Box 87463
Montgomery Village, MD 20886
Phone: 410-670-7577
Website: www.ehlers-danlos.com
E-mail: info@ehlers-danlos.com

Fibromyalgia Network
P.O. Box 31750
Tucson, AZ 85751-1750
Toll-Free: 800-853-2929
Phone: 520-290-5508
Fax: 520-290-5550
Website: www.fmnetnews.
iraherman.com
E-mail: inquiry@fmnetnews.com

*The Foundation for
Peripheral Neuropathy*
485 Half Day Rd., Ste. 350
Buffalo Grove, IL 60089
Toll-Free: 877-883-9942
Fax: 847-883-9960
Website: www.foundationforpn.
org
E-mail: info@TFFPN.org

The Hip Society
9400 W. Higgins Rd., Ste. 500
Rosemont, IL 60018
Phone: 847-698-1638
Fax: 847-823-0536
Website: www.hipsoc.org
E-mail: hip@aaos.org

*International RadioSurgery
Association (IRSA)*
P.O. Box 5186
Harrisburg, PA 17110
Phone: 717-260-9808
Fax: 717-260-9809
Website: www.irsa.org

*International Research
Foundation for RSD/CRPS*
1910 E. Busch Blvd.
Tampa, FL 33612
Phone: 813-995-5511
Website: www.rsdfoundation.org

*Interstitial Cystitis
Association (ICA)*
7918 Jones Branch Dr.
Ste. 300
McLean, VA 22102
Phone: 703-442-2070
Fax: 703-506-3266
Website: www.ichelp.org
E-mail: ICAmail@ichelp.org

Juvenile Diabetes Research Foundation (JDRF)
26 Bdwy.
14th Fl.
New York, NY 10004
Toll-Free: 800-533-CURE
(800-533-2873)
Fax: 212-785-9595
Website: www.jdrf.org
E-mail: info@jdrf.org

Model Systems Knowledge Translation Center (MSKTC)
American Institutes for Research (AIR)
1000 Thomas Jefferson St. N.W.
Washington, DC 20007
Phone: 202-403-5600
TTY: 877-334-3499
Website: www.msktc.org
E-mail: msktc@air.org

Mount Sinai Beth Israel
First Ave. at 16th St.
New York, NY 10003
Toll-Free: 877-620-9999
Phone: 212-420-2000
Website: www.mountsinai.org

Muscular Dystrophy Association (MDA)
222 S. Riverside Plaza
Ste. 1500
Chicago, IL 60606
Toll-Free: 800-572-1717
Website: www.mda.org

National Athletic Trainers Association (NATA)
1620 Valwood Pkwy
Ste. 115
Carrollton, TX 75006
Toll-Free: 800-879-6282
Phone: 214-637-6282
Fax: 214-637-2206
Website: www.nata.org

National Fibromyalgia Association (NFA)
3857 Birch St.
Ste. 312
Newport Beach, CA 92660
Website: www.fmaware.org
E-mail: nfa@fmaware.org

National Fibromyalgia Partnership, Inc. (NFP)
140 Zinn Way
Linden, VA 22642-5609
Website: www.fmpartnership.org

National Headache Foundation (MHF)
820 N. Orleans
Ste. 201
Chicago, IL 60610-3131
Phone: 312-274-2650
Website: www.headaches.org
E-mail: info@headaches.org

National Osteonecrosis Foundation
P.O. Box 518
Jarrettsville, MD 21084
Phone: 410-550-4001
Website: www.nonf.org

Neuropathy Association
60 E. 42nd St.
Ste. 942
New York, NY 10165
Phone: 212-692-0662
Fax: 212-692-0668
Website: www.neuropathy.org
E-mail: info@neuropathy.org

North American Spine Society (NASS)
7075 Veterans Blvd.
Burr Ridge, IL 60527
Toll-Free: 866-960-6277
Phone: 630-230-3600
Fax: 630-230-3700
Website: www.spine.org

Pedorthic Footcare Association (PFA)
P.O. Box 72184
Albany, GA 31708-2184
Phone: 229-389-3440
Fax: 888-563-0945
Website: www.pedorthics.org
E-mail: info@pedorthics.org

Phoenix Society for Burn Survivors
1835 RW Berends Dr. S.W.
Grand Rapids, MI 49519-4955
Toll-Free: 800-888-2876
Phone: 616-458-2773
Fax: 616-458-2831
Website: www.phoenix-society.
org
E-mail: info@phoenix-society.org

Reflex Sympathetic Dystrophy Syndrome Association (RSDSA)
99 Cherry St.
P.O. Box 502
Milford, CT 06460
Toll-Free: 877-662-7737
Phone: 203-877-3790
Fax: 203-882-8362
Website: www.rsds.org
E-mail: info@rsds.org

Sickle Cell Disease Association of America (SCDAA)
3700 Koppers St., Ste. 570
Baltimore, MD 21227
Toll-Free: 800-421-8453
Phone: 410-528-1555
Fax: 410-528-1495
Website: www.sicklecelldisease.org
E-mail: scdaa@www.
sicklecelldisease.org

Sleep HealthCenters
8381 Riverwalk Park Blvd.
Ste. 201
Ft Myers, FL 33919
Phone: 239-689-4758
Website: www.
sleephealthcenter.com
E-mail: info@provent.net

Spondylitis Association of America
P.O. Box 5872
Sherman Oaks, CA 91413
Toll-Free: 800-777-8189
Phone: 818-892-1616
Fax: 818-892-1611
Website: www.spondylitis.org
E-mail: info@spondylitis.org

TNA—Facial Pain Association
408 W. University Ave.
Ste. 402
Gainesville, FL 32601
Toll-Free: 800-923-3608
Phone: 352-384-3600
Fax: 352-384-3606
Website: www.fpa-support.org
E-mail: info@tna-support.org

University of California, San Diego
Student Health Services
9500 Gilman Dr.
La Jolla, CA 92093-0039
Phone: 858-534-3300
Fax: 858-534-7545
Website: www.wellness.ucsd.edu
E-mail: studenthealth@ucsd.edu

University of California, San Francisco
Medical Center
505 Parnassus Ave.
San Francisco, CA 94143
Toll-Free: 888-689-UCSF
(888-689-8273)
Phone: 415-476-1000
Website: www.ucsfhealth.org
E-mail: referral.center@ucsf.edu

University of Michigan Health System
1500 E. Medical Center Dr.
Ann Arbor, MI 48109
Toll-Free: 800-211-8181
Phone: 734-936-6666
Website: www.med.umich.edu

Urology Care Foundation
1000 Corporate Blvd.
Linthicum, MD 21090
Toll-Free: 800-828-7866
Phone: 410-689-3700
Fax: 410-689-3998
Website: www.urologyhealth.org
E-mail: info@
UrologyCareFoundation.org

Index

Index